Pediatric Prevention of Atherosclerotic Cardiovascular Disease

Pediatric Prevention
of Atherosclerotic
Cardiovascular Disease

EDITED BY

Ronald M. Lauer, MD

Trudy L. Burns, MPH, PhD

and Stephen R. Daniels, MD, PhD

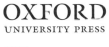

OXFORD
UNIVERSITY PRESS

2006

OXFORD
UNIVERSITY PRESS

Oxford University Press, Inc., publishes works that further
Oxford University's objective of excellence
in research, scholarship, and education.

Oxford   New York
Auckland   Cape Town   Dar es Salaam   Hong Kong   Karachi
Kuala Lumpur   Madrid   Melbourne   Mexico City   Nairobi
New Delhi   Shanghai   Taipei   Toronto

With offices in
Argentina   Austria   Brazil   Chile   Czech Republic   France   Greece
Guatemala   Hungary   Italy   Japan   Poland   Portugal   Singapore
South Korea   Switzerland   Thailand   Turkey   Ukraine   Vietnam

Published by Oxford University Press, Inc.
198 Madison Avenue, New York, New York 10016

www.oup.com

Oxford is a registered trademark of Oxford University Press

Library of Congress Cataloging-in-Publication Data
Pediatric prevention of atherosclerotic cardiovascular disease / edited
by Ronald M. Lauer, Trudy L. Burns, and Stephen R. Daniels.
p. ; cm.
Includes bibliographical references and index.
ISBN-13: 978-0-19-515065-0
ISBN-10: 0-19-515065-1
1. Atherosclerosis in children—Prevention.   2. Atherosclerosis in
Children—Risk factors.   I. Lauer, Ronald M., 1930-   .   II. Burns,
Trudy L.   III. Daniels, Stephen R.
[DNLM: 1. Arteriosclerosis—epidemiology—Adolescent.   2. Arterio-
sclerosis—epidemiology—Child. 3.   Arteriosclerosis—prevention &
control—Adolescent.   4. Arteriosclerosis—prevention & control—Child.
5. Risk Factors.   WG 550 P371 2006]
RJ426.A82P43 2006
618.92'136—dc22   2005026505

9 8 76 5 4 3 2 1

Printed in the United State of America
on acid-free paper

PREFACE

The most common cause of premature death in the United States and in many of the world's countries is atherosclerotic cardiovascular disease, which includes coronary heart disease, peripheral vascular disease, and stroke. The consequence of the current worldwide epidemic of obesity in both children and adults is likely to be an increase in the incidence of cardiovascular disease and other disorders. For most of the twentieth century and into the present, individuals in public health and medicine have found ways to respond to the challenge of preventing the development of infectious diseases, thus minimizing infectious disease–associated morbidity and mortality in children and adults. There is now clear pathologic and epidemiologic evidence that the atherosclerotic process begins during childhood (see Fig. 1.1 in Chapter 1), when primordial prevention may be initiated. This evidence raises a new challenge for pediatricians, pediatric cardiologists and other pediatric health care providers. This book focuses on the concept that if we are to change the course of atherosclerotic cardiovascular disease development, efforts must begin during childhood and adolescence.

Most of the referrals to a disease entity in this book are to cardiovascular disease, which is to be interpreted as atherosclerotic cardiovascular disease. There are less frequent referrals to atherosclerosis or the atherosclerotic process, and Chapters 2, 3, and 4 focus more specifically on coronary heart disease that results from the occlusion of arteries supplying blood to the heart.

The prevalence of various forms of cardiovascular disease mortality in the United States is presented in Figure P.1. Traditionally, pediatricians and pediatric cardiologists have focused their attention on congenital heart disease, which makes up 0.4% of the total. While this emphasis remains important because congenital heart disease is associated with the highest mortality of any congenital defects, we should also remember that coronary heart disease (54%), stroke (18%), congestive heart failure (6%), and high blood pressure (5%) make up the bulk of cardiovascular mortality, which causes the greatest disease burden in our society. Strong evidence suggests that genetic and environmental factors, as well as gene–environment interaction effects, are involved in the etiology of these complex diseases.

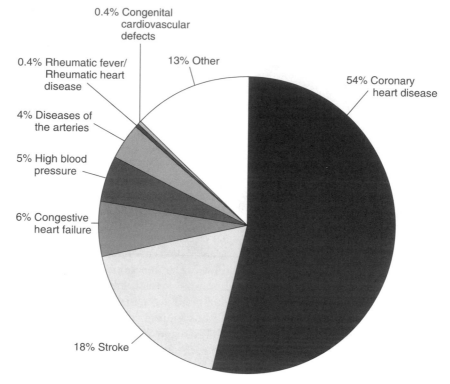

0.4% Congenital
cardiovascular
defects

0.4% Rheumatic fever/
Rheumatic heart
disease

13% Other

54% Coronary
heart disease

4% Diseases of
the arteries

5% High blood
pressure

6% Congestive
heart failure

18% Stroke

FIGURE P.1.
Percentage breakdown of deaths from cardiovascular diseases. United States: 2001.
Source: American Heart Association. Heart Disease and Stroke Statistics. Dallas, TX.
http://www.americanheart.org/presenter.jhtml?identifier=1200026 Statistics Update,
accessed January 2006.

In adults, high cholesterol, high blood pressure levels, diabetes, obesity, and smoking have been shown to be predictive of cardiovascular disease resulting in morbidity and mortality. These risk factors in children and adolescents track into adult age when the atherosclerotic process is advanced. There are few studies that have followed children with risk factors for cardiovascular disease into adulthood. There are no studies that have followed children or adolescents to firm cardiovascular outcomes such as myocardial infarction or stroke. Some studies have been able to establish the relationship between risk factors in childhood and intermediate or surrogate outcomes such as the presence of coronary artery calcium or increased carotid artery intimal–medial thickness. Studies performed over the last 25 to 30 years in young people have produced epidemiologic findings that can now be applied to clinical practice. In several of the chapters of this book the data from studies of children and adolescents in the United States and abroad are addressed, including data from the Bogalusa Heart Study, the Muscatine Study, the Dietary Intervention Study in Children (DISC), the Pathobiologic Determinants of Atherosclerosis in Youth (PDAY) Study, and the Special Turku Coronary Risk Factor Intervention Project for Children Study from Finland, among others.

In this book we merge epidemiology and pathophysiology with descriptions of risk factors in childhood and adolescence and how they affect blood vessels and the heart. The causes of high cholesterol, high blood pressure, diabetes, obesity, and smoking in children and adolescents are described here, and their management is discussed. The epidemiologic evidence serves as the underpinning of recommendations for clinical practice, thus establishing an evidence-based approach to prevention of cardiovascular disease in children, adolescents, and young adults. The organization of the book makes clear the most up-to-date clinical recommendations from the National High Blood Pressure Education Program, the National Cholesterol Education Program, the American Academy of Pediatrics, and the American Heart Association, while also presenting the results of epidemiologic studies that support the clinical recommendations. This combination provides the reader with both the science and application of pediatric preventive cardiology. For example, the epidemiologic evidence regarding the distributions of body mass index, blood pressure, and cholesterol is used to determine which children are at risk for the development of future cardiovascular disease. These percentile cut points are then used in clinical practice to determine which patients should have closer follow-up and which patients require treatment with lifestyle changes or pharmaceutical agents. Areas where additional epidemiologic evidence is needed before clinical applications can be developed are also addressed.

This book will be of interest to health professionals who practice preventive cardiology in children, adolescents, and young adults, providing a clear and concise approach to populations of children and individual patients. The book will also be of interest to school nurses and school administrators who are committed to developing a healthful school environment with appropriate attention to school lunches and physical activity. Those who teach epidemiology and public health will now have as a resource a complete discussion of pediatric atherosclerotic cardiovascular disease epidemiology. The book will also be useful to medical historians, as it provides an historical perspective on the development of knowledge regarding risk of cardiovascular disease in children, adolescents, and young adults, and on the application of that knowledge in clinical practice.

ACKNOWLEDGMENTS

We would like to thank the many authors who contributed their knowledge to the chapters in this book. Its quality is a tribute to the care with which they prepared and revised their chapters, and it was a pleasure to work with them. Throughout our careers we have all profited immensely from discussions of prevention concepts with teachers, colleagues, students, and patients.

We are grateful to Ms. Jenevive McLandsborough, Department of Pediatrics, The University of Iowa, for her invaluable technical assistance and coordination of communications with the contributing authors of the chapters in this book. We also appreciate the guidance and suggestions of our editors Mr. Jeffrey House and Ms. Carrie Pederson at Oxford University Press from the conceptualization process to preparation of the final manuscript. The final editing process was expertly facilitated by Ms. Regan Hofmann and Ms. Nancy Wolitzer at Oxford.

Institutions participating in the Pathobiological Determinants of Atherosclerosis in Youth (PDAY) Study (Chapter 1) and the supporting grants from the National Heart, Lung, and Blood Institute of the National Institutes of Health include the following:

- University of Alabama, Birmingham, AL, HL-33733, HL 33728
- Albany Medical College, Albany, NY, HL 33765
- Baylor College of Medicine, Houston, TX, HL 33750
- University of Chicago, Chicago, IL, HL-33740, HL 45715
- The University of Illinois, Chicago, IL, HL 33758
- Louisiana State University Medical Center, New Orleans, LA, HL-33746, HL 45720
- University of Maryland, Baltimore, MD, HL-33752, HL 45693
- Medical College of Georgia, Augusta, GA, HL 33772
- University of Nebraska Medical Center, Omaha, NE, HL 33778
- The Ohio State University, Columbus, OH, HL-33760, HL 45694
- Southwest Foundation for Biomedical Research, San Antonio, TX, HL 39913
- The University of Texas Health Science Center at San Antonio, San Antonio, TX, HL-33749, HL 45719

• Vanderbilt University, Nashville, TN, HL-33770, HL 45718
• West Virginia University Health Sciences Center, Morgantown, WV, HL 33748

The work of the Chicago Heart Association Detection Project in Industry (Chapters 2 and 3) was accomplished thanks to the invaluable cooperation of the many Chicago area companies and organizations, their officers, staff, and employees whose volunteer efforts made the project possible. Acknowledgement is also gratefully extended to all those in the Chicago Heart Association —staff and volunteers—serving the project. We are also grateful for the indispensable contributions of the many colleagues in the 22 clinical centers in 18 cities across the United States where the 361,662 men in the Multiple Risk Factor Intervention Trial (MRFIT) were screened and where the serum cholesterol analyses were conducted. We also thank the staff at the MRFIT Coordinating Center, Division of Biometry, School of Public Health, University of Minnesota, where the analyses of the MRFIT data were performed. The Chicago research was supported by the American Heart Association and its Chicago and Illinois affiliates; the Chicago Health Research Foundation; the Illinois Regional Medical Program; the National Heart, Lung, and Blood Institute; and private donors. The MRFIT investigation was a collaborative research effort undertaken with National Heart, Lung, and Blood Institute contract and grant support.

Preparation of Chapter 4 was supported in part by two research grants from the National Institutes of Health, HL 46292 and HL 48050. Material in Chapter 7 is adapted from the Report of the Expert Panel on Blood Cholesterol in Children and Adolescents of the National Cholesterol Education Program (1991). Preparation of Chapter 12 was supported in part by a research grant from the National Institutes of Health, HD 29569. Preparation of Chapter 14 was supported in part by a research grant from the National Institutes of Health, DK 60476.

I (RML) would like to thank my wife Eileen and my family for their continued encouragement, understanding, and patience during my academic career. I also gratefully acknowledge my many colleagues and the field staff for their numerous contributions and continuing efforts; the school nurses, teachers, administrators, and school board for their enthusiastic endorsement; and the children and families of Muscatine, Iowa, for their loyalty to and participation in The Muscatine Study since its initiation in 1970.

I (TLB) would like to thank my parents, Alfred and Albertine Burns, who created an atmosphere that encouraged learning for me, my sister Susan, and my brother Wayne, and who continue to encourage us in our careers.

I (SRD) would like to acknowledge my father, Robert Daniels, who inspired me to become a clinical investigator and fostered a love for academic medicine. I also thank my wife Dee, who has been a source of encouragement and who has put up with endless hours of my being away from home to work on improving the health of children.

Finally, we (TLB and SRD) would like to acknowledge our co-editor Dr. Ronald M. Lauer for his invaluable contributions as a personal mentor and his stimulating discussions about atherosclerotic cardiovascular disease epidemiology and prevention.

CONTENTS

CONTRIBUTORS

Mary Lober Aquilino, PhD, RN, FNP
Department of Community and
   Behavioral Health
College of Public Health
University of Iowa
Iowa City, Iowa

Esther M. Baker, MA
Department of Community and
   Behavioral Health
College of Public Health
University of Iowa
Iowa City, Iowa

Laura E. Beane Freeman, PhD
Division of Cancer Prevention
National Cancer Institute
National Institutes of Health
Bethesda, Maryland

Robert I. Berkowitz, MD
Department of Child and Adolescent
   Psychiatry
The Children's Hospital
   of Philadelphia, and
Department of Psychiatry, Weight
   and Eating Disorder Program
University of Pennsylvania School
   of Medicine
Philadelphia, Pennsylvania

Lawrence F. Bielak, DDS, MPH
Department of Epidemiology
School of Public Health
University of Michigan
Ann Arbor, Michigan

Trudy L. Burns, MPH, PhD
Public Health Genetics
Center for Statistical Genetics
   Research
College of Public Health
University of Iowa
Iowa City, Iowa

William R. Clarke, PhD
Department of Biostatistics
College of Public Health
University of Iowa
Iowa City, Iowa

Stephen R. Daniels, MD, PhD
Department of Pediatrics
University of Colorado School of
   Medicine, and
The Children's Hospital
Denver, Colorado

Martha L. Daviglus, MD, PhD
Department of Preventive Medicine
Feinberg School of Medicine
Northwestern University
Chicago, Illinois

Patricia H. Davis, MD
Department of Neurology
Division of Cerebrovascular
  Diseases
Carver College of Medicine
University of Iowa
Iowa City, Iowa

Jeffrey D. Dawson, ScD
Department of Biostatistics
College of Public Health
University of Iowa
Iowa City, Iowa

Patricia A. Donohoue, MD
Department of Pediatrics
Division of Pediatric Endocrinology
Carver College of Medicine
University of Iowa
Iowa City, Iowa

Lynn E. Eberly, PhD
Division of Biostatistics
School of Public Health
University of Minnesota
Minneapolis, Minnesota

Daniel B. Garside, MA
Department of Preventive Medicine
Feinberg School of Medicine
Northwestern University
Chicago, Illinois

Cynthia M. Goody, PhD, RD, LD
Diabetes Educator
HyVee, Inc.
Iowa City, Iowa

Philip Greenland, MD
Department of Preventive
  Medicine
Feinberg School of Medicine
Northwestern University
Chicago, Illinois

Ronald M. Lauer, MD
Department of Pediatrics
Division of Pediatric Cardiology
Carver College of Medicine
University of Iowa
Iowa City, Iowa

John B. Lowe, DrPH, FAHPA,
  FAAHB
Department of Community
  and Behavioral Health
College of Public Health
University of Iowa
Iowa City, Iowa

Russell V. Luepker, MD, MS
Division of Epidemiology
  and Community Health
School of Public Health
University of Minnesota
Minneapolis, Minnesota

Leslie A. Lytle, PhD, RD
Division of Epidemiology
  and Community Health
School of Public Health
University of Minnesota
Minneapolis, Minnesota

Larry T. Mahoney, MD
Department of Pediatrics
Division of Pediatric Cardiology
Carver College of Medicine
University of Iowa
Iowa City, Iowa

Henry C. McGill, Jr., MD
Department of Physiology
 and Medicine
Southwest Foundation
 for Biomedical Research
San Antonio, Texas

C. Alex McMahan, PhD
Department of Pathology
The University of Texas Health
 Science Center
San Antonio, Texas

James D. Neaton, PhD
Division of Biostatistics
School of Public Health
University of Minnesota
Minneapolis, Minnesota

Patricia A. Peyser, PhD
Department of Epidemiology
School of Public Health
University of Michigan
Ann Arbor, Michigan

Brian E. Saelens, PhD
Department of Pediatrics
Division of Behavioral Medicine
 and Clinical Psychology
Cincinnati Children's Hospital
 Medical Center, and
University of Cincinnati College
 of Medicine
Cincinnati, Ohio

Linda Snetselaar, PhD, RD
Department of Epidemiology
College of Public Health
University of Iowa
Iowa City, Iowa

Jeremiah Stamler, MD
Department of Preventive Medicine
Feinberg School of Medicine
Northwestern University
Chicago, Illinois

Michael Tansey, MD
Department of Pediatrics
Division of Pediatric Endocrinology
Carver College of Medicine
University of Iowa
Iowa City, Iowa

Andrew M. Tershakovec, MD
Director, Clinical Development
U.S. Human Health Division
Merck and Co., Inc.
West Point, Pennsylvania

Eva Tsalikian, MD
Department of Pediatrics
Division of Pediatric Endocrinology
Carver College of Medicine
University of Iowa
Iowa City, Iowa

Linda Van Horn, PhD, RD
Department of Preventive Medicine
Feinberg School of Medicine
Northwestern University
Chicago, Illinois

Eileen Vincent, MS, RD
Department of Preventive Medicine
Feinberg School of Medicine
Northwestern University
Chicago, Illinois

Lingfeng Yang, MS
Department of Biostatistics and
Epidemiology
School of Medicine
University of Pennsylvania
Philadelphia, Pennsylvania

INTRODUCTION

Jeremiah Stamler

■ LONG-TERM STRATEGIC CONSIDERATIONS
UNDERLYING THE CARDIOVASCULAR
DISEASE PREVENTION EFFORT

About a half-century ago, medical statesmen leading the new "heart" movement
recognized that the onslaught of the major adult cardiovascular diseases (CVD),
especially coronary heart disease (CHD), was epidemic, and that lessons from
earlier struggles against epidemic diseases had to be applied to cope with mass
CVD. In the late 1950s and early 1960s, initial strategic approaches to CVD prevention and control were advanced. By 1970, specific emphasis was placed on
the need for population-wide endeavors, i.e., to be effective and end the epidemic,
CVD prevention required a two-pronged approach: (1) recommendations to the
entire population for primary prevention through improvement of lifestyles,
based on a growing recognition that most adults in Western countries are at risk
due to adverse lifestyles; and (2) special complementary efforts by public health
and clinical medicine to achieve early detection, evaluation, and sustained treatment of individuals (and families) at higher risk.

The essence of the population-wide strategy was set down in the 1970 Report of the Inter-Society Commission for Heart Disease Resources (1970): "The
Commission recommends that a strategy of primary prevention of premature
atherosclerotic diseases be adopted as long-term national policy for the United
States and to implement this strategy that adequate resources of money and
manpower be committed to accomplish: changes in diet to prevent or control
hypercholesterolemia, obesity, hypertension and diabetes; elimination of cigarette smoking; and pharmacologic control of elevated blood pressure."

Such strategic emphases were endorsed in the United States by the federal
government, major voluntary health agencies (e.g., American Heart Association,

xxi

American Diabetes Association, American Cancer Society), and organizations of
health professionals, including the many medical and other health professional
organizations represented in the Inter-Society Commission for Heart Disease
Resources, the National High Blood Pressure Education Program, and the National
Cholesterol Education Program. Similar positive developments occurred in several other Western countries plagued by the coronary epidemic, and in the World
Health Organization (WHO). Reflecting this broad support, considerable progress
was registered from the 1960s on in implementation of these recommendations.
In the United States, for example, multiple sets of trend data showed:

- improvements in nutrition including decreased intake of total fat, saturated fat, and cholesterol;
- progressive declines in adult average serum cholesterol (antedating statin use)
  from about 235–240 mg/dL in the 1950s to about 200–205 mg/dL in the latter 1990s, with probable achievement of the national health goal for the year
  2000 of an adult population average level no greater than 200 mg/dL;
- progressive increases in the percentage of individuals with dyslipidemia
  detected, treated, and controlled;
- evidence by the early 1990s of a modest fall in adult systolic/diastolic blood
  pressure (SBP/DBP) independent of antihypertensive drug use, reasonably attributable to improved dietary patterns, particularly in people with
  a history of high blood pressure;
- progressive increases in the percentage of hypertensive people detected,
  treated, and controlled;
- progressive falls in the percentage of the population smoking cigarettes;
- progressive increases in the percentage of the population engaged in leisure time physical activity; and
- progressive declines in CHD, stroke, all CVD, and all cause mortality rates,
  with resultant increases in life expectancy, a "bottom-line" achievement.

By the turn of the century, however, it was clear that these advances, although
impressive and meaningful, were generally less than agreed-on goals. For example, U.S. population surveys indicated that total fat intake was down on
average from its high point of 38%–42% of kilocalories to about 33%; the goal
was less than 30%, however. Similarly, for saturated fatty acids, there was a decline from about 17% of kilocalories to about 11%, but the goal was less than
10%. Also, dietary cholesterol was down from an average of about 700 mg/day
to about 300, but the goal was less than 300 mg/day.

    For several areas, the available trend data give little or no evidence of progress;
there are even indications of retrogression.

- There is little, if any, evidence of lower salt intake by the general population, despite repeated recommendations for reduction from an average
  level of about 9 g NaCl per day to less than 6 g per day.

• As of the 1990s there was no clear sign of improvement in the long-standing adverse trend of sequentially higher average blood pressure levels with age, from young adulthood through middle age. For women and men of all ethnicities, this trend results in a transformation from favorable levels in youth (e.g., average SBP/DBP 116/70 mmHg) to pre-hypertensive (SBP 130–139 and/or DBP 80–89 mmHg) or high (SBP 140+ and/or DBP 90+ mmHg) average levels in middle and older age.

• The decline in percentage of the population who are currently smoking leveled off or ceased, especially among women (with evidence among teenagers of an increase, particularly among girls).

• An unremitting increase in the average body weight for every population stratum (children, youth, young and middle-aged adults, male and female, of all ethnicities) was documented, along with an accelerated rise to epidemic levels in the proportions of overweight and obese individuals.

• Corresponding increases occurred in the incidence and prevalence of diabetes, particularly type 2 diabetes (traditionally called "maturity onset"), not only among adults but also among children and youth.

• An increased proportion of meals were eaten out or brought in. These meals had larger portion sizes, and the calorie, macronutrient, and salt content was more adverse than that of meals prepared at home.

• There was little or no evidence of an increase in the proportion of the population engaged in regular, frequent leisure-time physical activity. And a steady decline took place nationwide in the availability and use of physical training resources in public schools.

These shortfalls in reducing risk have resulted in less favorable outcomes in morbidity and mortality. There is also evidence of disparity among ethnic groups and by socioeconomic status. In the 1990s (compared to the 1960s, 1970s, and 1980s) the rate of decline in coronary mortality slowed and the decline in stroke mortality leveled off (i.e., ceased), despite multiple advances and contributions of high-tech cardiovascular medical care. Also, multiple sets of evidence indicate that for lower socioeconomic (SES) strata of all ethnic backgrounds (African-American, Hispanic-American, non-Hispanic white American), the shortfalls and unfavorable trends in lifestyles, lifestyle-related risk factors, and mortality are even worse than for individuals from higher SES strata (e.g., those less educated compared with those more educated, or lower income compared with higher income).

These decade-long experiences in the effort to control epidemic CVD—the accomplishments, their limitations, the shortfalls—all make clear that reassessment, refinement, and elaboration of fundamental strategies are in order, to review and reconsider the nature and scope of resources needed to effectively implement sound long-term strategy. In particular, a fresh, in-depth look at the strategy of "primordial prevention" (a World Health Organization term), through which favorable patterns for all lifestyles and all major lifestyle-related risk factors among progressively increasing proportions of the population can be achieved, from early conception to birth, weaning, and throughout childhood is essential. These patterns can then be maintained for decades thereafter.

Why has there been less than optimum success in the prevention of CVD morbidity and mortality? One key factor is the inadequate attention paid to primordial prevention beginning in childhood. Comprehensive, new population-based data show that favorable levels of all the readily measured major CVD risk factors in young adulthood lead to extraordinarily low, nonepidemic long-term CVD mortality rates and substantially lower rates of cancers, other medical causes of death, and all-cause mortality—i.e., sizable increases in life expectancy. These data also show that the prevalence of this favorable low-risk profile is low everywhere. For example, it is less than 10% among young adult American men and about 20% among young adult American women, and even lower for middle-aged and older men and women. The inference is virtually self-evident: a progressive increase in the proportion of the population, first and foremost among its younger strata, is at low risk through effective primordial prevention is crucial to achieving population-wide progress against the CVD epidemic and to ending that epidemic in the next decades. To accomplish this it is necessary to better understand the early etiopathogenesis of atherosclerotic disease and the genesis of behaviors that lead to a poorer risk profile. Through such understanding, effective preventive strategies can be implemented early in life leading to lower risk profiles in young adulthood and further reductions of CVD morbidity and mortality.

In the last few years, this emphasis has been formally noted at the official national policy level in the United States, but much remains to be done to make it a living, breathing reality at all levels in all countries. This book makes available to clinicians, other health professionals, policymakers, and the public a wealth of materials for effective implementation of preventive and other complementary strategies to achieve this goal.

REFERENCE

Inter-Society Commission for Heart Disease Resources, Atherosclerosis Study Group and Epidemiology Study Group. 1970. "Primary Prevention of the Atherosclerotic Diseases." *Circulation* 42:A55–A95.

PART I

Origins of Cardiovascular Disease

CHAPTER 1

Pathology of Atherosclerosis in Youth and the Cardiovascular Risk Factors

Henry C. McGill, Jr. and C. Alex McMahan

Atherosclerosis, the arterial lesion underlying most forms of adult cardiovascular disease, was formerly considered an inevitable consequence of aging. Studies of the past half-century dispelled the notion of inevitability and showed that atherosclerosis resulted from the interaction between a genetic substrate and a number of environmental agents, a model now applicable to many common chronic diseases. Application of this knowledge to control the epidemic of atherosclerotic disease that developed in the first half of the twentieth century, particularly coronary heart disease, became a major public health goal of the latter half of that century and remains so today. Most efforts are directed at middle-aged and older adults, but there is now evidence that primary prevention should begin earlier in life. Atherosclerosis begins in childhood and progresses through adolescence and young adulthood to result in clinically manifest disease many years later. The rate of progression during those preclinical stages is affected by the same conditions, commonly known as risk factors, that predict the probability of adult clinical atherosclerotic disease. Long-range primary prevention will be most effective if control of these risk factors begins in youth.

■ NATURAL HISTORY OF ATHEROSCLEROSIS

The natural history of atherosclerosis is outlined in Figure 1.1 (McGill et al., 1963). The earliest morphological change clearly identified as atherosclerosis is the *fatty streak*, an accumulation of lipid-filled macrophages ("foam cells") in the intima of large muscular and elastic arteries. The predominant lipids are cholesterol and its esters. With age, lipid continues to accumulate in macrophages, adjacent smooth muscle cells, and extracellular spaces. Smooth muscle cells and connective tissue proliferate to encapsulate the lipid and form the *fibrous plaque*. Fibrous plaques undergo a variety of complications, the most serious of which is rupture of the overlying cap, an event that exposes the blood to the lipid-rich debris of the plaque core and precipitates formation of a thrombus and rapid occlusion of the arterial lumen. Vascularization may lead to hemorrhage within the plaque, resulting in rapid swelling and arterial occlusion. Atrophy of the underlying media may weaken the artery wall and lead to an aneurysm. Calcification causes few if any further complications and may even stabilize the plaque. As indicated in Figure 1.1, the resulting clinical syndrome depends on the location of the affected artery. Detailed gross and microscopic characteristics of these stages in the progression of atherosclerosis have been thoroughly described and illustrated in publications of the Committee on Vascular Lesions of the Council on Arteriosclerosis, American Heart Association (Stary et al., 1994, 1995).

▦ Fate of the Fatty Streak

The evolution of the fatty streak into the fibrous plaque and other advanced lesions has been a controversial issue in the pathogenesis of atherosclerosis because many fatty streaks, particularly those in the thoracic aorta, do not become fibrous plaques. Fatty streaks occur in the aorta of almost every child over the age of 3 years and vary only slightly in extent among young persons of all populations, regardless of the severity of atherosclerosis in adults from those populations (McGill, 1968). In contrast, fatty streaks appear in the coronary arteries of adolescents and young adults later in life than they appear in the aorta (Strong et al., 1999) and their distribution in a coronary artery in young persons is similar to that of fibrous plaques in older persons (Montenegro and Eggen, 1968; McGill et al., 2000a). The average extent of coronary artery fatty streaks in young persons from a population is associated with the extent of coronary fibrous plaques and the incidence of coronary heart disease in older persons from that same population (McGill, 1968).

Chemical, physiochemical, histologic, and electron microscopic studies of fatty streaks and fibrous plaques have shown that they contain similar tissue elements, and differ only in the proportions of each component. Furthermore, examination of lesions in a large number of children, adolescents, and young adults has led to identification of a lesion that has gross and microscopic characteristics common to both fatty streaks and fibrous plaques (Stary et al., 1994; Wissler et al., 1996). This lesion is interpreted as representing a transition from fatty streaks to fibrous plaques and has been termed the *raised fatty streak, fatty plaque, transitional lesion,* or *intermediate lesion*. Thus, little doubt remains that the fatty streak of childhood, an apparently innocuous cluster of macrophage

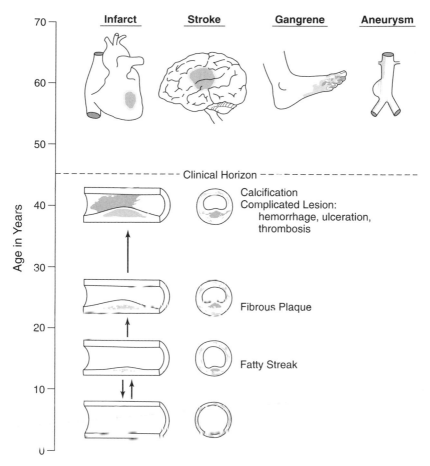

FIGURE 1.1
Natural history of atherosclerosis. (Reproduced from McGill et al., 1963.)

foam cells in the arterial intima, can in some individuals and at some arterial sites progress to an advanced atherosclerotic lesion.

■ Vulnerable Plaques

The qualities of fibrous plaques that lead to plaque rupture are more important than the size of the plaque. A thin fibrous cap, a large lipid pool, collagen degradation, loss of smooth muscle, and macrophage activity are associated with the susceptibility of a plaque to rupture (Lee and Libby, 1997), an event that precipitates thrombosis and infarction. Although plaque rupture and thrombosis are rare before age 35, characteristics of the vulnerable plaque are present in the coronary arteries of some young persons in the third and fourth decades of life.

■ Relation of Atherosclerosis to Clinical Disease

There is enormous variability among individuals within any population in the extent and severity of atherosclerotic lesions and in the rate at which lesions progress. There is also great variability in average extent and severity of atherosclerosis among populations. Coronary heart disease rates become high in populations in which the average extent of fibrous plaques and other advanced lesions approaches about 30% of the intimal surface of the coronary arteries (Tejada et al., 1968).

■ Molecular Biology of Atherosclerosis

Plausible molecular and cellular mechanisms now explain the origin of the fatty streak and its progression to a clinically significant lesion under certain conditions. Macrophages stationed in all tissues, including the arterial wall, possess a variety of receptors that enable them to participate in host defenses and to remove apoptotic cellular debris. Some of these receptors allow macrophages to engulf low-density lipoprotein (LDL) that has been oxidatively modified after passage through the endothelium and the macrophages become lipid-filled foam cells (Steinberg, 1997). Continued uptake and recruitment of macrophages leads to the grossly visible fatty streak. A variety of conditions can accelerate this process: higher LDL concentration, more rapid oxidation of LDL, and inability of macrophages to discharge ingested debris. Furthermore, lipid-filled macrophages secrete cytokines that stimulate an inflammatory reaction in the adjacent tissues (Wang et al., 1996). The inflammatory reaction, together with the continued accumulation of lipid, converts the original fatty streak into a transitional lesion and to the mature fibrous plaque. These observations suggest that the progression of atherosclerosis is an active process; that it can be accelerated or retarded by physiologic conditions; and that lesions may even be caused to regress if those physiologic conditions are changed.

■ RISK FACTORS FOR THE ATHEROSCLEROTIC DISEASES

Nearly 50 years ago, epidemiologic studies showed that a few characteristics predicted the probability of a person developing coronary heart disease, stroke, or peripheral arterial disease in a subsequent 5- to 10-year interval. These characteristics became known as *risk factors*. Higher risk of atherosclerotic disease was associated with age, male sex, high total serum cholesterol concentration, high LDL cholesterol concentration, low high-density lipoprotein (HDL) cholesterol concentration, hypertension, smoking, obesity, and diabetes (Pooling Project Research Group, 1978). These same risk factors were also associated with the extent and severity of atherosclerosis in persons over 35 years of age (Solberg and Strong, 1983). In the past 30 years, clinical trials have shown that modification of risk factors by either lifestyle changes or drugs, or both, reduced the risk of clinical disease and retarded the progression of atherosclerosis in adults (Steinberg and Gotto, 1999).

In the 1970s, epidemiologic surveys showed that children and adolescents varied in their serum lipid concentrations and blood pressure levels, although the average values and ranges were lower than those of adults (Lauer et al., 1975; Berenson, 1977). These observations suggested that the risk factors for adult coronary heart disease might influence the rate of progression of atherosclerosis in childhood and young adulthood, and that long-range prevention might be possible if begun early in life. Whether these childhood traits predicted risk of adult atherosclerotic disease, and whether they should be controlled by hygienic measures, became a controversial issue. The only direct evidence linking an adult risk factor with atherosclerosis in youth were rare case reports of advanced atherosclerosis and myocardial infarction in young persons with homozygous familial hypercholesterolemia (Sprecher et al., 1984). Noninvasive methods of reliably evaluating atherosclerosis in living persons were not available. A controlled clinical trial of lifestyle modification beginning in childhood with an end point of atherosclerotic disease in middle age appeared not to be feasible. Comparison of risk factors measured during life with atherosclerosis measured after death showed associations in a limited number of cases (Berenson et al., 1992), but a larger number of cases and a broader range of variables were needed for conclusive results. This need led to a major effort to relate the adult coronary heart disease risk factors, as they occurred in youth, to the preclinical lesions of atherosclerosis.

▪ PATHOBIOLOGICAL DETERMINANTS OF ATHEROSCLEROSIS IN YOUTH

In 1985, a group of investigators organized a multicenter cooperative study of the relation of the risk factor variables in adolescents and young adults to atherosclerosis, Pathobiological Determinants of Atherosclerosis in Youth (PDAY) (Wissler, 1991). Fifteen cooperating centers adopted a standard operating protocol and manual of procedures to collect specimens and information and submit them to central laboratories for analysis. A statistical coordinating center received all data pertaining to each case. Detailed descriptions of methods and results have been presented in a number of publications (McGill et al., 1995, 1997, 1998, 2000a, 2000b, 2000c, 2001; Strong et al., 1999).

■ Study Subjects

Study subjects were persons 15 through 34 years of age who died of external causes (accident, homicide, or suicide) within 72 hours after injury and were autopsied in cooperating forensic laboratories. Age and race were obtained from the death certificate. Persons of race other than black or white and those with congenital heart disease, Down syndrome, the acquired immune deficiency syndrome, or hepatitis were excluded. Between June 1, 1987, and August 31, 1994, 2876 acceptable cases were collected. Of these, 48% were white and 52% were black; 76% were men and 24% were women. The major cause of death among whites was accidents; among blacks, homicide. The distribution of causes of death among accidents, homicides, and suicides was consistent with national statistics for sex, race, and age groups. Analyses showed no differences in associations of atherosclerotic lesions with age, sex, race, or risk factors by cause of death, and therefore all causes of death were pooled for statistical analyses.

■ Dissecting and Preserving Arteries

PDAY investigators bisected the aorta longitudinally and fixed the left half in 10% neutral buffered formalin. They opened the right coronary artery longitudinally and fixed it in the same manner. They perfused the left main and left anterior descending (LAD) coronary artery with 10% buffered formalin at a pressure of about 100 mmHg (130 cm H_2O) and dissected them from the heart. A central laboratory stained the aortas and right coronary arteries with Sudan IV and packaged them in plastic bags. Abdominal aortas from 2833 cases and right coronary arteries from 2788 cases were available. Of the cases having data on all risk factors, 1458 abdominal aortas and 1427 right coronary arteries were available.

In another central laboratory, a technician cut a 5–mm transverse block from the fixed LAD coronary artery distal to the flow divider of the left main and left circumflex arteries. Sections from the proximal half were stained with oil red O (ORO), and sections from the distal half were stained with Gomori-trichrome aldehyde fuchsin (GTAF). Of the cases having data on all risk factors, microscopic sections of the LAD were available for 760 cases.

■ Gross Lesions of Atherosclerosis

Three pathologists independently estimated the extent of intimal surface area of the right coronary artery and abdominal aorta involved with fatty streaks, fibrous plaques, and other complicated lesions. Because complicated lesions (rupture, hemorrhage, and calcification) were uncommon in this age group, the area involved by complicated lesions was combined with that involved by fibrous plaques and termed *raised lesions*. The consensus grade was the average of the grades of the three pathologists. Agreement among and within pathologists was good (McGill et al., 1997). The thoracic aorta was much less likely to develop advanced atherosclerotic lesions than the abdominal aorta (Strong et al., 1999), an observation consistent with the low incidence of clinically significant lesions in the thoracic aortas of adults. Therefore, the analyses involving aortic lesions focused on those in the abdominal aorta.

The involvement with fatty streaks was divided into involvement with flat and with raised fatty streaks (McGill et al., 2000b). The raised fatty streak represents the gross classification of the intermediate or transitional lesion, that is, a lesion with microscopic characteristics suggesting it is in the process of becoming a fibrous plaque.

■ Microscopic Qualities of Coronary Atherosclerosis

Two pathologists graded GTAF- and ORO-stained sections of the LAD coronary artery using the American Heart Association (AHA) classification system (Stary et al., 1995). Differences were resolved by discussion and a consensus grade was reached. Grade 0 designated a normal artery with no intimal lipid and with or without adaptive intimal thickening. A grade 1 lesion, corresponding to a gross fatty streak, showed isolated macrophage foam cells containing lipid. A grade 2 lesion showed numerous lipid containing macrophage foam cells and fine particles of extracellular lipid, but no pools of extracellular lipid, and also corresponded to a gross fatty streak. A grade 3 lesion showed numerous macrophage foam cells and one or more pools of extracellular lipid, but no well defined core of lipid, and corresponded to an intermediate or transitional lesion. A grade 4 lesion showed numerous macrophage foam cells plus a well-defined core of extracellular lipid covered by normal intima. A grade 5 lesion showed one or more cores of extracellular lipid plus a reactive fibrous cap, vascularization, or calcification. Grade 6 lesions, characterized by an intimal surface defect, were not encountered in the PDAY sample. Grade 4 to 6 lesions corresponded to fibrous plaques and complicated plaques, which are grouped together in analyses of gross lesions as raised lesions. Grade 4 and 5 lesions have characteristics considered markers for the vulnerable plaque (Lee and Libby, 1997; Libby, 2001).

■ Stenosis of the Left Anterior Descending Coronary Artery

Stenosis of the LAD coronary was assessed by a combination of computerized morphometry and microscopic examination. In the GTAF sections, the length of the external elastic lamina (EEL) and the medial and intimal cross-sectional areas were measured. The EEL was assumed to be a circle and the maximum potential lumen area was calculated by subtracting the measured medial area from the area within the EEL. A case was classified as having atherosclerotic steno-sis if the AHA grade was 3 or greater and the ratio of intimal area to maximum potential lumen area was ≥40%. Cases with grade 0, 1, or 2 lesions were consid-ered to have adaptive intimal thickening, a normal structure that did not repre-sent atherosclerotic stenosis.

■ Risk Factor Assessment

Table 1.1 summarizes the methods of measuring coronary heart disease risk fac-tors and the prevalence of each risk factor by 10-year age groups. Criteria for unfavorable lipoprotein values were based on the recommendation of the Na-tional Cholesterol Education Program (1993): LDL cholesterol ≥130 mg/dL; HDL cholesterol <35 mg/dL. Because the fasting status of these autopsied individuals was not known, triglyceride data would not be interpretable. Therefore, the non-HDL cholesterol concentration was used as a risk factor by assuming that an LDL cholesterol concentration of 130 mg/dL was approximately equal to a non-HDL cholesterol of 160 mg/dL (Grundy, 2001). The serum thiocyanate concentration is a reliable objective indicator of smoking. Because some individuals dying of trauma receive large quantities of fluids immediately prior to death, all data from serum were excluded if the serum cholesterol concentration was <100 mg/dL. Mean arterial blood pressure was estimated using the intimal thickness of the small renal arteries and an algorithm established in previous studies in which premortem blood pressures were available. Body mass index (BMI) was com-puted from weight and body length measured at autopsy. Subjects were classi-fied as obese if the BMI was >30 kg/m². An additional measure of adiposity was the thickness of the panniculus adiposus, measured midway between the xiphoid process and the umbilicus. A glycohemoglobin concentration ≥8% indicated an average blood glucose concentration ≥150 mg/dL for several weeks prior to death, and indicated the presence of impaired glucose tolerance and probably diabetes mellitus. The average lipoprotein levels were comparable to those reported for young U.S. living populations (Donahue et al., 1989). The prevalence rates of obesity (Troiano et al., 1995) and hypertension (National Heart, Lung, and Blood Institute, 1985) were also similar to those reported for living populations. The prevalence of smoking was higher than that in most reports from this period (Centers for Disease Control, 1992), probably because smoking is associated with accidents and suicides and because we used an objective indicator of smoking.

■ RISK FACTORS AND ATHEROSCLEROSIS IN YOUTH

Figure 1.2 illustrates quantitatively the progression of atherosclerosis that was indicated schematically in Figure 1.1. It shows the extent of fatty streaks and raised

TABLE 1.1

Risk factors, samples, analysis, risk classification criteria, numbers of cases, and prevalence of risk factors in PDAY cases by 10-year age group

				Age			
				15 to 24 years		25 to 34 years	
Risk Factor	Sample	Analysis	Criterion for Presence of Risk Factor	n	Prevalence %	n	Prevalence %
Non-HDL cholesterol	Serum	Total cholesterol less HDL cholesterol	≥160 mg/dL	717	22.0	789	33.5
HDL cholesterol	Serum	Cholesterol after precipitation of apo-B lipoproteins	<35 mg/dL	717	18.7	789	18.8
Smoking	Serum	Thiocyanate	≥90 μmol/L	717	35.2	789	52.0
Hypertension	Renal arteries	Intimal thickness and algorithm to estimate mean arterial pressure	≥110 mmHg	1358	14.3	1475	16.7
Obesity	Measured at autopsy	Body mass index = weight (kg)/height (m)²	>30 kg/m²	1375	11.8	1488	16.2
Hyperglycemia	Red blood cells	% glycohemoglobin	≥8%	1237	4.0	1307	4.5

HDL, high-density lipoprotein; PDAY, Pathological Determinants of Atherosclerosis in Youth.

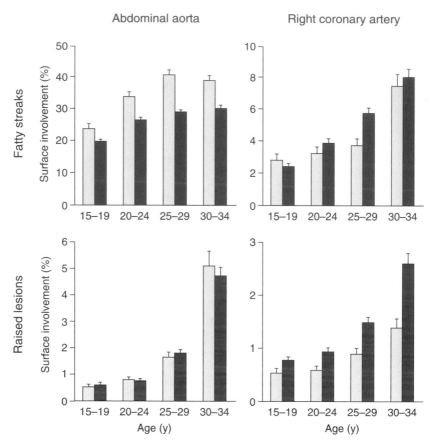

FIGURE 1.2

Mean extent of fatty streaks (top panels) and raised lesions (lower panels) in women (gray bars) and men (black bars) in the abdominal aorta (left panels) and right coronary artery (right panels) by 5-year age group. The mean values are adjusted for race but not for risk factors. Numbers of cases: men, 15–19, 455; 20–24, 569; 25–29, 613; 30–34, 466; women, 15–19, 140; 20–24, 169; 25–29, 176; 30–34, 177. ⊤ above the bars represents the standard error.

lesions in the abdominal aorta (left panels) and in the right coronary artery (right panels) by 5-year age group and sex. There were minor differences between blacks and whites and the means are adjusted for race, but not for other risk factors. In the abdominal aorta, women have slightly more extensive fatty streaks than men (upper left panel), but a similar extent of raised lesions (lower left panel) as men throughout the 15- to 34-year age span. The lessening or reversal of the increase in fatty streaks with age is due to the replacement of fatty streaks with raised lesions. In the right coronary artery, the extent of fatty streaks was about equal in women and men (upper right panel), but men had almost double the extent of raised lesions as women (lower right panel) through the 15- to 34-year age span.

Figure 1.3 shows the prevalence of AHA grade 4 and 5 lesions and of atherosclerotic stenosis ≥40% in microscopic sections of the LAD coronary artery by 5-year age group and sex. Both measures of atherosclerosis showed age and sex differences similar to those for gross raised lesions in the right coronary artery. No women had atherosclerotic stenosis ≥40% before age 25, and women had about half the prevalence of grade 4 and 5 lesions and of atherosclerotic stenosis ≥40% as men in the 30- to 34-year age group. Because AHA grade 4 and 5 lesions had characteristics that make them vulnerable to rupture, a substantial proportion of young people had coronary artery lesions that are vulnerable to rupture and thrombosis and have the potential to precipitate coronary heart disease.

Young men and women developed the advanced lesions of atherosclerosis in the abdominal aorta at about the same rate, but young men developed advanced

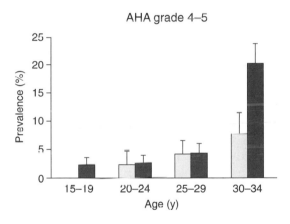

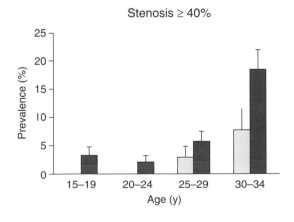

FIGURE 1.3
Prevalence of American Heart Association (AHA) grade 4 and 5 lesions (top panel) and of atherosclerotic stenosis ≥40% (lower panel) in the left anterior descending coronary artery of women (gray bars) and of men (black bars). The prevalence rates are adjusted for race but not for risk factors. Numbers of cases: men, 15–19, 127; 20–24, 149; 25–29, 157; 30–34, 128; women, 15–19, 36; 20–24, 42; 25–29, 70; 30–34, 51. T above the bars represents the standard error. (Reproduced from McGill et al., 2000c.)

lesions of the coronary arteries (measured both grossly and microscopically) much more rapidly than young women. Women lagged behind men in the progression of coronary atherosclerosis by about 10 years. This sex difference is consistent with the lower rate of clinically manifest coronary heart disease in middle-aged women compared to that in middle-aged men.

▦ Effects of Risk Factors on Atherosclerosis in Youth

Table 1.2 presents the effects of the risk factors on the gross extent of fatty streaks and raised lesions as ratios of the percent intimal surface involved in subjects with a risk factor (as defined in Table 1.1) to the percent involvement in subjects without the risk factor by 10-year age groups. Table 1.3 presents risk factor effects on microscopic lesion grade and atherosclerotic stenosis in the LAD coronary artery as odds ratios for the same risk factors. In both Tables 1.2 and 1.3, the effect of each risk factor is adjusted for the effects of all other risk factors measured. Some of the effects may be biologically important even though they are not statistically significant.

▦ Male Sex

The excess of advanced coronary atherosclerosis among men, already seen in Figures 1.2 and 1.3, was again demonstrated both in extent of raised lesions (Table 1.2, Fig. 1.2) and in microscopic qualities (Table 1.3, Fig. 1.3). The sex difference began in the teenage years and was twofold or greater by the early 30s, presaging the higher risk of coronary heart disease among middle-aged men. The excess of raised lesions in men occurred only in the coronary arteries and there was no sex difference in the aorta. The sex effect was not due to differences in other risk factors because the analyses adjusted for those effects (McGill et al., 1997).

▦ Non-HDL Cholesterol Concentration

The effect of a high non-HDL cholesterol concentration on fatty streaks and raised lesions in both the abdominal aorta and the right coronary artery, and on the microscopic qualities of LAD coronary artery atherosclerosis, is consistent with the large body of experimental, epidemiologic, and clinical evidence relating blood concentrations of apo-B-containing lipoproteins to atherosclerosis and risk of coronary heart disease (Stamler et al., 1993). The non-HDL cholesterol effect is apparent in these data by the late teenage years, and probably is present at even earlier ages (Berenson et al., 1998). The significance of this association for subsequent risk of coronary heart disease is supported by long-term follow-up of serum cholesterol levels in youth (Klag et al., 1993; Stamler et al., 2000).

TABLE 1.2
Ratio of percent intimal surface area involved for cases with a risk factor to involvement for cases without the risk factor by 10-year age group (± SE)*

Risk Factor	Group	Lesion	Abdominal Aorta		Right Coronary Artery	
			15 to 24 years	25 to 34 years	15 to 24 years	25 to 34 years
Male sex	All	Fatty streaks	**0.87 ± 0.07**†	**0.76 ± 0.07**	**1.37 ± 0.18**	**1.29 ± 0.13**
		Raised lesions	0.93 ± 0.19	0.89 ± 0.15	1.56 ± 0.23	1.77 ± 0.20
Non-HDL cholesterol	All	Fatty streaks	1.27 ± 0.07	1.32 ± 0.05	1.35 ± 0.20	1.83 ± 0.19
		Raised lesions	0.96 ± 0.15	1.50 ± 0.17	1.23 ± 0.19	1.85 ± 0.23
HDL cholesterol	All	Fatty streaks	1.12 ± 0.06	1.27 ± 0.06	1.03 ± 0.14	1.59 ± 0.18
		Raised lesions	0.89 ± 0.15	1.15 ± 0.14	1.03 ± 0.15	1.15 ± 0.14
Smoking	All	Fatty streaks	1.15 ± 0.05	1.10 ± 0.04	0.99 ± 0.12	0.95 ± 0.09
		Raised lesions	1.15 ± 0.15	2.68 ± 0.34	1.07 ± 0.13	1.14 ± 0.11
Hypertension	Whites	Fatty streaks	1.02 ± 0.09	0.93 ± 0.08	1.22 ± 0.26	1.29 ± 0.22
		Raised lesions	0.72 ± 0.23	1.14 ± 0.22	0.91 ± 0.21	1.72 ± 0.33
	Blacks	Fatty streaks	1.05 ± 0.07	0.95 ± 0.05	1.22 ± 0.21	1.28 ± 0.16
		Raised lesions	1.29 ± 0.27	1.87 ± 0.30	1.35 ± 0.27	2.44 ± 0.41
Obesity	Men	Fatty streaks	1.09 ± 0.08	1.11 ± 0.07	**2.03 ± 0.38**	**1.36 ± 0.17**
		Raised lesions	1.06 ± 0.21	0.80 ± 0.16	**1.58 ± 0.32**	**1.53 ± 0.22**
	Women	Fatty streaks	0.88 ± 0.10	0.91 ± 0.09	1.04 ± 0.26	0.75 ± 0.22
		Raised lesions	1.19 ± 0.33	0.89 ± 0.24	1.06 ± 0.28	1.08 ± 0.26
Hyperglycemia	All	Fatty streaks	0.93 ± 0.13	**0.80 ± 0.08**	1.69 ± 0.51	1.32 ± 0.28
		Raised lesions	0.94 ± 0.34	1.62 ± 0.37	1.52 ± 0.51	**2.29 ± 0.53**

*Ratios <1.00 indicate that cases with the risk factor had a lower percent of surface area involved than cases without the risk factor. Ratios >1.00 indicate that cases with the risk factor had a higher percent of surface area involved than cases without the risk factor. See Table 1.1 for risk factor definitions and number of cases. HDL, high-density lipoprotein.
†Bold typeface indicates a ratio significantly different from 1.00 ($p < 0.05$).

TABLE 1.3
Odds ratios and 95% confidence intervals (CI) for risk factor effects on the left anterior descending coronary artery*

Risk Factor	Group	AHA Grade (2–3 vs.0–1)		AHA Grade (4–5 vs. 0–1)		Atherosclerotic Stenosis ≥40%	
		Odds Ratio	95% CI	Odds Ratio	95% CI	Odds Ratio	95% CI
Male sex	All	2.75†	1.48–5.10	4.01	1.52–10.58	3.27	1.11–9.64
Non-HDL cholesterol	All	2.04	1.39–3.01	2.78	1.40–5.52	3.09	1.60–5.96
HDL cholesterol	All	1.64	1.04–2.59	1.89	0.86–4.15	1.39	0.64–3.01
Smoking	All	1.42	0.99–2.04	1.11	0.52–2.39	0.87	0.45–1.66
Hypertension	All	1.28	0.78–2.10	2.15	0.95–4.90	1.33	0.58–3.01
Obesity	Men	1.96	1.10–3.50	5.15	2.14–12.39	3.31	1.51–7.26
	Women	0.60	0.20–1.72	0.40	0.06–2.80	0.56	0.08–4.20
Hyperglycemia	All	1.72	0.79–3.76	2.55	0.53–12.25	1.52	0.42–5.50

*Odds ratios <1.00 indicate that cases with the risk factor had lower odds of American Heart Association (AHA) grade 2–3 or 4–5, or stenosis ≥40%, than cases without the risk factor. Odds ratios >1.00 indicate that cases with the risk factor had higher odds of AHA grade 2–3 or 4–5, or stenosis ≥40%, than cases without the risk factor.
†Bold typeface indicates an odds ratio for which the 95% CI does not include 1.00.

HDL Cholesterol Concentration

A low HDL cholesterol concentration showed a consistent association with more extensive and more advanced lesions in both the abdominal aorta and coronary arteries. This observation is consistent with the association of low HDL cholesterol with coronary heart disease (Miller and Miller, 1975).

Smoking

Smoking was associated with a much greater extent of lesions in the abdominal aorta, but not in the right coronary artery. This selective effect of smoking on the abdominal aorta began by age 15 and was concentrated on the dorsolateral aspect of the aorta just proximal to its bifurcation (McGill et al., 2000a). The strength of the association and the location of the maximal effect are consistent with the well-known predisposition of smokers to abdominal aortic aneurysms (Auerbach and Garfinkel, 1980). There was a nonsignificant trend toward a higher microscopic grade of atherosclerosis in the LAD coronary artery, a forerunner of the atherogenic effect of smoking after age 35 (Strong and Richards, 1976) and of its subsequent effect on the risk of coronary heart disease

Hypertension

Hypertension, long known as a risk factor for adult coronary heart disease (Master et al., 1939), had little effect on fatty streaks and was associated primarily with extent of coronary artery raised lesions, with the association being somewhat stronger in black subjects. Thus, hypertension appears primarily to accelerate the conversion of fatty streaks to fibrous plaques. Hypertension also was associated with larger diameters of the right and LAD coronary arteries and with larger cross-sectional intimal and medial areas of the LAD coronary artery (McGill et al., 1998), an observation suggesting that arterial walls are hypertrophied in association with hypertension at this early age.

Obesity

A remarkable feature of obesity was its strong effect on fatty streaks and raised lesions in the right coronary artery, and on microscopic grade of atherosclerosis in the LAD coronary artery of men but not of women. Obesity is associated with clinical coronary heart disease in older women, but the relative risk of coronary heart disease for obese women is slightly lower than the relative risk for obese men (Calle et al., 1999). Obesity may be augmenting atherosclerosis in women after age 35, or it may be increasing the risk of coronary heart disease by mechanisms other than accelerating atherosclerosis. Central (abdominal) obesity is widely considered to confer a greater risk than noncentral obesity (Stern and Haffner, 1986). Among obese men (BMI > 30 kg/m^2), those with a thick panniculus adiposus had more extensive involvement with raised lesions. In women with a thick panniculus adiposus, there was a nonsignificant trend for obese women to have more extensive fatty streaks.

Although the effect of obesity on lesions in men is not accounted for by the association of obesity with other risk factors measured in this study, new risk factor variables are emerging. Potential intervening variables include C-reactive protein (Ford et al., 2001), insulin resistance (Steinberger et al., 2001), and fibrinogen (Cook et al., 1999), all of which are associated with both coronary heart disease and obesity. The effect of obesity on atherosclerosis in young men is consistent with recent reports of long-term follow-up of obese children (Must et al., 1992; Gunnell et al., 1998).

▪ Hyperglycemia

Hyperglycemia, as measured by postmortem glycohemoglobin, was strongly associated with more extensive raised lesions of both the abdominal aorta and the right coronary artery. There was a positive trend for its association with the microscopic qualities of coronary atherosclerosis, but it was not significant, probably because of the smaller number of cases. This association is consistent with the greatly increased risk of coronary heart disease among diabetics and suggests that glycemic control, even in the early stages of diabetes, may be important for the prevention of macrovascular as well as microvascular disease (Haffner et al., 1990).

▪ Is a Favorable Lipoprotein Profile Sufficient?

Programs to prevent the atherosclerotic diseases have focused on control of hypercholesterolemia because of the strength of its association with atherosclerotic disease, because there are plausible physiologic mechanisms that account for the association, and because there are safe and effective drugs that lower serum cholesterol. This emphasis has been justified by the results of clinical trials showing that lowering blood cholesterol decreased coronary heart disease risk (Sacks, 1998). As a result, control of the other risk factors has sometimes been neglected. The effects of the nonlipid risk factors were investigated in PDAY cases with a favorable lipoprotein profile—that is, with non-HDL cholesterol <160 mg/dL, and HDL cholesterol ≥35 mg/dL. Figure 1.4 shows the combined effects of the four nonlipid risk factors on raised lesions of the right coronary artery in

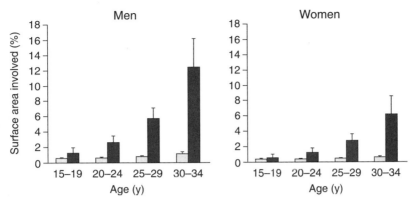

FIGURE 1.4

Mean extent of raised lesions in the right coronary arteries of men (left panel) and women (right panel) with a favorable lipoprotein profile and no nonlipid risk factors (gray bars) compared with extent involvement in men and women also with a favorable lipoprotein profile and all of the nonlipid risk factors (smoking, hypertension, obesity, and hyperglycemia) (black bars) by 5-year age group. T above the bars represents the standard error.

men and women with a favorable lipoprotein profile. By age 30 to 34, men who had hypertension, obesity, smoking, and hyperglycemia had over 10-fold the extent of raised lesions compared to those without nonlipid risk factors, even though they had a favorable lipoprotein profile. Among women, the effect was less because obesity was not associated with raised lesions in women. These results show that control of all the risk factors is important for effective long-range prevention of atherosclerosis in youth.

Combined Risk Factor Effects: Risk Level

Individuals often have more than one risk factor, and the effects on atherosclerotic lesions are cumulative. In the PDAY cases, 22.4% had no risk factors; 42.7% had one risk factor; 26.2% had two risk factors; 6.9% had three risk factors; and 1.8% had four or more risk factors. Figure 1.5 shows the extent of involvement for individuals with no risk factors compared with the extent involvement for individuals with one, two, three, or four or more risk factors for both fatty streaks and raised lesions in the right coronary arteries of men and women. As the number of risk factors increased, the extent of involvement with fatty streaks and raised lesions increased. Within each sex, individuals with no risk factors showed less than a twofold increase in extent of raised lesions between 15 to 19 and 30 to 34 years of age, whereas those with four or more risk factors showed a greater

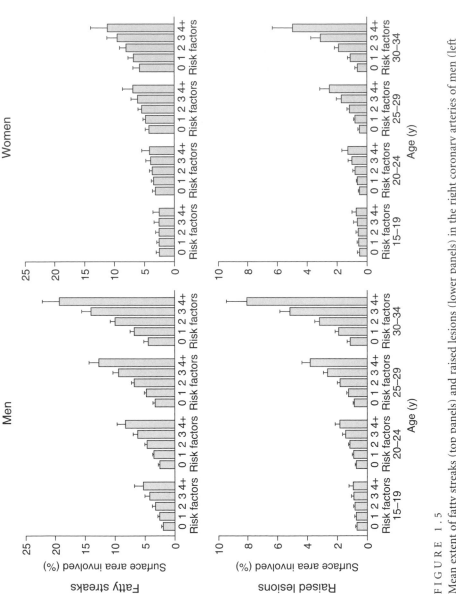

FIGURE 1.5

Mean extent of fatty streaks (top panels) and raised lesions (lower panels) in the right coronary arteries of men (left panels) and women (right panels) by number of risk factors present and 5-year age group. Means are adjusted for race. T above the bars represents the standard error.

than sixfold increase in extent of raised lesions over the same age span. This cumulative effect of multiple risk factors is similar to that reported from the Bogalusa Heart Study, which included younger subjects (Berenson et al., 1998). These comparisons show the ultimate potential for preventing or delaying the progression of atherosclerosis in young people and for retarding the onset of clinical coronary heart disease (and other atherosclerotic diseases) in later life. Although risk factor effects vary in magnitude, no established risk factor can be safely ignored.

These results reinforce the importance of controlling *all* the risk factors beginning in childhood and adolescence, as emphasized in American Heart Association reports in 1992 and 2002 (Strong et al., 1992; Williams et al., 2002). These results also suggest that more aggressive intervention is indicated for individuals with multiple risk factors, as is done in considering risk and interventions in older individuals.

Locations within Arteries That Are Vulnerable to Atherosclerosis

As pointed out with respect to the thoracic aorta, the propensity to develop lesions varies by artery. This propensity also varies within an artery. In the abdominal aorta, lesions are most likely to develop on the dorsolateral aspect of the aorta just proximal to its bifurcation (McGill et al., 2000a). This location is most responsive to the effect of smoking on the abdominal aorta and the effect begins by age 15. In the right coronary artery, the first 2 cm are more likely to develop lesions than the remainder of the artery. The risk factor effects on these sites where lesions are likely to develop are about 25% greater than effects estimated for an entire artery. Because only a small part of an artery needs to be involved to cause clinical disease, some of these young adults are probably closer to the clinical disease threshold than we might anticipate on the basis of the results for an entire artery.

Effects on Transitional or Intermediate Lesions

The effects of risk factors on the raised fatty streak (also known as an intermediate lesion), a gross lesion interpreted as representing the transition between the flat fatty streak and the fibrous plaque, were similar to the effects on raised lesions. However, these effects were observed at younger ages than the ages at which effects on raised lesions are seen (McGill et al., 2000b). While some investigators have questioned the importance of the fatty streak, the microscopic qualities associated with the raised fatty streak indicate that it is a lesion progressing to a raised lesion, which in turn is directly related to clinical disease.

▓ Underestimation of Risk Factor Effects

The strength of the associations of risk factors and atherosclerotic lesions reported from the PDAY study are probably underestimates of the true strengths of the associations. Measurement errors in the risk factors are expected to reduce the observed association of the risk factors with lesions. Also, because there is substantial within-subject biologic variation in the risk factor variables measured in serum, the single measurement available for each subject in this study reflects the long-term average less precisely than multiple measurements that are possible in living subjects. Hemodilution or hemoconcentration, either of which occurs in some subjects, introduces additional variation. These sources of additional variation are expected to reduce the observed association of the risk factors measured in serum with atherosclerotic lesions.

We would expect to find a lower prevalence of advanced lesions and stenosis in the LAD coronary artery because we assessed lesions and stenosis at only one arterial site. Stary reported the prevalence of coronary artery lesions in 1160 persons from birth to 29 years of age using a grading system similar to the AHA system (Stary, 1989). For comparable age and sex groups, the prevalence of advanced lesions (AHA grade 4 or 5) we found in PDAY cases is about one-quarter to one-half the prevalence reported by Stary in multiple coronary artery sections.

As pointed out above, estimates of risk factor effects based on measurement of atherosclerosis in the most vulnerable regions of an artery are about 25% greater than estimates of risk factor effects on atherosclerosis in entire arterial segments as presented here (McGill et al., 2000a).

▓ SUMMARY: IMPLICATIONS OF RESULTS FROM PATHOLOGIC STUDIES FOR PRIMARY PREVENTION

* *Atherosclerosis begins in childhood.*
    Atherosclerosis appears in the first decade of life and, in a population with a high rate of atherosclerotic disease in middle age, progresses rapidly during adolescence and young adulthood. Atherosclerotic lesions are present in almost all aortas and about half the right coronary arteries by the late teens (15 to 19 years) and increase in extent and severity through the early thirties (30 to 34 years). Furthermore, a substantial proportion of young people have coronary artery lesions that are vulnerable to rupture and thrombosis and have the potential to precipitate coronary heart disease.
* *Risk factors accelerate the progression of atherosclerosis in youth.*
    The extent and severity of atherosclerosis in young people, assessed by both gross and microscopic criteria, are associated with the same risk factors as coronary heart disease in middle-aged and older adults. Although

risk factor effects vary in magnitude, no established risk factor can be safely ignored. The risk factor effects are cumulative, and the more risk factors an individual has, the greater the likelihood of progressing atherosclerosis and the greater the need for intervention.

• *There is potential for primary prevention.*

The differences between young men and women in extent and severity of advanced atherosclerotic lesions, observed some 20 years before the occurrence of the well-known difference between middle-aged men and women in susceptibility to coronary heart disease, support the concept that retarding the progression of atherosclerosis by risk factor modification in young people will delay the onset of clinical coronary heart disease. The limited increase in extent of coronary artery raised lesions between 15 and 34 years of age in the absence of any risk factors, compared to the extent of lesions for those with risk factors, illustrates the potential for primary prevention.

• *Intervention should begin early.*

The rapid increase in raised lesions at about age 25 suggests that risk factor control should be initiated prior to that age. The results of the pathology studies regarding fatty streaks and intermediate lesions suggest intervention at an even younger age. This conclusion is consistent with the observation that serum cholesterol levels in young adults predict coronary heart disease risk in middle age (Klag et al., 1993; Stamler et al., 2000). The earlier all of the cardiovascular risk factors are controlled, as recommended by the American Heart Association in 1992 and 2002 (Strong et al., 1992; Williams et al., 2002), the greater the potential for deferring the onset of coronary heart disease. Prevention of adult coronary heart disease is, indeed, a pediatric problem (Van Horn and Greenland, 1997).

■ REFERENCES

Auerbach, O., and L. Garfinkel. 1980. Atherosclerosis and Aneurysm of Aorta in Relation to Smoking Habits and Age. *Chest* 78:805–9.

Berenson, G.S. 1977. Risk Factors in Children—The Early Natural History of Atherosclerosis. In: *Atherosclerosis IV; International Symposium on Atherosclerosis, 4th, Tokyo, Japan, 1976, Proceedings.* Edited by G. Schettler, Y. Goto, Y. Hata, and G. Klose. Berlin: Springer-Verlag, pp. 489–97.

Berenson, G.S., S.R. Srinivasan, W. Bao, W.P. Newman, III, R.E. Tracy, and W.A. Wattigney, for the Bogalusa Heart Study. 1998. Association between Multiple Cardiovascular Risk Factors and Atherosclerosis in Children and Young Adults. *N Engl J Med* 338:1650–6.

Berenson, G.S., W.A. Wattigney, R.E. Tracy, W.P. Newman, III, S.R. Srinivasan, L.S. Webber, E.R. Dalferes, Jr., and J.P. Strong. 1992. Atherosclerosis of the Aorta and Coronary Arteries and Cardiovascular Risk Factors in Persons Aged 6 to 30 Years and Studied at Necropsy (The Bogalusa Heart Study). *Am J Cardiol* 70:851–8.

Calle, E.E., M.J. Thun, J.M. Petrelli, C. Rodriguez, and C.W. Heath, Jr. 1999. Body-Mass Index and Mortality in a Prospective Cohort of U.S. Adults. *N Engl J Med* 341:1097–105.

Centers for Disease Control. 1992. Tobacco, Alcohol, and Other Drug Use Among High School Students—United States, 1991. *Morb Mortal Wkly Rep* 41:698–703.

Cook, D.G., P.H. Whincup, G. Miller, I.M. Carey, F.J. Adshead, O. Papacosta, M. Walker, and D. Howarth. 1999. Fibrinogen and Factor VII Levels are Related to Adiposity but Not to Fetal Growth or Social Class in Children Aged 10–11 Years. *Am J Epidemiol* 150: 727–36.

Donahue, R.P., D.R. Jacobs, Jr., S. Sidney, L.E. Wagenknecht, J.J. Albers and S.B. Hulley. 1989. Distribution of Lipoproteins and Apolipoproteins in Young Adults. The CARDIA Study. *Arteriosclerosis* 9:656–64.

Ford, E.S., D.A. Galuska, C. Gillespie, J.C. Will, W.H. Giles, and W.H. Dietz. 2001. C-Reactive Protein and Body Mass Index in Children: Findings from the Third National Health and Nutrition Examination Survey, 1988–1994. *J Pediatr* 138:486–92.

Grundy, S.M. 2001. Non-High-Density Lipoprotein Cholesterol Level as Potential Risk Predictor and Therapy Target. *Arch Intern Med* 161:1379–90.

Gunnell, D.J., S.J. Frankel, K. Nanchahal, T.J. Peters, and G.D. Smith. 1998. Childhood Obesity and Adult Cardiovascular Mortality: A 57-year Follow-up Study Based on the Boyd Orr Cohort. *Am J Clin Nutr* 67:1111–8.

Haffner, S.M., M.P. Stern, H.P. Hazuda, B.D. Mitchell, and J.K. Patterson. 1990. Cardiovascular Risk Factors in Confirmed Prediabetic Individuals. Does the Clock for Coronary Heart Disease Start Ticking Before the Onset of Clinical Diabetes? *JAMA* 263:2893–8.

Klag, M.J., D.E. Ford, L.A. Mead, J. He, P.K. Whelton, K-Y. Liang, and D.M. Levine. 1993. Serum Cholesterol in Young Men and Subsequent Cardiovascular Disease. *N Engl J Med* 328:313–8.

Lauer, R.M., W.E. Connor, P.E. Leaverton, M.A. Reiter, and W.R. Clarke. 1975. Coronary Heart Disease Risk Factors in School Children: The Muscatine Study. *J Pediatr* 86:697–706.

Lee, R.T., and P. Libby. 1997. The Unstable Atheroma. *Arterioscler Thromb Vasc Biol* 17:1859–67.

Libby, P. 2001. Current Concepts of the Pathogenesis of the Acute Coronary Syndromes. *Circulation* 104:365–72.

Master, A.M., S. Dack, and H.L. Jaffe. 1939. Age, Sex and Hypertension in Myocardial Infarction Due to Coronary Occlusion. *Arch Intern Med* 64:767–86.

McGill, Jr., H.C. 1968. Fatty Streaks in the Coronary Arteries and Aorta. *Lab Invest* 18:560–4.

McGill, Jr., H.C., J.C. Geer, and J.P. Strong. 1963. Natural History of Human Atherosclerotic Lesions. In: *Atherosclerosis and Its Origin.* Edited by M. Sandler and G.H. Bourne. New York: Academic Press, pp. 39–65.

McGill, Jr., H.C., C.A. McMahan, E.E. Herderick, R.E. Tracy, G.T. Malcom, A.W. Zieske, J.P. Strong, for the PDAY Research Group. 2000a. Effects of Coronary Heart Disease Risk Factors on Atherosclerosis of Selected Regions of the Aorta and Right Coronary Artery. *Arterioscler Thromb Vasc Biol* 20:836–45.

McGill, Jr., H.C., C.A. McMahan, G.T. Malcom, M.C. Oalmann, J. P. Strong, and the Pathobiological Determinants of Atherosclerosis in Youth (PDAY) Research Group. 1995. Relation of Glycohemoglobin and Adiposity to Atherosclerosis in Youth. *Arterioscler Thromb Vasc Biol* 15:431–40.

McGill, Jr., H.C., C.A. McMahan, G.T. Malcom, M.C. Oalmann, J.P. Strong, for the PDAY Research Group. 1997. Effects of Serum Lipoproteins and Smoking on Atherosclerosis in Young Men and Women. *Arterioscler Thromb Vasc Biol* 17:95–106.

McGill, Jr., H.C., C.A. McMahan, R.E. Tracy, M.C. Oalmann, J.F. Cornhill, E.E. Herderick, and J.P. Strong, for the Pathobiological Determinants of Atherosclerosis in Youth (PDAY) Research Group. 1998. Relation of a Postmortem Renal Index of Hypertension to Atherosclerosis and Coronary Artery Size in Young Men and Women. *Arterioscler Thromb Vasc Biol* 18:1108–18.

McGill, Jr., H. C., C.A. McMahan, A.W. Zieske, G.T. Malcom, R.E. Tracy, and J.P. Strong, for the Pathobiological Determinants of Atherosclerosis in Youth (PDAY) Research

Group. 2001. Effects of Nonlipid Risk Factors on Atherosclerosis in Youth with a Favorable Lipoprotein Profile. *Circulation* 103:1546–50.

McGill, Jr., H.C., C.A. McMahan, A.W. Zieske, G.D. Sloop, J.V. Walcott, D.A. Troxclair, G.T. Malcom, R.E. Tracy, M.C. Oalmann, J.P. Strong, for the Pathobiological Determinants of Atherosclerosis in Youth (PDAY) Study. 2000b. Associations of Coronary Heart Disease Risk Factors with the Intermediate Lesion of Atherosclerosis in Youth. *Arterioscler Thromb Vasc Biol* 20:1998–2004.

McGill, Jr., H.C, C.A. McMahan, A.W. Zieske, R.E. Tracy, G.T. Malcom, E.E. Herderick, and J.P. Strong, for the Pathobiological Determinants of Atherosclerosis in Youth (PDAY) Research Group. 2000c. Association of Coronary Heart Disease Risk Factors with Microscopic Qualities of Coronary Atherosclerosis in Youth. *Circulation* 102:374–9.

Miller, G.J., and N.E. Miller. 1975. Plasma-High-Density-Lipoprotein Concentration and Development of Ischaemic Heart-Disease. *Lancet* 305:16–9.

Montenegro, M.R., and D.A. Eggen. 1968. Topography of Atherosclerosis in the Coronary Arteries. *Lab Invest* 18:586–93.

Must, A., P.F. Jacques, G.E. Dallal, C.J. Bajema and W.H. Dietz. 1992. Long-Term Morbidity and Mortality of Overweight Adolescents: A Follow-Up of the Harvard Growth Study of 1922 to 1935. *N Engl J Med* 327:1350–5.

National Cholesterol Education Program. 1993. Summary of the Second Report of the National Cholesterol Education Program (NCEP) Expert Panel on Detection, Evaluation, and Treatment of High Blood Cholesterol in Adults (Adult Treatment Panel II). *JAMA* 269:3015–23.

National Heart, Lung, and Blood Institute [U. S.]. 1985. Hypertension Prevalence and the Status of Awareness, Treatment, and Control in the United States: Final Report of the Subcommittee on Definition and Prevalence of the 1984 Joint National Committee. *Hypertension* 7:457- 68.

Pooling Project Research Group. 1978. Relationship of Blood Pressure, Serum Cholesterol, Smoking Habit, Relative Weight and ECG Abnormalities to Incidence of Major Coronary Events: Final Report of the Pooling Project. *J Chron Dis* 31:201–306.

Sacks, F.M. 1998. Why Cholesterol as a Central Theme in Coronary Artery Disease? *Am J Cardiol* 82:14T–17T.

Solberg, L.A., and J.P. Strong. 1983. Risk Factors and Atherosclerotic Lesions: A Review of Autopsy Studies. *Arteriosclerosis* 3:187 98.

Sprecher, D.L., F.J. Schaefer, K.M. Kent, R.E. Gregg, L.A. Zech, J.M. Hoeg, B. McManus, W.C. Roberts and H.B. Brewer, Jr. 1984. Cardiovascular Features of Homozygous Familial Hypercholesterolemia: Analysis of 16 Patients. *Am J Cardiol* 54:20–30.

Stamler, J., M.L. Daviglus, D.B. Garside, A.R. Dyer, P. Greenland, and J.D. Neaton. 2000. Relationship of Baseline Serum Cholesterol Levels in 3 Large Cohorts of Younger Men to Long-Term Coronary, Cardiovascular, and All-Cause Mortality and to Longevity. *JAMA* 284:311–8.

Stamler, J., R. Stamler, W.V. Brown, A.M. Gotto, P. Greenland, S. Grundy, M. Hegsted, R.V. Luepker, J.D. Neaton, D. Steinberg, N. Stone, L, Van Horn, and R.W. Wissler. 1993. Serum Cholesterol: Doing the Right Thing. *Circulation* 88:1954–60.

Stary, H.C. 1989. Evolution and Progression of Atherosclerotic Lesions in Coronary Arteries of Children and Young Adults. *Arteriosclerosis* Supplement I 9:I-19–I-32.

Stary, H.C., A.B. Chandler, R.E. Dinsmore, V. Fuster, S. Glagov, W. Insull, Jr., M.E. Rosenfeld, C.J. Schwartz, W.D. Wagner, and R.W. Wissler. 1995. A Definition of Advanced Types of Atherosclerotic Lesions and a Histological Classification of Atherosclerosis: A Report from the Committee on Vascular Lesions of the Council on Arteriosclerosis, American Heart Association. *Arterioscler Thromb Vasc Biol* 15:1512–31.

Stary, H.C., A.B. Chandler, S. Glagov, J.R. Guyton, W. Insull, Jr., M.E. Rosenfeld, S.A. Schaffer, C.J. Schwartz, W.D. Wagner, and R.W. Wissler. 1994. A Definition of Initial,

Fatty Streak, and Intermediate Lesions of Atherosclerosis: A Report from the Committee on Vascular Lesions of the Council on Arteriosclerosis, American Heart Association. *Circulation* 89:2462–78.

Steinberg, D. 1997. Lewis A. Conner Memorial Lecture: Oxidative Modification of LDL and Atherogenesis. *Circulation* 95:1062–71.

Steinberg, D., and A.M. Gotto, Jr. 1999. Preventing Coronary Artery Disease by Lowering Cholesterol Levels: Fifty Years from Bench to Bedside. *JAMA* 282:2043–50.

Steinberger, J., A. Moran, C-P. Hong, D.R. Jacobs, Jr., and A.R. Sinaiko. 2001. Adiposity in Childhood Predicts Obesity and Insulin Resistance in Young Adulthood. *J Pediatr* 138: 469–73.

Stern, M.P., and S.M. Haffner. 1986. Body Fat Distribution and Hyperinsulinemia as Risk Factors for Diabetes and Cardiovascular Disease. *Arteriosclerosis* 6:123–30.

Strong, J.P., G.T. Malcom, C.A. McMahan, R.E. Tracy, W.P. Newman, III, E.E. Herderick, and J.F. Cornhill, for the Pathobiological Determinants of Atherosclerosis in Youth Research Group. 1999. Prevalence and Extent of Atherosclerosis in Adolescents and Young Adults: Implications for Prevention from the Pathobiological Determinants of Atherosclerosis in Youth Study. *JAMA* 281:727–35.

Strong, J.P., and M.L. Richards. 1976. Cigarette Smoking and Atherosclerosis in Autopsied Men. *Atherosclerosis* 23:451–76.

Strong, W.B., R.J. Deckelbaum, S.S. Gidding, R-E.W. Kavey, R. Washington, J.H. Wilmore, and C.L. Perry. 1992. Integrated Cardiovascular Health Promotion in Childhood: A Statement for Health Professionals from the Subcommittee on Atherosclerosis and Hypertension in Childhood of the Council on Cardiovascular Disease in the Young, American Heart Association. *Circulation* 85:1638–50.

Tejada, C., J.P. Strong, M.R. Montenegro, C. Restrepo, and L.A. Solberg. 1968. Distribution of Coronary and Aortic Atherosclerosis by Geographic Location, Race, and Sex. *Lab Invest* 18:509–26.

Troiano, R.P., K.M. Flegal, R.J. Kuczmarski, S.M. Campbell, and C.L. Johnson. 1995. Overweight Prevalence and Trends for Children and Adolescents: The National Health and Nutrition Examination Surveys, 1963 to 1991. *Arch Pediatric Adolesc Med* 149:1085–91.

Van Horn, L., and P. Greenland. 1997. "Prevention of Coronary Artery Disease Is a Pediatric Problem." *JAMA* 278:1779–80.

Wang, N., I. Tabas, R. Winchester, S. Ravalli, L.E. Rabbani, and A. Tall. 1996. Interleukin 8 Is Induced by Cholesterol Loading of Macrophages and Expressed by Macrophage Foam Cells in Human Atheroma. *J Biol Chem* 271:8837–42.

Williams C.L., L.L. Hayman, S.R. Daniels, T.N. Robinson, J. Steinberger, S. Paridon, and T. Bazzarre. 2002. Cardiovascular Health in Childhood: A Statement for Health Professionals from the Committee on Atherosclerosis, Hypertension, and Obesity in the Young (AHOY) of the Council on Cardiovascular Disease in the Young, American Heart Association. *Circulation* 106:143–160.

Wissler, R. W. 1991. USA Multicenter Study of the Pathobiology of Atherosclerosis in Youth. *Ann NY Acad Sci* 623:26–39.

Wissler, R.W., L. Hiltscher, T. Oinuma, and the PDAY Research Group. 1996. The Lesions of Atherosclerosis in the Young. From Fatty Streaks to Intermediate Lesions. In: *Atherosclerosis and Coronary Artery Disease, Volume 1*. Edited by V. Fuster, R. Ross, and E. J. Topol. Philadelphia: Lippincott-Raven, pp. 475–89.

CHAPTER 2

The Major Adult Cardiovascular Diseases: A Global Historical Perspective

Jeremiah Stamler, James D. Neaton, Daniel B. Garside, and Martha L. Daviglus

The major adult cardiovascular diseases (CVD) have their nutritional, metabolic, and pathophysiologic beginnings early in life. The epidemic onslaught of these diseases is due to multiple adverse environmental exposures, particularly adverse lifestyles, from preconception on, in populations of general genetic susceptibility (related to evolution of the human species).

▓ EARLY CLINICAL PATHOLOGIC INVESTIGATION

Starting in the late nineteenth century, pathologic studies showed that early cholesterol lipid–laden atherosclerotic lesions (aortic, coronary) can occur in the first and second decades of life (Hueper, 1944, 1945; Katz and Stamler, 1953). Linked with clinical investigation, such studies demonstrated that younger people with diseases producing endogenous hypercholesterolemia are prone to atherosclerotic lesions early in life. These diseases associated with elevated plasma cholesterol, include genetic hyperbetalipoproteinemia, hypothyroidism, biliary obstruction, nephrosis, and type 1 diabetes (Katz and Stamler, 1953). These observations, on otherwise unrelated diseases involving diverse endogenous metabolic abnormalities producing hypercholesterolemia, fostered the inference that serum cholesterol was importantly related to the large accumulations of cholesterol (especially esterified cholesterol) in early intimal atherosclerotic plaques. Such findings laid the foundation for the conclusion early in the twentieth century that atherosclerosis is a specific disease entity among the several arterioscleroses (the generic designation). The hallmark of atherosclerosis is abnormal accumulations of cholesterol-laden lipids in the arterial intima-media (Marchand, 1904, Katz and Stamler, 1953). These concepts were reinforced in the early years after World War II by ultracentrifugal analyses identifying essential familial xanthomatosis as genetically transmitted hyperbetalipoproteinemia. The rare individuals homozygous for this abnormality, hence with very high levels of serum low-density lipoprotein cholesterol (LDL-C), were found to develop early, severe atherosclerosis and consequent severe coronary heart disease (CHD) that was often fatal before age 15 (Gofman et al., 1950; Thannhauser, 1950; Katz and Stamler, 1953).

■ CLINICAL CARDIOLOGY

The importance of adverse serum cholesterol levels in the pathogenesis of premature CHD was underscored by case series data from clinical cardiology. By the middle decades of the twentieth century, there was extensive evidence that average levels of serum total cholesterol (TC) and LDL-C were much higher among cases than among controls, especially at younger ages, (Boas et al., 1948; Katz and Stamler, 1953; Gertler and White, 1954; Katz et al., 1958; Lawry et al., 1957). With the subsequent development of coronary angiography, multiple clinical studies linked dyslipidemia to severity of coronary lesions, especially in younger people (Pearson, 1984). Other traits such as high blood pressure and diabetes mellitus were also related to CHD. An important advance during the first decades of the twentieth century was the demonstration by clinicians in France and the United Sates that severe high blood pressure and its complications could be controlled with diets markedly reduced in salt (NaCl) (Ambard and Beaujard, 1904; Allen and Sherrill, 1922; Kempner, 1948; Stamler, 1997).

■ ANIMAL EXPERIMENTATION

This mounting knowledge base from pathologic and clinical research was concordant with findings from animal experimentation. During the period from 1908 to 1912, a group of young investigators in St. Petersburg, Russia serendipitously produced atherosclerotic lesions for the first time, by feeding meats, eggs, and milk to rabbits. They quickly showed that the critical offending dietary ingredient, the "materia pecans," as Anitschkow dubbed it, was the cholesterol in these foods (Anitschkow, 1933; Katz and Stamler, 1953; Katz et al., 1958). After World War II, animal experimentation burgeoned in the United States and many other countries. The animal model was expanded to include several species (avian and mammalian; herbivorous, carnivorous, omnivorous, including nonhuman primates), with cholesterol feeding virtually a *sine qua non* to achieve the altered serum cholesterol-lipoprotein patterns essential for significant atherogenesis. Lesions were produced in young animals, yielding data that helped lay to rest the notion, widely current for decades, that atherosclerosis was an inevitable consequence of "normal" aging (Katz and Stamler, 1953). It was also shown that once excess cholesterol was added to the diet, producing dyslipidemia, multiple other factors influenced the process, including other dietary components, for example, amount and type of neutral fat, blood pressure level, and hormones (thyroid, estrogenic, etc.). In several species, mammalian and avian, salt intake was shown to relate directly to blood pressure (Meneely, 1967; Meneely and Battarbee, 1976; Laragh and Pecker, 1983; Tobian, 1991; Denton et al., 1995; Stamler, 1997). The experimental coproduction of diet-induced dyslipidemia and increased blood pressure resulted in aggravated atherogenesis.

■ POPULATION-BASED EPIDEMIOLOGIC RESEARCH

The stream of epidemiologic evidence also originated in the late nineteenth and early twentieth century with studies on "geographic pathology" (the original terminology) done mainly by physicians from metropolitan countries sent to work in imperial colonies of Africa, Asia, and Latin America. On the basis of clinical observations and postmortem examinations, they reported that severe atherosclerotic disease was rare among the rural and urban populations of these countries, in contrast to its commonality among people in their home countries and in affluent upper-class individuals with "Western" lifestyles in the colonies. In the years just before and after World War II, reviews of such studies, linked to results of cholesterol feeding experiments in rabbits, produced meaningful scientific generalizations (Raab, 1932; Rosenthal, 1934; Snapper, 1941; Katz and Stamler, 1953; Katz et al., 1958; Stamler, 1966; Stamler, 1967). They underscored the key role of dietary patterns in producing atherosclerotic disease and in accounting for cross-population contrasts. These reviews particularly emphasized the adverse role of high animal product intake, i.e., high cholesterol and animal fat intake, prevailing in Europe and North America. These nutritional patterns were implicated as related to both adverse serum cholesterol and blood pressure levels. After World War II, epidemiologic research expanded in the United States and several other countries, encompassing both cross-population and within-population studies.

■ CROSS-POPULATION STUDIES AFTER WORLD WAR II

Comparisons have involved populations both across and within countries (Keys and White, 1956; Inter-Society Commission for Heart Disease Resources, 1970;

Stamler, 1966, 1967, 1978, 1979, 1989, 1992, 1994, 1995, 1997; Stamler et al., 1993b, 1994, 1997, 1999, 2000, 2002, 2003). International investigations involving young adults include three significant analyses of postmortem findings: the Kyushu (Japan) and Minnesota (U.S.) autopsy study; the assessments of coronary atherosclerosis in American and Asian (Korean, Vietnamese) soldiers killed in battle; and the International Atherosclerosis Project (IAP). In addition, multiple analyses were done of international data relating national per capita averages for dietary variables, particularly dietary lipids, to age- and sex-specific CHD, CVD, and all cause mortality rates. Nutrient data were derived from national food balance sheets available from the United Nations Food and Agriculture Organization (FAO); mortality data were obtained from the World Health Organization (WHO) (Stamler, 1979; Stamler, 1989).

The mid-twentieth century Kyushu–Minnesota age- and sex-specific comparisons of coronary atherosclerosis showed that occurrence of lesions was greater in American than in Japanese individuals from young adulthood on, with a conspicuous sex differential for American decedents (more atherosclerosis in men than women), but not for Japanese (i.e., both men and women just above zero for lesions) (Kimura, 1956). A similar contrast for men was found between American and Asian soldiers killed in Korea and Vietnam (Enos et al., 1953; Rogot and Hrubec, 1989).

The IAP researchers conducted analyses on microscopic as well as gross characteristics of early atherosclerotic lesions in coronary arteries of younger decedents from several countries of contrasting economic development. The data indicated that even in these "juvenile" lesions, cellular pathology was more advanced in younger decedents from more affluent countries than in those from poorer, economically developing countries (McGill, 1968; McGill et al., 2000).

All these international studies related their findings on atherosclerosis across populations to differences in lifestyles, particularly habitual dietary patterns, most particularly dietary lipid consumption. This link between dietary lipid (especially cholesterol and saturated fat) and atherogenesis has also been shown repeatedly in the analyses of FAO-WHO data. These invariably show high-order associations between national per capita averages of dietary lipids (cholesterol, saturated fats, combined dietary lipid scores) and age- and sex-specific national CHD mortality rates, including for younger age groups (e.g., 35 to 44 years) (Stamler, 1979, 1989). Also, national trends of these dietary variables over time relate to national trends of CHD mortality (Byington et al., 1979).

Considered together, the results of these international studies support the concept of a significant three-way relationship among diet (particularly dietary lipids), serum lipids (particularly TC and LDL-C), and atherogenesis (Stamler, 1967, 1979, 1989; Inter-Society Commission for Heart Disease Resources, 1970). The international cross-population analyses from the prospective Seven Countries and Ni-Hon-San studies of middle-aged men have yielded concordant findings (Inter-Society Commission for Heart Disease Resources, 1970; Keys, 1970, 1980; Kagan et al., 1974; Marmot et al., 1975; Worth et al., 1975; Stamler, 1979,

1989). Further, the cross-population analyses for 52 samples (about 200 men and women per sample) in 32 countries worldwide conducted by the INTERSALT Study showed a significant association between median 24-hour Na excretion (index of salt intake) and several blood pressure indices, including the upward slope of systolic (SBP) and diastolic blood pressure (DBP) from ages 20 to 60 (INTERSALT Cooperative Research Group, 1988; Elliott et al., 1996; Stamler, 1997). The INTERSALT samples included four isolated population groups with low salt intake. In accordance with many prior reports, their average SBP/DBP was low at every age, there was little or no evidence of higher average blood pressure at older ages, and hypertension was rare or nonexistent (Shaper, 1974; Page et al., 1974; Page et al., 1981; Mancilha-Carvalho et al., 1989; Stamler, 1997). Studies in migrants and populations in transition have shown that these "exceptional" blood pressure patterns are attributable to environmental factors, not population genetics.

Other cross-population comparisons have focused on contrasting samples within a country. One example is the study of an American Zen Buddhist group eating vegetarian fare (Sacks et al., 1975). Compared to age- and sex-matched people from the general population eating the usual American diet, average serum lipids and blood pressures were lower for the vegetarians. These differences were in part attributable to the fact that the vegetarians were leaner. More favorable levels of nutrient intake also contributed to lower risk factor levels. Several other studies reported lower blood pressure in vegetarians than in omnivores in Western industrialized countries (Sacks et al., 1974; Sacks and Kass, 1988). Further, the markedly different eating patterns among vegetarian Seventh Day Adventists in California were shown to be associated with more favorable serum lipid levels and lower CHD rates from young adulthood on, compared to those for age and sex-matched people from the general California population (Walden et al., 1964; Phillips et al., 1978; Fraser, 1986).

■ WITHIN-POPULATION STUDIES AFTER WORLD WAR II

Within-population studies, especially long-term prospective investigations, have also been important. Among the "first generation" of these studies, most dealt with men who were middle-aged at baseline. The studies included the Albany and Los Angeles civil servant, the Chicago Peoples Gas and Western Electric, the Framingham and Tecumseh community, Midwest railroad, and Minnesota business- and professional-men studies (American Public Health Association Symposium, 1957; Inter-Society Commission for Heart Disease Resources, 1970; Pooling Project Research Group, 1978). The prospective findings of these studies were assessed jointly in analyses by the national cooperative Pooling Project for over 8200 men of baseline ages 40 to 59 with 8.6 years of follow-up. They demonstrated significant, continuous, graded, strong, independent relationships of three readily measured traits—serum cholesterol, blood pressure, and cigarette smoking—to incidence of first major coronary events (Inter-Society Commission for Heart Disease Resources, 1970; Pooling Project Research Group, 1978). The findings from these studies formed the basis for the concept of major CVD risk factors. Traits amenable to prevention and control, common in the general population, were shown repeatedly to be related prospectively, independently, strongly, and significantly to CVD risk. Expert groups judged these factors to be causative (Inter-Society Commission for Heart Disease Resources, 1970). The initial definition of major risk factors identified four as meeting all these criteria: adverse levels of serum cholesterol and blood pressure, cigarette smoking (the easily measured triad), and adverse diet. Based on the consequences of the years-long waxing obesity epidemic, overweight/obesity and diabetes were recently added to this set (Eckel and Krauss, 1998; National Heart, Lung, and Blood Institute [NHLBI], 1998a; National Cholesterol Education Program [NCEP], 2001, 2002). Increased obesity among children and youth and the related concurrent increase in the occurrence of type 2 diabetes at early ages have made it all too clear that "maturity-onset" diabetes is an anachronistic term (Sinha et al., 2002).

Use of multiple logistic regression coefficients for serum cholesterol, blood pressure, and cigarette smoking to stratify the Pooling Project cohort into quintiles of risk yielded data showing marked continuous gradation in CHD rates across the quintiles, with risk low in quintile one and several-fold higher risk in quintile five. Men with adverse levels of any two or all three major risk factors were shown to be at particularly greater risk. Moreover, use of this method yielded high-level agreement between predicted and observed risk when coefficients from one set of cohorts were applied to predict risk in another cohort (Pooling Project Research Group, 1978). For the youngest stratum, ages 40 to 44 at baseline, body mass index (BMI) was also independently related to risk. Long-term prospective analyses of data from individual men in the Seven Countries Study produced concordant results (Mariotti et al., 1986).

These U.S. cohorts consisted of men with American lifestyles that were common in that era. Most individuals had adverse eating patterns and were sedentary and overweight, and about half smoked cigarettes. Therefore, for prospective analytic purposes there were too few persons with favorable levels for all these traits (serum cholesterol <200 mg/dL *and* SBP/DBP ≤120/≤80 mmHg *and* non-smoking *and* BMI <25.0 kg/ m², *and* no history of diabetes or heart attack). While no such low risk subcohort of adequate size could be identified, the low estimated CHD rate for the Pooling Project men in the lowest quintile of calculated risk indicated the importance of low-risk status.

Among these and other first-generation studies, only the Chicago Western Electric (WE) study collected high-quality baseline data on nutrient intake for individual participants (Paul et al., 1963; Shekelle et al., 1981; Stamler et al., 1993a). At baseline, there was a significant association between dietary lipids and serum total cholesterol (Keys et al., 1965; Hegsted et al., 1993; Clarke et al., 1997).

The prospective data showed that serum cholesterol, blood pressure, smoking, BMI, and dietary cholesterol all related independently to risk of death from CHD (also CVD and all causes). This finding has been confirmed by several other prospective studies (Shekelle et al., 1981; Stamler and Shekelle, 1988; Stamler et al., 1993a). Therefore, the adverse dietary pattern prevailing in the United States in the mid-decades of the twentieth century, including ≥40% of kilocalories from total fat, ≥16% of kilocalories from saturated fatty acids, and ≥700 mg cholesterol/day (average intakes recorded for the WE men in 1957–59), was appropriately designated one of the major CHD risk factors.

INTERSALT analyses showed that daily sodium and alcohol intake (especially heavy drinking, ≥300 ml/week) and BMI were independently related to blood pressure. Daily potassium intake had an inverse relation to blood pressure. These associations were less strong for younger (ages 20 to 39) than older (ages 40 to 59) adults (INTERSALT Cooperative Research Group, 1988; 1989; Stamler, 1997). The level of these variables was more adverse among less educated persons than among more educated persons, and higher blood pressure levels were found among less than among more educated participants (Stamler et al., 1992). The importance of multiple dietary factors in accounting for this inverse association between education and blood pressure has been underscored by recent data from the INTERMAP Study (Stamler, 2003). With four 24-hour dietary recalls and two timed 24-hour urine collections done for all 2195 U.S. participants, several dietary variables were shown to account for higher blood pressure of those less educated, including Na, K, and BMI (as in INTERSALT), as well as vegetable protein, Keys dietary lipid score, Mg, Ca, P, and Fe (all with intakes putatively more adverse in those with less education) (Stamler et al., 2003). Concordantly, several dietary variables, such as lower BMI, lower salt and Na/K intake, higher phosphorus and magnesium intake, accounted for lower SBP/DBP levels in southern middle-aged Chinese men and women compared to their northern counterparts (Zhao et al., 2004). Further, prospective data from the WE study indicate that multiple dietary variables affect blood pressure slopes during middle age: there is less rise in blood pressure with greater intake of vegetable protein, antioxidants, fruits, and vegetables and with less intake of cholesterol, saturated fats, and meats, and less or no weight gain (Stamler et al., 2002; Miura et al., 2004).

Important within-population long-term prospective studies of teenagers and young adults were also initiated soon after World War II. One of the first of these used college entrance medical examination findings for students at Harvard and Penn Universities Several traits in these young men predisposed them to high blood pressure later in life (Paffenbarger et al., 1968; 1983). Blood pressure, body mass, physical inactivity, and cigarette smoking during their youth (serum cholesterol was not measured) were independently related to the risk of mortality from CHD and CVD (Thorne et al., 1968; Paffenbarger et al., 1978). The findings on blood pressure, body mass and risk were concordant with long-term data on younger adults from life insurance actuarial analyses (Society of

Actuaries, 1959). Similarly, for Johns Hopkins University medical students, average serum cholesterol level during the years at school was found to relate strongly to CHD risk over the next 40 years (Klag et al., 1993). For middle-aged men a common "shorthand" formula has been that 1% higher serum cholesterol leads to 2% higher CHD risk. For young adults (at least men) the Johns Hopkins data indicate that the equation is about 1 to 5, meaning that for each 1% increase in serum cholesterol, CHD risk is higher by 5%.

The Pathobiological Determinants of Atherosclerosis in Youth (PDAY) Study of U.S. young adult decedents (see Chapter 1) has also reported strong relations of dyslipidemia, postmortem markers of adverse blood pressure, and other major risk factors to atherosclerosis early in life (McGill et al., 2000).

The Bogalusa (Louisiana) and Muscatine (Iowa) prospective studies (see Chapters 4 and 5), based on follow-up of cohorts of school children into adulthood, generated comprehensive data concordant with results reviewed above on the three-way relation among lifestyles (adverse diet patterns, sedentary habits, and smoking), and lifestyle-related major risk factors (serum cholesterol, blood pressure, BMI, diabetes) and risk of CVD (Lauer et al., 1975; Lauer and Shekelle, 1980; Berenson et al., 1980; Berenson, 1986).

Beginning in the 1990s, a body of evidence progressively emerged that went an important step further to define the role of early life traits in influencing adult CVD risk. Studies have shown that fetal intrauterine nutrient status and dietary factors during the early postpartum years may relate to subsequent levels of major CVD risk factors (Barker, 1998). For example, authors of a study of 1147 English infants found a significant inverse relation of birth weight to SBP at age 4 (Law et al., 1993). They reported that 1 kg higher birth weight was associated with SBP at age 4 lower on average by almost 3 mmHg. Further, a significant positive relation was found between weight at age 4 and SBP at age 4: weight 1 kg higher was associated with SBP 1.5 mmHg higher on average. In addition, a study in the Philippines reported an inverse relation of birth weight to adolescent SBP level of boys, and a direct relation of adverse maternal nutrition during pregnancy to adolescent blood pressure of offspring (Adair et al., 2001). Indices of intrauterine fetal nutritional status have also been found to be associated with major risk factor levels in middle age (Barker, 1998). The obvious implication of such findings, assuming they reflect independent etiologically significant relationships, is that primary CVD prevention begins with conception and preconception.

The Chicago Heart Association Detection Project in Industry and the Multiple Risk Factor Intervention Trial

For younger adults, precise estimates of the impact of readily measured major risk factors on CHD are now available from two studies with large samples and long prospective follow-up: the Chicago Heart Association Detection Project in Industry (CHA) and the Multiple Risk Factor Intervention Trial (MRFIT) (Stamler et al., 1993a). Among younger men in these two cohorts, the relation of baseline serum cholesterol to long-term risk of CHD death was continuous, graded, strong, and independent of other risk factors, with hazard ratios (HRs) 3.3 and greater for men with levels ≥240 mg/dL compared to those with optimal levels (<160 mg/dL) (Table 2.1). Data for younger CHA women were based on only 35 CHD deaths; however, the trend was similar to that for men.

For the large cohort of younger men in the MRFIT ($n = 72,566$, ages 35 to 39 years at baseline), the relation of SBP to 25–year risk of CHD death was also continuous, graded, strong, and independent of other risk factors, with HRs of 1.5 for those who were pre-hypertensive and about 5.0 for men with stage 2 hypertension (Table 2.1). For the smaller cohort of younger CHA men ($n = 10,752$, ages 18 to 39 years at baseline), the HRs followed a similar pattern. For younger CHA women ($n = 7335$) there was no evidence of an association. This is almost certainly an artifact attributable to the few CHD deaths, since multiple other data sets, including a recent meta-analysis with large numbers of CHD deaths in younger women, show that blood pressure relates to CHD at least as strongly in women as in men (Prospective Studies Collaboration, 2002).

The association between cigarette smoking and CHD death was also continuous, strong, and independent of other risk factors (Table 2.1). Baseline BMI was directly related to baseline blood pressure and serum cholesterol, as well as to prevalence of diabetes in younger CHA men and women. With control for these four major risk factors, the significant HRs of 1.8 for CHA men and 3.0 for CHA women with BMI ≥30.0 (obese) compared to women with BMI <25.0 kg/m² (non-overweight) demonstrated an independent influence of BMI on CHD risk (Table 2.1). In these younger CHA cohorts surveyed in 1967–73, before the epidemic of obesity took off, the proportions of obese were still relatively low (12% and 6%), hence prevalence rates of diabetes were low (1%). No CHD deaths occurred in the 64 diabetic women. In both cohorts of younger men, diabetes was strongly related to CHD risk (Table 2.1).

The large size of the MRFIT cohort made possible an in-depth 50-strata categorical analysis of CHD HRs for the 72,566 men, classified by five intervals of baseline serum cholesterol and SBP and by smoking status (Table 2.2). In general, for both nonsmokers and smokers at baseline, the higher the serum cholesterol, the greater the HRs in every blood pressure group. Similarly, for both nonsmokers and smokers, across the blood pressure groups, HRs were generally graded within each of the five serum cholesterol strata. The highest HR, 68.9, was, as expected, for smokers with serum cholesterol ≥240 mg/dL (stratum 5) and SBP ≥160 mmHg (stratum 5). Only 5215 men were in the cell with an HR of 1.00, i.e., only 7% of these younger adult men ages 35 to 39 were low risk, based on these cut points. Clearly, even in younger adulthood, virtually this entire cohort was already at increased risk of varying degrees, that is, coronary-prone. This finding emphasizes the population-wide epidemic nature of the CVD problem.

TABLE 2.1

Relation of major risk factors considered singly to long-term risk of death from coronary heart disease in men and women, baseline ages 18 to 39 years

Major Risk Factor Level	CHA Men Ages 18 to 39[a] Years			CHA Women Ages 18 to 39[a] Years			MRFIT Men Ages 35 to 39[b] Years		
	N	Death Rate[c]	Hazard Ratio[d]	N	Death Rate[c]	Hazard Ratio[d]	N	Death Ratio[c]	Hazard Ratio[e]
Baseline Serum Cholesterol (mg/dL)									
<160	2070	3.2	1.00	1919	1.1	1.00	6898	2.5	1.00
160–179	2297	5.5	1.89*	1857	0.6	0.64	11,616	3.0	1.16
180–199	2378	8.2	2.55***	1613	2.7	2.48	15,197	4.4	1.58**
200–219	1891	8.2	2.58***	1050	2.1	2.31	15,299	5.5	1.88***
220–239	1173	14.2	4.04***	537	2.3	2.14	10,901	8.2	2.65***
240–259	533	21.3	4.32***	201	0.9	1.21	6482	10.8	3.32***
260–279	245	29.3	6.83***	95	5.2	4.33	3550	15.3	4.42***
≥280	165	41.6	9.09***	63	6.0	4.01	2623	26.8	7.01***
<200	6741	5.8	1.00	5389	1.3	1.00	33,711	3.5	1.00
200–239	3063	10.4	1.63**	1586	2.1	1.57	26,200	6.6	1.66***
≥240	948	26.5	2.96***	360	3.1	1.80	12,655	15.3	3.33***
Cox coefficient (SE)	0.0132 (0.0015)***			0.0072 (0.0046)			0.0087 (0.0004)***		
HR for +35 mg/dL	1.59			1.29			1.36		
95% CI	1.44–1.76			0.94–1.77			1.32–1.39		
Baseline Systolic Blood Pressure (mmHg)									
≤120	2707	5.4	1.00	4066	1.5	1.0	25,704	3.6	1.00
121–129	3436[f]	8.0	1.31	2073[f]	1.3	0.77	19,692	5.3	1.37**
130–139	3681	9.5	1.35	1029	3.2	1.46	16,151	8.0	1.94***
140–159	928[g]	19.4	2.19***	167[g]	1.1	0.52	9714	13.0	2.79***
≥160							1305	26.7	5.19***

Cox coefficient (SE)	0.0124 (0.0037)***			−0.0003 (0.0121)			0.0268 (0.0017)***		
HR for +15 mmHg	1.20			1.00			1.49		
95% CI	1.08–1.34			0.70–1.42			1.42–1.57		

Baseline SBP/DBP (JNC 7 Criteria)

Normotensive	2592	5.4	1.00	3978	1.5	1.00	36,923	3.9	1.00
Prehypertensive	3232	7.3	1.20	1966	1.3	0.71	16,513	6.2	1.48***
Hypertension stage 1	3861	9.6	1.39	1162	3.1	1.38	15,251	10.2	2.21***
Hypertension stage 2	1067	18.7	2.15***	229	0.7	0.34	3879	22.1	4.29***

Baseline Cigarette Smoking (Cigarettes/Day)

Cox coefficient (SE)	0.0222 (0.0041)***			0.0423 (0.0123)***			0.0311 (0.0015)***		
HR for +20/day	1.56			2.33			1.86		
95% CI	1.33–1.83			1.44–3.77			1.76–1.98		
Never	3074	4.5	1.00	2832	0.6	1.00			
Nonsmoker							43,520	3.5	1.00
Former	2583	5.9	1.22	1215	1.2	1.85			
<20	1475	9.4	2.14**	1577	2.6	3.92**	14,405	8.2	1.70***
20–39	3301	14.9	2.77***	1606	3.1	5.14***	12,729	14.6	3.09***
≥40	319	14.9	2.76**	105	0.0	0.00	1912	18.2	4.56***

Baseline Body Mass Index (kg/m^2)[h]

<23.0	2063	6.1	1.00	4532	1.1	1.00	
23.0–24.9	2419	7.0	1.13	1240	1.6	1.38	
25.0–29.9	4978	8.9	1.20	1142	2.4	1.94	
30.0–34.9	1084	16.2	1.31**	293	5.0	3.31	
≥35.0	208	20.3	1.82	128	3.7	3.53	
<25.0	4482	6.5	1.00	5772	1.2	1.00	
25.0–29.9	4978	8.9	1.11	1142	2.4	1.75	
≥30.0	1292	16.9	1.75**	421	4.6	3.04*	
Cox coefficient	0.0465 (0.0164)**			0.0826 (0.0331)*			
HR for +4.0 kg/m^2	1.20			1.39			
95% CI	1.06–1.37			1.07–1.81			

(continued)

TABLE 2.1
(Continued)

Major Risk Factor Level	CHA Men Ages 18 to 39[a] Years			CHA Women Ages 18 to 39[a] Years			MRFIT Men Ages 35 to 39[b] Years		
	N	Death Rate[c]	Hazard Ratio[d]	N	Death Rate[c]	Hazard Ratio[d]	N	Death Ratio[c]	Hazard Ratio[e]
Baseline History of Diabetes (No/Yes)									
No	10,636	8.8	1.00	7,271	1.7	1.00	72,144	6.5	1.00
Yes	116	22.1	2.37	64	0.0	0.00	422	36.5	3.09***
Cox Coefficient (SE)	0.8635 (0.3844)*			i			1.1287 (0.1865)***		
HR for yes	2.37						3.09		
95% CI	1.12–5.04						2.14–4.46		

Length of follow-up was 30 years for CHA cohorts and 25 years for MRFIT. Number of CHD deaths: 271 CHA men; 35 CHA women; 1174 MRFIT men. CHA, Chicago Heart Association Detection Project in Industry; CHD, Coronary heart disease; CI, confidence interval; HR, hazard ratio; JNC, Joint National Committee; MRFIT, Multiple Risk Factor Interevention Trial; SBP/DBP, systolic and diastolic blood pressure.

[a]Excludes persons with history of myocardial infarction (MI) or major ECG abnormalities at baseline.
[b]Excludes men with history of MI at baseline.
[c]Per 10,000 person-years (age-adjusted for CHA cohorts); crude CHD death rate: CHA men, 25.2/1000 in 30 years; CHA women, 4.8/1000 in 30 years; MRFIT men, 16.2/1000 in 25 years.
[d]Adjusted for age, education, race, minor ECG abnormality, other major risk factors.
[e]Adjusted for age, race, other major risk factors.
[f]Systolic blood pressure 121 to 139 mmHg
[g]Includes people on antihypertensive drug treatment.
[h]Height and weight were not measured at MRFIT first screen.
[i]No CHD deaths in small subgroup with diabetes at baseline, hence not estimable.
[A]$p < 0.10$; *$p < 0.05$; **$p < 0.01$; ***$p < 0.001$.

TABLE 2.2

Hazard ratios for death from coronary heart disease, by baseline serum cholesterol and systolic blood pressure strata, and cigarette smoking status, for 72,566 men 35 to 39 years of age, with no history of myocardial infarction at baseline, Multiple Risk Factor Intervention Trial

	Systolic Blood Pressure (mmHg)				
Serum Cholesterol (mg/dL)	*≤120*	*121–129*	*130–139*	*140–159*	*≥160*
Nonsmokers at Baseline					
<180	1.0	1.8	3.9***	3.7**	7.8**
180–199	2.3*	2.6*	3.2**	5.2***	14.9***
200–219	2.9**	2.8*	2.8*	5.9***	6.4*
220–239	3.2**	2.8*	6.2***	8.8***	35.8***
≥240	3.9***	8.2***	12.9***	19.6***	23.6**
Smokers at Baseline					
<180	4.6***	3.2***	8.2***	12.5***	52.2***
180–199	7.0***	9.3***	10.3***	14.1***	43.5***
200–219	7.5***	12.1***	14.3***	22.0***	18.6***
220–239	10.5***	13.0***	19.6***	28.5***	64.3***
≥240	16.5***	25.3**	30.9***	46.1***	68.9***

Median follow-up 25 years; 1174 coronary heart disease (CHD) deaths. The hazard ratios are adjusted for age and race; the hazard ratio for the substratum of nonsmokers with serum cholesterol <180 mg/dL and SBP ≤120 mmHg was set at 1.00; only 5215 men met these three criteria (7.2% of the cohort). *p < 0.05; **p < 0.01; ***p < 0.001.

■ INTERVENTION STUDIES

By the late 1960s, results of dozens of metabolic ward-type experiments showed that several dietary factors influenced blood cholesterol. Saturated fats, cholesterol, and BMI had a direct relation, and polyunsaturated fats and water-soluble fiber were inversely associated (Keys et al., 1965; National Diet-Heart Study Research Group, 1968; Hegsted et al., 1993; Clarke et al., 1997). Later, higher dietary intake of trans fatty acids was also shown to relate to higher blood cholesterol.

The Rotterdam Trial showed that feeding newborns a diet lower than usual in salt resulted in significantly lower SBP by age 6 months (Hofman et al., 1983). Moreover, at follow-up 15 years later, this significant difference was still present even though there was no intervention beyond age 6 months (Geleijnse et al., 1997).

In the Dietary Intervention Study in Children (DISC) of 8- to 10-year-old children with dyslipidemia (see Chapters 8 and 11), long-term dietary counseling achieved limited improvement in lipid levels despite societal countervailing influences that limited adherence (DISC Writing Group, 1995). On the other hand, the New England boarding school trial demonstrated more favorable responses of teenage risk factor levels to improved dietary patterns effectively achieved in school dining rooms (Ellison et al., 1989). Similarly, in a community-wide Portuguese trial, effective intervention to reduce high NaCl intake (mainly from highly salted bread and dried cod fish) significantly lowered blood pressure (Forte et al., 1989). In the well-controlled Dietary Approaches to Stop Hypertension (DASH) feeding trials, blood pressures were significantly lowered by a "combination diet" and by substantial reduction in salt intake (Appel et al., 1997; NHLBI, 1998a; Sacks et al., 2001). The combination diet involved increased intakes of fruits, vegetables, whole grain products, legumes, nuts, and fat-free and low-fat dairy foods, and lower intake of red meats, other sources of saturated fats, egg yolks, total fats, and sweets. Blood pressures fell in both nonhypertensive and hypertensive participants, younger and older individuals, men and women, African-Americans and white Americans who were on the DASH diet. Serum levels of TC and LDL-C were also reduced by the diet, as expected, given the more favorable intake of dietary lipids and fiber (Harsha et al., 2004). In composition, this DASH diet was increased in potassium, magnesium, phosphorus, fiber, vitamins, protein (including vegetable protein), complex carbohydrates, and the ratio of polyunsaturated to saturated fatty acids, and reduced in total fat (to about 27% of kilocalories), saturated fatty acids (to about 9% of kilocalories), cholesterol (to <100 mg/1000 kcal), sugars, and Na/K. In DASH-2, the crossover design enabled demonstration of independent effects on blood pressure of two lower levels of Na intake, moderately lower (to about 100 mmol/day) and markedly lower (to about 50 mmol/day), compared to usual intake (about 150 mmol/day) with either usual U.S. fare or the DASH combination diet (Sacks et al., 2001). Findings from multiple trials indicate further that increases in intake of potassium and of vegetable protein lower blood pressure, as does greater leisure-time physical activity (Whelton et al., 2003). Improved eating patterns, with at least partial, sustained correction of overweight, influence plasma glucose levels favorably and prevent the usual increases with age during adulthood (Farinaro et al., 1977; Hu et al., 2001; Diabetes Prevention Program Research Group, 2002).

Data from trials demonstrating efficacy for CVD prevention of pharmacologic agents, particularly cholesterol-lowering statins and blood pressure–reducing thiazide-type diuretics, are further confirmation of the key etiologic role of major risk factors in the chain of causation (National High Blood Pressure Education Program [NHBPEP], 1993a, 1997; NCEP, 2001; NCEP, 2002; Chobanian et al., 2003).

SUMMARY

- Research findings regarding dietary patterns, serum cholesterol, blood pressure, cigarette smoking, BMI, and diabetes have served as the solid foundation for understanding the etiopathogenesis of CHD. This research has also led to recommendations on the prevention and control of epidemic CVD, particularly primary prevention (White et al., 1959; Page et al., 1961; Report of the Surgeon General's Advisory Committee, 1964; Inter-Society Commission for Heart Disease Resources, 1970; American Heart Association, 1980; World Health Organization [WHO], 1982, 1990a, 1990b, 1997; NCEP, 1988, 1990, 1991, 2001, 2002; U.S. Department of Health and Human Services [USDHHS], 1988, 1991, 1996, 1998, 1999; National Research Council, 1989; NHBPEP, 1993a, 1993b, 1997; Department of Health, 1994; Dietary Guidelines Advisory Committee, 1995a, 1995b, 2000a, 2000b; Eckel and Krauss, 1998; International Task Force for Prevention of Coronary Heart Disease, 1998; Krauss et al., 2000; Whelton et al., 2002; Chobanian et al., 2003).

• The new understanding of the impact of low risk, resulting from favorable levels of all major risk factors, is of critical importance, both theoretically and practically.

▬ REFERENCES

Adair, L.S., C.W. Kuzawa, and J. Borja. 2001. Maternal Energy Stores and Diet Composition during Pregnancy Program Adolescent Blood Pressure. *Circulation* 104:1034–39.

Allen, F.M., and J.W. Sherrill. 1922. The Treatment of Arterial Hypertension. *J Metabol Res* 2:429–545.

Ambard, L., and E. Beaujard. 1904. Causes of Arterial Hypertension [in French]. *Arch Gen Med* 1:520–33.

American Heart Association Committee Report. 1980. Risk Factors and Coronary Diseases. A Statement for Physicians. *Circulation* 62:449A–55A.

American Public Health Association Symposium. 1957. Measuring the Risk of Coronary Heart Disease in Adult Population Groups. *Am J Public Health* 47(Part 2):1–63.

Anitschkow, N. 1933. Experimental Arteriosclerosis in Animals. In: *Arteriosclerosis*. Edited by E.V. Cowdry. New York: MacMillan, pp. 271–322.

Appel, L.J., T.J. Moore, E. Obarzanck, W.M. Vollmer, L.P. Svetkey, F.M. Sacks, G.A. Bray, T.M. Vogt, J.A. Cutler, M.M. Windhauser, P.H. Lin, N. Karanja (DASH Collaborative Research Group). 1997. A Clinical Trial of the Effects of Dietary Patterns on Blood Pressure. *N Engl J Med* 336:1117–24.

Barker, D.J.P. 1998. *Mothers, Babies, and Health in Later Life*. Churchill Livingston: Edinburgh.

Berenson, G.S. 1986. *Causation of Cardiovascular Risk Factors in Children. Perspective on Cardiovascular Risk in Early Life*. New York: Raven.

Berenson, G.S., C.A. McMahan, A.W. Voors, L.S. Webber, S.R. Srinivasan, G.C. Frank, T.A. Foster, and C.V. Blonde (eds). 1980. *Cardiovascular Risk Factors in Children: The Early Natural History of Atherosclerosis and Essential Hypertension*. New York: Oxford University Press.

Boas, E.P., A.D. Parets, and D. Adlersberg. 1948. Hereditary Disturbance of Cholesterol Metabolism: A Factor in the Genesis of Arteriosclerosis. *Am Heart J* 35:611–22.

Byington, R., A.R. Dyer, D. Garside, K. Liu, D. Moss, J. Stamler, and Y. Tsong. 1979. Recent Trends of Major Coronary Risk Factors and CHD Mortality in the United States and Other Industrialized Countries. In: *Proceedings of the Conference on the Decline in Coronary Heart Disease Mortality*. Edited by R.J. Havlik and M. Feinleib. Washington, DC: National Institutes of Health, NIH Publication 79–1610, pp. 340–80.

Chobanian, A.V., G.L. Bakris, H.R. Black, W.C. Cushman, L.A. Green, J.L. Izzo, Jr., D.W. Jones, B.J. Materson, S. Oparil, J.T. Weight, Jr., and E.J. Roccella. Joint National Committee on Prevention, Detection, Evaluation, and Treatment of High Blood Pressure. National Heart, Lung, and Blood Institute. National High Blood Pressure Education Program Coordinating Committee. 2003. The Seventh Report of the Joint National Committee on Detection, Evaluation, and Treatment of High Blood Pressure (JNC VII). *Hypertension* 42:1206–52.

Clarke, R., C. Frost, R. Collins, P. Appleby, and R. Peto. 1997. Dietary Lipids and Blood Cholesterol: Quantitative Meta-Analysis of Metabolic Ward Studies. *BMJ* 314:112–7.

Denton, D., R. Weisinger, N.I. Mundy, E.J. Wickings, A. Dixon, P. Moisson, A.M. Pingard, R. Shade, D. Carey, R. Ardaillou, F. Paillard, J. Chapman, J. Thillet, and J.B. Michel. 1995. The Effect of Increased Salt Intake on Blood Pressure of Chimpanzees. *Nat Med* 1:1009–16.

Department of Health. 1994. Nutritional Aspects of Cardiovascular Disease. Reports of the Cardiovascular Review Group, Committee on Medical Aspects of Food Policy. London: Her Majesty's Stationary Office. Reports of Health and Social Subjects #46.

Diabetes Prevention Program Research Group. 2002. Reduction in the Incidence of Type 2 Diabetes with Lifestyle Intervention or Metformin. *N Engl J Med* 346:393–403.

Dietary Guidelines Advisory Committee. 1995a. *Dietary Guidelines for Americans*, 4th ed. U.S. Department of Agriculture, U.S. Department of Health and Human Services. Washington, DC: U.S. Government Printing Office.

Dietary Guidelines Advisory Committee. 1995b. *Report of the Dietary Guidelines Advisory Committee on the Dietary Guidelines for Americans.* Washington, DC: U.S. Government Printing Office.

Dietary Guidelines Advisory Committee. 2000a. *Report of the Dietary Guidelines Advisory Committee on the Dietary Guidelines for Americans.* Washington, DC: U.S. Government Printing Office.

Dietary Guidelines Advisory Committee. 2000b. *Scientific Rationale: 2000 Dietary Guidelines for Americans.* Washington, DC: U.S. Government Printing Office.

DISC Writing Group. 1995. The Efficacy and Safety of Lowering Dietary Intake of Fat and Cholesterol in Children with Elevated Low-Density Lipoprotein Cholesterol. The Dietary Intervention Study in Children (DISC). *JAMA* 273:1429–35.

Eckel, R.H., and R.M. Krauss. 1998. American Heart Association Call to Action: Obesity as a Major Risk Factor for Coronary Heart Disease. *Circulation* 97:2099–100.

Elliott, P.E., J. Stamler, R. Nichols, A.R. Dyer, R. Stamler, H. Kesteloot, and M. Marmot for the INTERSALT Cooperative Research Group. 1996. INTERSALT Revisited: Further Analyses of 24 Hour Sodium Excretion and Blood Pressure Within and Across Populations. *BMJ* 312:1249–53.

Ellison, R.C., A.L. Capper, W.P. Stephenson, R.J. Goldberg, D.W. Hosmer, Jr., K.F. Humphrey, J.K. Ockene, W.J. Gamble, J.C. Witschi, and F.J. Stare. 1989. Effects on Blood Pressure of a Decrease in Sodium Use in Institutional Food Preparation: the Exeter-Andover Project. *J Clin Epidemiol* 42:201–8.

Enos, Jr., W.F., R.H. Holmes, and J. Beyer. 1953. Coronary Disease among United States Soldiers Killed in Action in Korea. *JAMA* 152:1090–3.

Farinaro, E., J. Stamler, M. Upton, L. Mojonnier, Y. Hall, D. Moss, and D.M. Berkson. 1977. Plasma Glucose Levels: Long-Term Effect of Diet in the Chicago Coronary Prevention Evaluation Program. *Ann Intern Med* 86:147–54.

Forte, J.G., J.M. Miguel, M.J. Miguel, F. DePadua, and G. Rose. 1989. Salt and Blood Pressure: A Community Trial. *J Hum Hypertens* 3:179–84.

Fraser, G.E. 1986. *Preventive Cardiology.* New York: Oxford University Press.

Geleijnse, J.M., A. Hofman, J.C. Witteman, A.A. Hazebroek, H.A. Valkenburg, and D.E. Grobee. 1997. Long-Term Effects of Neonatal Sodium Restriction on Blood Pressure. *Hypertension* 29:913–7 (erratum: *Hypertension* 1997;29:1211).

Gertler, M.M., and P.D. White. 1954. *Coronary Heart Disease in Young Adults. A Multi-disciplinary Study.* Cambridge, MA: Harvard University Press.

Gofman, J.W., H.B. Jones, F. Lindgren, T.P. Lyon, H.A. Elliott, and B. Strisower. 1950. Blood Lipids and Human Atherosclerosis. *Circulation* 2:161–78.

Harsha, D.W., F.M. Sacks, E. Obarzanek, L.P. Svetkey, P-H. Lin, G.A. Bray, M. Arckin, P.R. Conlin, E.R. Miller, III, and L.J. Appel. 2004. Effect of Dietary Sodium Intake on Blood Lipids. Results from the DASH-Sodium Trial. *Hypertension* 43:393–8.

Hegsted, D.M., L.M. Austman, J.A. Johnson, and G.E. Dallal. 1993. Dietary Fat and Serum Lipids: An Evaluation of the Experimental Data. *Am J Clin Nutr* 57:875–83.

Hofman, A., A. Hazebroek, and H.A. Valkenburg. 1983. A Randomized Trial of Sodium Intake and Blood Pressure in Newborn Infants. *JAMA* 250:370–3.

Hu, F.B., J.A.E. Manson, M.J. Stampfer, G. Colditz, S. Liu, C.G. Solomon, and W.C. Willett. 2001. Diet, Lifestyle, and the Risk of Type 2 Diabetes Mellitus in Women. *N Engl J Med* 345:790–7.

Hueper, W.C. 1944. Arteriosclerosis. *Arch Pathol* 38:162–81, 245–85, 350–64.

Hueper, W.C. 1945. Arteriosclerosis. *Arch Pathol* 39:51–65, 117–31, 187–216.

International Task Force for Prevention of Coronary Heart Disease in Cooperation with the International Atherosclerosis Society. 1998. Coronary Heart Disease: Reducing the Risk. The Scientific Background for Primary and Secondary Prevention of Coronary Heart Disease. *Nutr Metab Cardiol Dis* 8:205–71.

INTERSALT Cooperative Research Group. 1988. INTERSALT: An International Study of Electrolyte Excretion and Blood Pressure. Results for 24–Hour Urinary Sodium and Potassium Excretion. *BMJ* 297:319–28.

INTERSALT Cooperative Research Group (P. Elliott, guest ed.). 1989. The INTERSALT Study. An International Co-operative Study of Electrolyte Excretion and Blood Pressure: Further Results. *J Hum Hypertens* 3:279–407.

Inter-Society Commission for Heart Disease Resources, Atherosclerosis Study Group and Epidemiology Study Group. 1970. Primary Prevention of the Atherosclerotic Diseases. *Circulation* 42:A55–A95.

Kagan, A., B.R. Harris, W. Winkelstein, Jr., K.G. Johnson, H. Kato, S.L. Syme, G.G. Rhoads, M.I. Gay, M.Z. Nichaman, H.B. Hamilton, and J. Tillotson. 1974. Epidemiologic Studies of Coronary Heart Disease and Stroke in Japanese Men Living in Japan, Hawaii and California: Demographic, Physical, Dietary and Biochemical Characteristics (Ni-Hon-San Study). *J Chron Dis* 27:345–64.

Katz, L.N., and J. Stamler. 1953. *Experimental Atherosclerosis.* Springfield, IL: Charles C. Thomas.

Katz, L.N., J. Stamler, and R. Pick. 1958. *Nutrition and Atherosclerosis.* Philadelphia: Lea and Febiger.

Kempner, W. 1948. Treatment of Hypertensive Vascular Disease with a Rice Diet. *Am J Med* 4:545–77.

Keys, A. (ed). 1970. Coronary Heart Disease in Seven Countries. American Heart Association Monograph #29. *Circulation* 41:I-1–I-211.

Keys, A. 1980. *Seven Countries: A Multinational Analysis of Death and Coronary Heart Disease.* Cambridge, MA: Harvard University Press.

Keys, A., J.T. Anderson, and F. Grande. 1965. Serum Cholesterol Response to Changes in the Diet. *Metabolism* 14:747–87.

Keys, A., and P.D. White (eds). 1956. *World Trends in Cardiology: Cardiovascular Epidemiology. Selected Papers from Second World Congress and Twenty-Seventh Annual Scientific Sessions of the American Heart Association.* New York: Hoeber-Harper.

Kimura, N. 1956. Analysis of 10,000 Postmortem Examinations in Japan. In: *World Trends in Cardiology: Cardiovascular Epidemiology.* Edited by A. Keys and P.D. White. New York: Hoeber-Harper, pp. 22–33.

Klag, M.J., D.E. Ford, L.A. Mead, J. He, P.K. Whelton, K-Y. Liang, and D.M. Levine. 1993.

Serum Cholesterol in Young Men and Subsequent Cardiovascular Disease. *N Engl J Med* 328:313–8.

Krauss, R.M., R.H. Eckel, B. Howard, S.R. Daniels, R.J. Deckelbaum, J.W. Erdman, Jr., P. Kris-Etherton, I.J. Goldberg, T.A. Kotchen, A.H. Lichtenstein, W.E. Mitch, R. Mullis, K. Robinson, J. Wylie-Rosett, S. St. Jeor, J. Suttie, D.L. Tribble, and T.L. Bazzarre. 2000. AHA Dietary Guidelines. A Statement for Healthcare Professionals from the Nutrition Committee of the American Heart Association. *Circulation* 102:2284–99.

Laragh, J.H., and M.S. Pecker. 1983. Dietary Sodium and Essential Hypertension: Some Myths, Hopes, and Truths. *Ann Intern Med* 98:735–43.

Lauer, R.M., W.E. Connor, P.E. Leaverton, M.A. Reiter, and W.R. Clarke. 1975. Coronary Heart Disease Risk Factors in School Children. *J Pediatr* 86:697–706.

Lauer, R.M., and R.B. Shekelle (ed). 1980. *Childhood Prevention of Atherosclerosis and Hypertension.* New York: Raven Press.

Law, C.M., M. de Swiet, C. Osmond, P.M. Fayers, D.J. Barker, A.M. Cruddles, and C.H. Fall. 1993. Initiation of Hypertension in Utero and its Amplification Throughout Life. *BMJ* 306:24–27.

Lawry, E.Y., G.V. Mann, A. Peterson, A.P. Wysocki, R. O'Connell, and F.J. Stare. 1957. Cholesterol and β-Lipoproteins in the Serum of Americans: Well Persons and Those with Coronary Heart Disease. *Am J Med* 22:605–23.

Mancilha-Carvalho, J.J., R.G. Baruzzi, P.F. Howard, N. Poulter, M.P. Alpers, L.J. Franco, L.F. Marcopito, V.J. Spooner, A.R. Dyer, P. Elliott, J. Stamler, and R. Stamler. 1989. Blood Pressure in Four Remote Populations in the INTERSALT Study. *Hypertension* 14:238–46.

Marchand, F. 1904. Über arteriosklerose (atherosklerose). *Verhandl d 21. Kongr fur Inn Med* 21:23.

Mariotti, S., R. Capocaccia, G. Farchi, A. Menotti, A. Verdecchia, and A. Keys. 1986. Age, Period, Cohort, and Geographical Area Effects on the Relationship between Risk Factors and Coronary Heart Disease Mortality: 15–Year Follow-Up of the European Cohorts of the Seven Countries Study. *J Chron Dis* 39:229–42.

Marmot, M.G., S.L. Syme, A. Kagan, H. Kato, J.B. Cohen, and J. Belsky. 1975. Epidemiology Studies of Coronary Heart Disease and Stroke in Japanese Men Living in Japan, Hawaii and California: Prevalence of Coronary and Hypertensive Heart Disease and Associated Risk Factors. *Am J Epidemiol* 102:514–25.

McGill, Jr., H.C. (ed). 1968. *The Geographic Pathology of Atherosclerosis.* Baltimore: Williams and Wilkins.

McGill, Jr., H.C., C.A. MacMahan, E.E. Herderick, G.T. Malcom, R.E. Tracy, and J.P. Strong for the Pathobiological Determinants of Atherosclerosis in Youth (PDAY) Research Group. 2000. Origin of Atherosclerosis in Childhood and Adolescence. *Am J Clin Nutr* 72(Suppl):1307S–15S.

Meneely, G.R. 1967. The Experimental Epidemiology of Sodium Chloride Toxicity in the Rat. In: *The Epidemiology of Hypertension.* Edited by J. Stamler, R. Stamler, and T.N. Pullman. New York: Grune and Stratton, pp. 240–6.

Meneely, G.R., and H.D. Battarbee. 1976. High Sodium-Low Potassium Environment and Hypertension. *Am J Cardiol* 38:768–85.

Miura, K., P. Greenland, J. Stamler, K. Liu, M.L. Daviglus, and H. Nakagawa. 2004. Relation of Vegetable, Fruit, and Meat Intake to 7-Year Blood Pressure Change in Middle-Aged Men. The Chicago Western Electric Study. *Am J Epidemiol* 159:572–80.

[NCEP] National Cholesterol Education Program. 1988. Report of the NCEP Expert Panel on Detection, Evaluation, and Treatment of High Blood Cholesterol in Adults. *Arch Intern Med* 148:36–69.

[NCEP] National Cholesterol Education Program. 1990. Report of the Expert Panel on Population Strategies for Blood Cholesterol Reduction. Washington, DC: U.S. Department of Health and Human Services, Public Health Services. NIH Publication No. 90-3046.

[NCEP] National Cholesterol Education Program. 1991. Report of the Expert Panel on Blood Cholesterol Levels in Children and Adolescents. Washington, DC: National Institutes of Health, National Heart, Lung, and Blood Institute. NIH Publication No. 91-2732.

[NCEP] National Cholesterol Education Program. 2001. Adult Treatment Panel III (ATP III). Executive Summary of the Third Report of the National Cholesterol Education Program Expert Panel on Detection, Evaluation, and Treatment of High Blood Cholesterol in Adults. *JAMA* 285:2486–97.

[NCEP] National Cholesterol Education Program. 2002. Third Report of the National Cholesterol Education Program Expert Panel on Detection, Evaluation, and Treatment of High Blood Cholesterol in Adults (Adult Treatment Panel III). Washington, DC: National Institutes of Health. NIH Publication No. 02-5215.

National Diet-Heart Study Research Group. 1968. The National Diet-Heart Study Final Report. *Circulation* 37:I-1-I-428.

[NHLBI] National Heart, Lung, and Blood Institute. 1998a. The DASH Diet. Washington, DC: U.S. Department of Health and Human Services, Public Health Service, National Institutes of Health. NIH Publication No. 01-4082.

[NHBPEP] National High Blood Pressure Education Program. 1993a. The Fifth Report of the Joint National Committee on Detection, Evaluation, and Treatment of High Blood Pressure (JNC V). *Arch Intern Med* 153:154–83.

[NHBPEP] National High Blood Pressure Education Program Working Group. 1993b. National High Blood Pressure Education Program Working Group Report on Primary Prevention of Hypertension. *Arch Intern Med* 153:186–208.

[NHBPEP] National High Blood Pressure Education Program. 1997. The Sixth Report of the Joint National Committee on Detection, Evaluation, and Treatment of High Blood Pressure (JNC VI). *Arch Intern Med* 157:2413–46.

National Research Council, Committee on Diet and Health, Food and Nutrition Board, Commission on Life Sciences. 1989. Diet and Health—Implications for Reducing Chronic Disease. Washington, DC: National Academy Press.

[NHLBI] National Heart, Lung, and Blood Institute Obesity Education Initiative Expert Panel on the Identification, Evaluation, and Treatment of Overweight and Obesity in Adults. 1998b. Clinical Guidelines on the Identification, Evaluation, and Treatment of Overweight and Obesity in Adults: The Evidence Report. Washington, DC: National Institutes of Health. NIH Publication No. 98-4083.

Paffenbarger, R.S., M.C. Thorne, and A.L. Wing. 1968. Chronic Disease in Former College Students. VIII. Characteristics in Youth Predisposing to Hypertension in Later Years. *Am J Epidemiol* 88:25–32.

Paffenbarger, R.S., A.L. Wing, and R.T. Hyde. 1978. Physical Activity as an Index of Heart Attack Risk in College Alumni. *Am J Epidemiol* 108:161–75.

Paffenbarger, R.S., A.L. Wing, R.T. Hyde, and D.L. Jung. 1983. Physical Activity and Incidence of Hypertension in College Alumni. *Am J Epidemiol* 117:245–57.

Page, I.H., E.V. Allen, F.L. Chamberlain, A. Keys, J. Stamler, and F.J. Stare. 1961. Dietary Fat and its Relation to Heart Attacks and Strokes. *Circulation* 23:133–6.

Page, L.B., A. Damon, and R.C. Moellering. 1974. Antecedents of Cardiovascular Disease in Six Solomon Islands Societies. *Circulation* 49:1132–46.

Page, L.B., D.E. Vandevert, K. Nader, N.K. Lubin, and J.R. Page. 1981. Blood Pressure of Qash'Qai Pastoral Nomads in Iran in Relation to Culture, Diet, and Body Form. *Am J Clin Nutr* 34:527–38.

Paul, O., M.H. Lepper, W.H. Phelan, G.W. Dupertuis, A. MacMillan, H. McKean, and H. Park. 1963. A Longitudinal Study of Coronary Heart Disease. *Circulation* 28:20–31.

Pearson, T.A. 1984. Coronary Arteriography in the Study of the Epidemiology of Coronary Artery Disease. *Epidemiol Rev* 6:140–66.

Phillips, R., F. Lemon, and J. Kuzma. 1978. Coronary Heart Disease Mortality among Seventh-Day Adventists with Differing Dietary Habits: A Preliminary Report. *Am J Clin Nutr* 31:S191–S8.

Pooling Project Research Group. 1978. Relationship of Blood Pressure, Serum Cholesterol, Smoking Habit, Relative Weight and ECG Abnormalities to Incidence of Major Coronary Events: Final Report of the Pooling Project. *J Chron Dis* 31:201–306.

Prospective Studies Collaboration. 2002. Age-Specific Relevance of Usual Blood Pressure to Vascular Mortality: A Meta-Analysis of Individual Data for One Million Adults in 61 Prospective Studies. *Lancet* 360:1903–13.

Raab, W. 1932. Alimentare Faktoren in der Enstebung von Arteriosklerose and Hypertonie. *Med Klin* 28:487–521.

Report of the Surgeon General's Advisory Committee on Smoking and Health. 1964. Washington, DC: U.S. Department of Health, Education and Welfare.

Rogot, E., and Z. Hrubec. 1989. Trends in Mortality from Coronary Heart Disease and Stroke among U.S. Veterans: 1954–1979. *J Clin Epidemiol* 42:245–56.

Rosenthal, S.R. 1934. Studies in Atherosclerosis: Chemical, Experimental and Morphologic. *Arch Pathol* 18:473–506, 660–698, 827–842.

Sacks, F.M., W.P. Castelli, A. Donner, and E.H. Kass. 1975. Plasma Lipids and Lipoproteins in Vegetarians and Controls. *N Engl J Med* 292:1148–51.

Sacks, F.M., and E.H. Kass. 1988. Low Blood Pressure in Vegetarians: Effects of Specific Foods and Nutrients. *Am J Clin Nutr* 48:795–800.

Sacks, F.M., B. Rosner, and E.H. Kass. 1974. Blood Pressure in Vegetarians. *Am J Epidemiol* 100:390–8.

Sacks, F.M., L.P. Svetkey, W.M. Vollmer, L.J. Appel, G.A. Bray, D. Harsha, E. Obarzanek, P.R. Conlin, E.R. Miller, III, G.D. Simons-Morton, N. Karanja, and P.H. Lin for the DASH-Sodium Collaborative Research Group. 2001. Effects on Blood Pressure of Reduced Sodium and the Dietary Approaches to Stop Hypertension (DASH) Diet. *N Engl J Med* 344:3–10.

Shaper, A.G. 1974. Communities without Hypertension. In: *Cardiovascular Disease in the Tropics.* Edited by A.G. Shaper, M.S.R. Hutt, and Z. Fejfar. London: British Medical Association, pp. 77–83.

Shekelle, R.B., A.M. Shryock, O. Paul, M. Lepper, J. Stamler, S. Liu, and W.J. Raynor, Jr. 1981. Diet, Serum Cholesterol, and Death from Coronary Heart Disease. The Western Electric Study. *N Engl J Med* 304:65–70.

Sinha, R., G. Fisch, B. Teague, W.V. Tamborlane, B. Banyas, K. Allen, M. Savoye, V. Rieger, S. Taksali, G. Barbetta, R.S. Sherwin, and S. Caprio. 2002. Prevalence of Impaired Glucose Tolerance among Children and Adolescents with Marked Obesity. *N Engl J Med* 346:802–10.

Snapper, I. 1941. *Chinese Lessons to Western Medicine.* New York: Interscience.

Society of Actuaries. 1959. *Build and Blood Pressure Study.* Chicago: Society of Actuaries.

Stamler, J. 1966. Nutrition, Metabolism and Atherosclerosis – A Review of Data and Theories, and a Discussion of Controversial Questions. In: *Controversy in Internal Medicine.* Edited by F.J. Ingelfinger, A.L. Relman, and M. Finland. Philadelphia: WB Saunders, pp. 27–59.

Stamler, J. 1967. *Lectures on Preventive Cardiology.* New York: Grune and Stratton.

Stamler, J. 1978. George Lyman Duff Memorial Lecture. Lifestyles, Major Fisk Factors, Proof and Public Policy. *Circulation* 58:3–19.

Stamler, J. 1979. Population Studies. In: *Nutrition, Lipids, and Coronary Heart Disease—A Global View.* Edited by R.I. Levy, B.M. Rifkind, B.H. Dennis, and N.D. Ernst. New York: Raven Press, pp. 25–88.

Stamler, J. 1989. Opportunities and Pitfalls in International Comparisons Related to Patterns, Trends and Determinants of CHD Mortality. *Int J Epidemiol* 18(Suppl 1):S3–S18.

Stamler, J. 1992. Established Major Coronary Risk Factors. In: *Coronary Heart Disease Epi-*

demiology: From Aetiology to Public Health. Edited by M. Marmot and P. Elliott. New York: Oxford University Press, pp. 35–66.

Stamler, J. 1994. Assessing Diets to Improve World Health: Nutritional Research on Disease Causation in Populations. *Am J Clin Nutr* 59:146S–56S.

Stamler, J. 1995. Potential for Prevention of Major Adult Cardiovascular Disease. In: *Lessons for Science from the Seven Countries Study: A 35–Year Collaborative Experience in Cardiovascular Disease Epidemiology*. Edited by H. Toshima, Y. Koga, J.H. Blackburn, and A. Keys. Tokyo: Springer-Verlag, pp. 195–235.

Stamler, J. 1997. The INTERSALT Study: Background, Methods, Findings, and Implications. *Am J Clin Nutr* 65(Suppl):626S–42S.

Stamler, J. (guest ed.). 2003. INTERMAP. International Study of Macro- and Micro-nutrients and Blood Pressure. *J Hum Hypertens* 17:585–775.

Stamler, J., A.W. Caggiula, J.A. Cutler, T.A. Dolecek, G.A. Grandits, M.O. Kjelsberg, J.L. Tillotson (guest eds.). 1997. Dietary and Nutritional Methods and Findings: The Multiple Risk Factor Intervention Trial (MRFIT). *Am J Clin Nutr* 65 (Suppl):183S–402S.

Stamler, J., M.L. Daviglus, D.B. Garside, A.R. Dyer, P. Greenland, and J.D. Neaton. 2000. Relationship of Baseline Serum Cholesterol Levels in 3 Large Cohorts of Younger Men to Long-Term Coronary Cardiovascular, and All-Cause Mortality and to Longevity. *JAMA* 284:311–8.

Stamler, J, A.R. Dyer, R.B. Shekelle, J. Neaton, and R. Stamler. 1993a. Relationship of Baseline Major Risk Factors to Coronary and All-Cause Mortality, and to Longevity: Findings from Long Term Follow-Up of Chicago Cohorts. *Cardiology* 82:191–222.

Stamler, J., P. Elliott, L. Appel, Q. Chan, M. Buzzard, B. Dennis, A.R. Dyer, P. Elmer, P. Greenland, D. Jones, H. Kesteloot, L. Kuller, D. Labarthe, K. Liu, A. Moag-Stahlberg, M. Nichaman, A. Okayama, N. Okuda, C. Robertson, B. Rodriguez, M. Stevens, H. Ueshima, L. Van Horn, and B. Zhou for the INTERMAP Cooperative Research Group. 2003. Higher Blood Pressure in Middle-Aged American Adults with Less Education—Role of Multiple Dietary Factors: The INTERMAP Study. *J Hum Hypertens* 17: 655–64.

Stamler, J., K. Liu, K.J. Ruth, J. Pryer, and P. Greenland. 2002. Eight-Year Blood Pressure Change in Middle-Aged Men: Relationship to Multiple Nutrients. *Hypertension* 39:1000–6.

Stamler, J., and R. Shekelle. 1988. Dietary Cholesterol and Human Coronary Heart Disease. The Epidemiologic Evidence. *Arch Pathol Lab Med* 112:1032–40.

Stamler, J., R. Stamler, W.V. Brown, A.M. Gotto, P. Greenland, S. Grundy, M. Hegsted, R.V. Luepker, J.D. Neaton, D. Steinberg, N. Stone, L. Van Horn, and R.W. Wissler. 1993b. Serum Cholesterol: Doing the Right Thing. *Circulation* 88:1954–60.

Stamler, J., R. Stamler, W.V. Brown, A.M. Gotto, P. Greenland, S. Grundy, M. Hegsted, R.V. Luepker, J.D. Neaton, D. Steinberg, N. Stone, L. Van Horn, and R.W. Wissler. 1994. Reply to Letters to Editor on Editorial, Doing the Right Thing. *Circulation* 90:2573–7.

Stamler, J., R. Stamler, J.D. Neaton, D. Wentworth, M.L. Daviglus, D. Garside, A.R. Dyer, P. Greenland, and K. Liu. 1999. Low Risk Factor Profile and Long-Term Cardiovascular and Non-Cardiovascular Mortality and Life Expectancy: Findings for Five Large Cohorts of Young Adult and Middle-Aged Men and Women. *JAMA* 282:2012–8.

Stamler, R., M. Shipley, P. Elliott, A. Dyer, S. Sans, and J. Stamler on behalf of the INTERSALT Cooperative Research Group. 1992. Higher Blood Pressure in Adults with Less Education: Some Explanatory Factors. Findings of the INTERSALT Study. *Hypertension* 19:237–41.

Thannhauser, S.J. 1950. *Lipidoses: Diseases of the Cellular Lipid Metabolism*, 2nd ed. London, New York: Oxford.

Thorne, M.C., A.L. Wing, and R.S. Paffenbarger, Jr. 1968. Chronic Disease in Former College Students. VII. Early Precursors in Nonfatal Coronary Heart Disease. *Am J Epidemiol* 87:520–9.

Tobian, L. 1991. Salt and Hypertension: Lessons from Animal Models that Relate to Human Hypertension. *Hypertension* 17(Suppl I):I-52–I-58.

U.S. Department of Health and Human Services. 1988. The Surgeon General's Report on Nutrition and Health. Washington, DC: U.S. Government Printing Office.

U.S. Department of Health and Human Services. 1991. Healthy People 2000: National Health Promotion and Disease Prevention Objectives (Summary Report). Washington, DC: U.S. Government Printing Office, DHHS Publ. No.(PHS) 91–50213.

U.S. Department of Health and Human Services. 1996. Physical Activity and Health. A Report of the Surgeon General. Atlanta, GA: U.S. Department of Health and Human Services, Centers for Disease Control and Prevention, National Center for Chronic Disease Prevention and Health Promotion.

U.S. Department of Health and Human Services. 1998. U.S. Department of Health and Human Services, Office of Public Health and Science. Healthy People 2010 Objectives: Draft for Public Comment. Washington, DC.

U.S. Department of Health and Human Services. 1999. Healthy People 2000 Review, 1998–1999. Hyattsville, MD: U.S. Department of Health and Human Services, Centers for Disease Control and Prevention, National Center for Health Statistics. Publ. No. (PS) 99–1256.

Walden, R.T., L.E. Schaefer, F.R. Lemon, A. Aunshine, and E.L. Wynder. 1964. Effect of Environment on the Serum Cholesterol-Triglyceride Distribution among Seventh-Day Adventists. *Am J Med* 36:269–76.

Whelton, P.K., J. He, L.J. Appel, J.A. Culter, S. Havas, T.A. Kotchen, E.J. Roccella, R. Stout, C. Vallbona, M.C. Winston, and J. Karimbakas, for the National High Blood Pressure Education Program Coordinating Committee. 2002. Primary Prevention of Hypertension. Clinical and Public Health Advisory from the National High Blood Pressure Education Program. *JAMA* 288:1882–8.

Whelton, P.K., J. He, and G.T. Louis (eds). 2003. *Lifestyle Modification for the Prevention and Treatment of Hypertension.* New York: Marcel Dekker.

White, P.D., H.B. Sprague, J. Stamler, F.J. Stare, I.S. Wright, L.N. Katz, S.L. Levine, and I.H. Page. 1959. A Statement on Arteriosclerosis, Main Cause of Heart Attacks and Strokes. New York: National Health Education Council, Inc.

WHO Expert Committee Report. 1982. Prevention of Coronary Heart Disease. Geneva: World Health Organization. Technical Report Series, No. 678.

WHO Expert Committee Report. 1990a. Prevention in Childhood and Youth of Adult Cardiovascular Diseases: Time for Action. Geneva: World Health Organization. Technical Report Series, No. 792.

WHO Study Group Report. 1990b. Diet, Nutrition, and the Prevention of Chronic Diseases. Geneva: World Health Organization. Technical Report Series, No. 797.

[WHO] World Health Organization. 1997. Obesity: Preventing and Managing the Global Epidemic. Geneva: World Health Organization.

Worth, R.M., H. Kato, G.G. Rhoads, K. Kagan, and S.L. Syme. 1975. Epidemiologic Studies of Coronary Heart Disease and Stroke in Japanese Men Living in Japan, Hawaii, and California: Mortality. *Am J Epidemiol* 102:485–90.

Zhao, L., J. Stamler, L.L. Yan, B. Zhou, Y. Wu, K. Liu, M.L. Daviglus, B.H. Dennis, P. Elliott, H. Ueshima, J. Yang, L. Zhu, D. Guo for the INTERMAP Research Group. 2004. Blood Pressure Differences between Northern and Southern Chinese: Role of Dietary Factors—The INTERMAP Study. *Hypertension* 43:1–6.

CHAPTER **3**

Low-Risk Cardiovascular Status: Impact on Cardiovascular Mortality and Longevity

Jeremiah Stamler, Martha L. Daviglus, Daniel B. Garside, Philip Greenland, Lynn E. Eberly, Lingfeng Yang, and James D. Neaton

Decades of research document conclusions and concepts about the natural history, etiology, and prevention of cardiovascular disease (CVD). Key relevant factors include:

- Multiple aspects of lifestyle, first and foremost dietary patterns high in several macronutrients (total, saturated, and trans fatty acids, cholesterol, salt, sugars), high in caloric density (concentrated calories from fats and refined carbohydrates), and relatively low in specific micronutrients (e.g., K, Mg, Ca, P, folate), fiber, and the ratio of essential nutrients to calories; excessive intake of alcohol, for a proportion of the population; and low levels of habitual physical activity of work and leisure, resulting in epidemic levels of overweight and obesity.
- Cigarette smoking
- The readily measured, diet related major risk factors: adverse levels of serum total cholesterol (and its atherogenic fractions LDL-C, IDL-C, VLDL-C), adverse blood pressure levels, overweight–obesity, and diabetes. All of these factors are at the individual level environmentally and genetically determined.
- The importance for prevention of low risk status, i.e., favorable levels of all readily measured established major risk factors

• The need for a sustained, effective effort throughout the population (from conception on) to achieve progressive, substantial increases in the proportion of the population at low risk (all ages, both genders, all socioeconomic–ethnic strata), until most people are at low risk (instead of the present small minority).

For younger adults, precise estimates of the long-term impact of the readily measured major risk factors are now available from two prospective studies from the late 1960s and early 1970s that had large samples and long-term follow-up: the Chicago Heart Association Detection Project in Industry (CHA) Study (Stamler et al., 1975, 1979, 1993; Dyer et al., 1980; Cedres et al., 1982; Liu et al., 1982; Pan et al., 1986; Liao et al., 1987; Levine et al., 1989) and the Multiple Risk Factor Intervention Trial (MRFIT) Study (Sherwin et al., 1981; MRFIT Research Group, 1982; Neaton et al., 1984, 1987; Kannel et al., 1986; Stamler et al., 1986).

■ DEFINITION OF LOW-RISK STATUS

Low-risk younger adult participants (CHA men and CHA women baseline ages 18 to 39, and men baseline ages 35 to 39 screened for MRFIT) were defined as those with favorable levels of all readily measured major risk factors: serum cholesterol <200 mg/dL *and* systolic blood pressure/diastolic blood pressure (SBP/DBP) ≤120/≤80 mmHg *and* nonsmoking at baseline *and* body mass index (BMI) <25.0 kg/m² (BMI data available only for CHA) *and* no history of diagnosed diabetes or myocardial infarction *and* no major electrocardiographic (ECG) abnormalities (ECG data available only for CHA). Persons with a history at baseline of diagnosed myocardial infarction (heart attack) or major ECG abnormality were excluded from the cohorts for analyses here.

■ BASELINE DESCRIPTION OF LOW-RISK COHORT MEMBERS

The proportion of the cohort at low risk at baseline was uniformly low, only 5% for CHA men ages 18 to 39 years, 10% for MRFIT men ages 35 to 39, and 20% for CHA women ages 18 to 39 (Table 3.1). In contrast, for a majority of each cohort, two or more risk factors were at unfavorable or high levels (58% to 85%), and 15% to 32% already manifested high levels of two or more major risk factors. These findings indicate that unfavorable lifestyles, particularly unfavorable dietary patterns, are common among young adults.

Levels of all major risk factors were much lower for low risk than for non-low-risk subcohorts. For example, for CHA men, average serum total cholesterol was 163 vs. 191 mg/dL; SBP was 116 vs. 135 mmHg; current cigarette smoking, 0 vs. 50%; and BMI, 22.6 vs. 26.2 kg/m² (Table 3.1). Contrasts were even greater

TABLE 3.1

Young adult subcohorts (baseline ages 18 to 39), according to risk of cardiovascular and coronary heart disease: demographic data and baseline major risk factor levels

Cohort and Variables*	Low Risk†	All Others, Not Low Risk	Any Two or More Risk Factors Unfavorable or High‡	Any Two or More Risk Factors High**
No. of People				
CHA men	582	10,170	9144	3491
CHA women	1479	5856	4701	1062
MRFIT men	7163	65,403	42,282	14,120
% of Cohort				
CHA men	5.4	94.6	85.0	32.5
CHA women	20.2	79.8	64.1	14.5
MRFIT men	9.9	90.1	58.3	19.4
Age (years)				
CHA men	27.9	29.8	29.9	30.2
CHA women	25.3	27.1	27.3	28.8
MRFIT men	36.9	37.0	37.0	37.1
Serum Cholesterol (mg/dL)				
CHA men	162.9	191.3	193.2	204.4
CHA women	163.5	184.9	186.0	198.8
MRFIT men	171.8	209.5	222.2	239.6
SBP (mmHg)				
CHA men	115.6	135.4	136.8	145.0
CHA women	113.3	125.8	126.7	138.0
MRFIT men	112.5	128.0	130.6	136.9
Cigarette Smoking (%)				
CHA men	0.0	50.0	56.0	79.6
CHA women	0.0	56.0	70.0	85.3
MRFIT men	0.0	44.4	59.0	80.8
No. of Cigarettes/Day				
CHA men	0	10.6	11.8	17.3
CHA women	0	9.5	11.8	15.5
MRFIT men	0	11.3	15.1	21.1
Body Mass Index (kg/m²)				
CHA men	22.6	26.2	26.4	27.9
CHA women	20.9	23.3	23.6	26.5
MRFIT men	—	—	—	—

(*continued*)

TABLE 3.1
(*Continued*)

Cohort and Variables*	Low Risk†	All Others, Not Low Risk	Any Two or More Risk Factors Unfavorable or High‡	Any Two or More Risk Factors High**
Diabetes History (%)				
CHA men	0.0	1.1	1.3	2.5
CHA women	0.0	1.1	1.4	4.0
MRFIT men	0.0	0.6	0.9	1.4

BMI, body mass index; CHA, Chicago Heart Association Detection Project in Industry; DBP, diastolic blood pressure, MRFIT, Multiple Risk Factor Intervention Trial; SBP, systolic blood pressure.
*Excludes individuals with a history of myocardial infarction or (CHA cohorts only) major ECG abnormality at baseline.
†Criteria for low risk: *All* of the following: SBP ≤120 mmHg, DBP ≤80 mmHg, total cholesterol <200 mg/dL, nonsmoker, no diabetes, BMI <25.0 kg/m² (CHA cohorts only) at baseline.
‡Criteria for unfavorable or high risk (i.e., not low risk): any one or more of the following: SBP >120 mmHg, DBP >80 mmHg, total cholesterol ≥200 mg/dL, diabetes, BMI ≥25 kg/m² (CHA cohorts only), current cigarette smoking at baseline.
**Cut points for high risk: SBP ≥140 mmHg, DBP ≥90 mmHg, total cholesterol ≥240 mg/dL, diabetes, BMI ≥30 kg/m² (CHA cohorts only), cigarette smoking at baseline.

between the low-risk subcohort and subcohorts with any two or more risk factors that were unfavorable or high, and any two or more risk factors high.

■ FOLLOW-UP OF THE CHA AND MRFIT COHORTS

Analyses of the 25- to 30-year impact of low-risk status on coronary heart disease (CHD) and CVD mortality and longevity focused on three contrasts (Tables 3.2 and 3.3):

- Low-risk subcohort vs. not-low-risk subcohort
- Low-risk subcohort vs. subcohort with any two or more risk factor levels that were unfavorable or high (total cholesterol ≥200 mg/dL, SBP >120 and/or DBP >80 mmHg, cigarette smoking, BMI ≥25.0 kg/m², diabetes at baseline)
- Low-risk subcohort vs. subcohort with any two or more risk factor levels high (total cholesterol ≥240 mg/dL, SBP ≥140 and/or DBP ≥90 mmHg, cigarette smoking, BMI ≥30.0 kg/m², diabetes at baseline)

TABLE 3.2

Young adult subcohorts (baseline ages 18 to 39) according to risk: numbers of deaths and percent deceased by cause

Cohort and Variables*	Low Risk†	All Others, Not Low Risk	Any Two or More Risk Factors Unfavorable or High‡	Any Two or More Risk Factors High**
CHD Deaths††				
CHA men	1	270	264	165
CHA women	2	33	32	15
MRFIT men	18	1156	1008	628
CVD Deaths‡‡				
CHA men	4	383	372	232
CHA women	6	71	67	27
MRFIT men	23	1630	1399	868
All Deaths				
CHA men	33	1130	1073	567
CHA women	46	383	347	103
MRFIT men	191	4078	3250	1729
Deceased, CHD (%)				
CHA men	0.3	2.6	2.9	4.6
CHA women	0.2	0.5	0.6	1.2
MRFIT men	0.2	1.8	2.4	4.5
Deceased, CVD (%)				
CHA men	0.9	3.7	4.0	6.4
CHA women	0.4	1.2	1.3	2.1
MRFIT men	0.3	2.5	3.3	6.2
Deceased, All Causes (%)				
CHA men	6.4	11.0	11.6	15.7
CHA women	3.4	6.4	7.1	8.2
MRFIT men	2.7	6.2	7.7	12.3

BMI, body mass index; CHA, Chicago Heart Association Detection Project in Industry; CHD, coronary heart disease; CVD, cardiovascular disease; DBP, diastolic blood pressure; MRFIT, Multiple Risk Factor Intervention Trial; SBP, systolic blood pressure.

*Excludes individuals with a history of myocardial infarction or (CHA cohorts only) major ECG abnormality at baseline. For CHA men and women, ages 18 to 39 years at baseline, percent deceased is age adjusted by the direct method to the age distribution of all CHA men and women ages 18 to 39 (18–19, 20–24, 25–29, 30–34, 35–39) years. Follow-up for CHA men and women was an average of 30 years; for MRFIT men, a median of 25 years.

†Criteria for low risk: All of the following: SBP ≤120 mmHg, DBP ≤80 mmHg, total cholesterol <200 mg/dL, nonsmoker, no diabetes, BMI <25 kg/m² (CHA cohorts only) at baseline.

‡Criteria for unfavorable or high risk (i.e., not low risk): any one or more of the following: SBP >120 mmHg, DBP >80 mmHg, total cholesterol ≥200 mg/dL, diabetes, BMI ≥25 kg/m² (CHA cohorts only), current cigarette smoking at baseline.

**Cut points for high risk: SBP ≥140 mmHg, DBP ≥90 mmHg, total cholesterol ≥240 mg/dL, diabetes, BMI ≥30 kg/m² (CHA cohorts only), cigarette smoking at baseline.

††Coronary heart disease was defined as *International Classification of Diseases 8th Revision* (ICD-8) and *International Classification of Diseases 9th Revision* (ICD-9) codes 410.0–414.9 and *International Classification of Diseases 10th Revision* (ICD-10) codes I20.0–I25.9.

‡‡Cardiovascular disease mortality was defined as ICD-8/ICD-9 codes 390.0–459.9 and ICD-10 codes I00.0–I99.9.

TABLE 3.3

Young adult subcohorts (baseline ages 18 to 39) according to risk and long-term mortality: hazard ratio by cause of death and estimated greater longevity

| | Hazard Ratio and Estimated Greater Longevity† | | | | | | | | |
| | Low Risk vs. All Others | | | Low Risk vs. Those with Any Two or More Risk Factors Unfavorable or High | | | Low Risk vs. Those with Any Two or More Risk Factors High | | |
Cause of Death	CHA Men	CHA Women	MRFIT Men	CHA Men	CHA Women	MRFIT Men	CHA Men	CHA Women	MRFIT Men
Coronary heart disease‡	0.08**	0.30	0.14***	0.07**	0.25	0.11***	0.04**	0.13**	0.06***
Cardiovascular diseases††	0.22**	0.40*	0.13***	0.20**	0.34*	0.10***	0.12***	0.21***	0.05***
All causes	0.59***	0.55***	0.44***	0.56***	0.49***	0.35***	0.40***	0.40***	0.22***
Greater longevity (years)	+7.9	+6.4	+8.3	+8.6	+7.8	+10.6	+12.3	+11.4	+13.7

Excludes individuals with history of myocardial infarction or (for two CHA cohorts only) major ECG abnormality at baseline. For subcohort criteria, number of people, baseline average risk factor levels, number and percent deceased by cause, and abbreviations see Tables 3.1 and 3.2. CHA men and women were ages 18 to 39 years at baseline, follow-up was 30 years. Men screened for MRFIT were ages 35 to 39 years at baseline, follow-up was 25 years.

†Hazard ratio controlled for age and race; for the two CHA cohorts, also controlled for education and minor ECG abnormality. Cohort average age at baseline: CHA men 29.6 years; life expectancy for 30-year-old U.S. men (1990 U.S. life-table data) 44.1 years; CHA women 26.8 years; life expectancy for 27-year-old U.S. women (1990 U.S. Life Table) 53.0 years; MRFIT men 37.0 years; life expectancy for 37-year-old U.S. men (1990 U.S. life-table data) 37.8 years.

‡Coronary heart disease was defined as *International Classification of Diseases 8th Revision* (ICD-8) and *International Classification of Diseases 9th Revision* (ICD-9) codes 410.0–414.9 and *International Classification of Diseases 10th Revision* (ICD-10) codes I20.0–I25.9.

††Cardiovascular disease mortality was defined as ICD-8/ICD-9 codes 390.0–459.9 and ICD-10 codes I00.0–I99.9.

*p < 0.05; **p < 0.01; ***p < 0.001.

Compared to the not-low-risk group, the proportions of deaths due to CHD and CVD among low-risk subcohorts were much lower. For men, deaths were lower by 76% to 89%; for women, they were lower by 60% to 67% (Table 3.2). With the low proportions of deaths due to CHD for low-risk subcohorts, the usual sex differential in CHD mortality was virtually absent—i.e, the proportion dying from CHD was 0.3% for CHA men and 0.2% for CHA women. The proportions of low-risk persons deceased from all causes were lower than for persons not low risk, by 42% to 56%. These differences were even more marked for low-risk subcohorts compared to those with any two or more risk factors that were unfavorable or high, and to those with any two or more risk factors high.

The hazard ratios (HRs) estimated from Cox multivariate models lead to similar conclusions (Table 3.3). For low-risk younger adult men compared to all others, HRs for CHD and CVD range from 0.08 to 0.22, i.e., risk is lower by 78% to 92% for low-risk men; all-cause HRs are 0.44 and 0.59, or 41% to 56% lower. For low-risk younger adult women compared to all others, the risk of CHD or CVD mortality is lower by 60% to 70%; it is 45% lower for all-cause mortality. Compared to persons with unfavorable or high levels of any two or more risk factors, HRs for low-risk cohorts are indicative of even greater long-term benefits for low-risk status in young adulthood.

For the 582 younger adult low-risk CHA men, with an average follow-up of 30 years, among 33 deaths only one was from CHD and only four were from CVD (Table 3.2). The age-adjusted percent deceased was 0.3% (CHD) and 0.9% (CVD), compared to 2.6% and 3.7%, respectively, for all other CHA men. In terms of proportionate mortality for this low-risk subcohort, CHD accounted for only 5% of all deaths, and only 14% of deaths were due to CVD, whereas for the not-low-risk subcohort these percentages were 24% and 34%, respectively. For those with combinations of major risk factors unfavorable or high, these proportions were even higher.

The favorable data on all-cause mortality for low-risk persons in each of the three cohorts translate into estimated sizable increases in life expectancy compared to that of all others (Table 3.3). The estimates are 8 to 12 years greater longevity for low-risk men across the comparisons (all others and those with any two or more risk factors unfavorable or high). Favorable values for each risk factor contribute additively to these estimates of greater longevity for low-risk men. For the men in the CHA cohort with average age about 30 at baseline, a life expectancy of about 44 years is a reasonable estimate (U.S. life-table data, without correction for the "healthy worker effect"). Thus, when compared to men with any two or more risk factors unfavorable or high, the estimate of about 9 additional years of life expectancy for low-risk men is 20% greater longevity. Life expectancy estimates for low-risk younger adult MRFIT men and CHA women are similar to those for the CHA men.

All these advantages of low-risk status prevail across socioeconomic and ethnic strata. That is, for the inordinately small percentages of the cohorts at low risk despite less education/lower income, the usual adverse CHD/CVD/all-cause mortality rates associated with lower socioeconomic status (Stamler 1967; Marmot et al., 1984, 1986, 1991; Rose 1992; Davey Smith et al., 1996a, 1996b; Stamler and Hazuda, 1996; Stamler et al., 1996; Cooper et al., 2000) are markedly attenuated.

Data on the benefits of low risk have also been reported by the Nurses Health Study, based on a 14-year follow-up of 84,129 U.S. women ages 30 to 55 at baseline in 1976 (Stampfer et al., 2000). Since data were collected by questionnaire only (resulting in no measured values for serum total cholesterol, blood pressure, or BMI), alternative criteria were used to define low risk, i.e., all of the following:

- Not smoking
- BMI (based on reported weight and height) <25.0 kg/m^2
- Engaged in moderate to vigorous physical activity for at lease one-half hour/ day
- Scored in the highest 40% of the cohort for diet high in cereal fiber, marine omega-3 fatty acids, folate, and ratio of polyunsaturated to saturated fatty acids
- Low intake of trans fatty acids, low glycemic load
- Average alcohol intake at lease half a drink/day

Only 3% of the cohort met these criteria. For these low risk women compared to all other women, the relative risk of a major CHD event (1128 events total, 296 fatal and 832 nonfatal) was 0.17 (95% confidence interval [CI] 0.07–0.41), with control for age, family history, diagnosed high blood pressure or serum total cholesterol, and menopausal status (Stampfer et al., 2000).

IMPLICATIONS OF LOW RISK

For the small minority of young adult Americans at low risk for CVD, all of the foregoing findings are underestimates of favorable long-term mortality experience because the people defined as low risk in these studies were identified from a set of measurements at only a single point in time. Therefore, some people are likely to have been misclassified (MacMahon et al, 1990; Stamler 1997; Lewington et al., 2002). Underestimation also results from the fact that low risk as defined here includes ex-smokers, with hazard ratios above optimal, and people with serum cholesterol 160 to 199 mg/dL, i.e., with favorable but not optimal levels. Finally, the definition of low risk does not include information on less readily measured risk factors, such as diet and physical activity, nor does it include data on genetic predisposition.

Despite these limitations in defining low-risk younger men, long-term CHD death rates were lower for this group than for all others by 86% (MRFIT) to 92% (CHA), and life expectancy was estimated to be greater by about 8 years. For younger women in the CHA cohort, the data are qualitatively similar (based on few CHD or CVD deaths). For the large cohort of women ages 30 to 55 at baseline in the Nurses Health Study, with 1128 major CHD events in 14 years, results are fully concordant with the MRFIT and CHA data, with risk lower by 83%, based on alternative low-risk criteria. Thus, results of these long-term, large-scale studies refute the oft-repeated notion that the easily measured major risk factors account for "only about 50%" of CHD risk. On the contrary, with CHD rates as much as 92% lower for low-risk younger adults compared to all others, and with quantitatively concordant findings for middle-aged men and women of these cohorts (Stamler et al., 1999, 2005a), we can conclude that the major risk factors account overwhelmingly for the CHD-CVD epidemic—that is, for both the high-risk status of the population as a whole and the commonality of individuals at high risk. Among individuals with favorable and optimal levels of all readily measured major risk factors (plus no history of myocardial infarction), CHD-CVD is uncommon. Practically, these data underscore the importance of using low risk, not population average risk, as the gold standard for risk assessment. Moreover, they emphasize the importance of primary prevention of all major risk factors through improvement of lifestyles to increase the proportion of the population at low risk.

However useful other components of strategy may be, they are not enough to end this epidemic. Ongoing, comprehensive, "early" detection, evaluation, and treatment of people with unfavorable and high levels of major risk factors (the high-risk arm of the strategy) are late, defensive, and reactive, not proactive. Pharmacologic treatment of risk factors is costly, is accompanied by side effects, and in most cases is incapable of achieving optimal levels. Only the practice throughout the population of comprehensive, primary prevention of CHD-CVD, so that most people are and remain at low risk from conception through older age, can conquer this epidemic.

■ PERSPECTIVE

Knowledge is currently extant on how to achieve population-wide favorable average serum cholesterol, plasma glucose, and blood pressure levels at all ages, as well as prevent the usual substantial rises from youth through middle age that result in conversion from favorable to adverse average levels. High serum cholesterol and blood pressure levels can be reduced to favorable or optimal levels by safe nutritional means.

Since the late 1980s, data from population-based epidemiologic research and results from the two Dietary Approaches to Stop Hypertension (DASH) feeding trials (see Chapter 2) have made it clear that it is entirely possible to lower average blood pressure levels through improved eating patterns. These patterns, as exemplified by the DASH combination diet, include increased intake of fruits, vegetables, whole grains, legumes, and fat-free and low-fat dairy products; decreased intake of red meats, other foods high in saturated fats and cholesterol, sweets; substantially reduced salt intake (to about 50 mmol/day Na, 2900 mg

NaCl/day); and prevention or control of heavy alcohol intake and of overweight. The DASH combination diet, with total fat about 26% kcal, saturated fatty acids about 7%, monounsaturated fatty acids about 9%, polyunsaturated fatty acids about 8%, dietary cholesterol about 260 mg/day, and fiber over 20 g/day, also lowers serum cholesterol (Stamler et al. 2005; also see Chapter 2). Since it is high in total protein, vitamins, minerals (other than Na), and other essential nutrients, it is highly nutritious, with a high ratio of nutrients to calories and low caloric density, thus favorable for weight control with optimal nutrition.

■ SUMMARY

- For younger adults, as for middle-aged population cohorts, low-risk status is associated with low death rates from CHD and all CVD compared to rates for all other persons, with estimated life expectancy greater by several years.
- Low risk is defined by serum total cholesterol <200 mg/dL *and* SBP ≤120 mmHg *and* DBP ≤80 mmHg *and* BMI <25.0 kg/m^2 *and* freedom from diabetes *and* nonsmoking in persons without history or evidence of definite CHD or CVD.
- Low-risk status is the exception, not the rule, among younger adults
- This rarity of low risk and commonality of unfavorable and high risk in the young adult population is due overwhelmingly to adverse lifestyles.
- It is fully possible to increase the proportion of the population at low risk—among younger as well as older adults of both genders from all major ethnic and socioeconomic strata—just as it has been possible to achieve marked sustained decreases year after year in CHD and CVD death rates, as recorded from the mid-1960s to the late 1980s.
- An important goal is to increase the proportion of the population at low risk throughout life, until low risk people are the overwhelming majority. This can be achieved by improving lifestyles, from the time of preconception to birth and through school age to young adulthood.

■ REFERENCES

Cedres, B.L., K. Liu, J. Stamler, A.R. Dyer, R. Stamler, D.M. Berkson, O. Paul, M. Lepper, H.A. Lindberg, J. Marquardt, E. Stevens, J.A. Schoenberger, R.B. Shekelle, P. Collette, and D. Garside. 1982. Independent Contribution of Electrocardiographic Abnormalities to Risk of Death from Coronary Heart Disease, Cardiovascular Diseases and All Causes. Findings of Three Chicago Epidemiologic Studies. *Circulation* 65:146–53.
Cooper, R., J. Cutler, P. Desvigne-Nickens, S.P. Fortmann, L. Friedman, R. Havlik, G. Hogelin, J. Marler, P. McGovern, G. Morosco, L. Mosca, T. Pearson, J. Stamler, D. Stryer, and T. Thom. 2000. Trends and Disparities in Coronary Heart Disease, Stroke,

and Other Cardiovascular Diseases in the United States: Findings of the National Conference on Cardiovascular Disease Prevention. *Circulation* 102:3137–47.

Davey Smith, G., J.D. Neaton, D. Wentworth, R. Stamler, and J. Stamler. 1996a. Socioeconomic Differentials in Mortality Risk Among Men Screened for the Multiple Risk Factor Intervention Trial: I. White Men. *Am J Public Health* 86:486–96.

Davey Smith, G., J.D. Neaton, D. Wentworth, R. Stamler, and J. Stamler. 1996b. Socioeconomic Differentials in Mortality Risk among Men Screened for the Multiple Risk Factor Intervention Trial: II. Black Men. *Am J Public Health* 86:497–504.

Dyer, A.R., V. Persky, J. Stamler, O. Paul, R.B. Shekelle, D.M. Berkson, M. Lepper, J.A. Schoenberger, and H.A. Lindberg. 1980. Heart Rate as a Prognostic Factor for Coronary Heart Disease and Mortality: Findings in Three Chicago Epidemiologic Studies. *Am J Epidemiol* 112:736–49.

Kannel, W.B., J.D. Neaton, D. Wentworth, H.E. Thomas, J. Stamler, S.B. Hulley, and M.O. Kjelsberg. 1986. Overall and Coronary Heart Disease Mortality Rates in Relation to Major Risk Factors in 325,348 Men Screened for the Multiple Risk Factor Intervention Trial (MRFIT). *Am Heart J* 112:825–36.

Levine, W., A.R. Dyer, R.B. Shekelle, J.A. Schoenberger, and J. Stamler. 1989. Serum Uric Acid and 11.5-Year Mortality of Middle-Aged Women: Findings of the Chicago Heart Association Detection Project in Industry. *J Clin Epidemiol* 42:257–67.

Lewington, S., R. Clarke, N. Qizilbash, R. Peto, and R. Collins (Prospective Studies Collaboration). 2002. Age-Specific Relevance of Usual Blood Pressure to Vascular Mortality. A Meta-Analysis of Individual Data for One Million Adults in 61 Prospective Studies. *Lancet* 360:1903–13.

Liao, Y., K. Liu, A. Dyer, J.A. Schoenberger, R.B. Shekelle, P. Collette, and J. Stamler. 1987. Sex Differential in the Relationship of Electrocardiographic ST-T Abnormalities to Risk of Coronary Death: 11.5 Year Follow-Up Findings of the Chicago Heart Association Detection Project in Industry. *Circulation* 75:347–52.

Liu, K., L.B. Cedres, J. Stamler, A. Dyer, R. Stamler, S. Nanas, D.M. Berkson, O. Paul, M. Lepper, H.A. Lindberg, J. Marquardt, E. Stevens, J.A. Schoenberger, R.B. Shekelle, P. Collette, S. Shekelle, and D. Garside. 1982. Relationship of Education to Major Risk Factors and Death from Coronary Heart Disease, Cardiovascular Disease and All Causes. Findings of Three Chicago Epidemiologic Studies. *Circulation* 66:1308–14.

MacMahon, S., R. Peto, J. Cutler, R. Collins, P. Sorlie, J. Neaton, R. Abbott, J. Godwin, A. Dyer, and J. Stamler. 1990. Blood Pressure, Stroke, and Coronary Heart Disease. Part 1: Prolonged Differences in Blood Pressure: Prospective Observational Studies Corrected for the Regression Dilution Bias. *Lancet* 335:765–74.

Marmot, M.G. and M.E. McDowall. 1986. Mortality Decline and Widening Social Inequalities. *Lancet* 2:274–6.

Marmot, M.G., M.J. Shipley, and G. Rose. 1984. Inequalities in Death—Specific Explanations of a General Pattern. *Lancet* 1:1003–6.

Marmot, M.G., G.D. Smite, S. Stansfield, C. Patel, F. North, J. Head, I. White, E. Brunner, and A. Feeney. 1991. Health Inequalities among British Civil Servants: The Whitehall II Study. *Lancet* 337:1387–93.

Multiple Risk Factor Intervention Trial Research Group. 1982. Multiple Risk Factor Intervention Trial—Risk Factor Changes and Mortality Results. *JAMA* 248:1465–77. Also reprinted as a Landmark Article in *JAMA* in 1997 (277:582–94) with commentary by A.M. Gotto, Jr.: The Multiple Risk Factor Intervention Trial (MRFIT). A Return to a Landmark Trial. *JAMA* 277:595–7.

Neaton, J.D., R.H. Grimm, and J.A. Cutler. 1987. Recruitment of Participants for the Multiple Risk Factor Intervention Trial. *Controlled Clin Trials* 8:41S–53S.

Neaton, J.D., L.H. Kuller, D. Wentworth, and N.O. Borhani. 1984. Total and Cardiovascular Mortality in Relation to Cigarette Smoking, Serum Cholesterol Concentration, and

Diastolic Blood Pressure among Black and White Males Followed For Five Years. *Am Heart J* 108:759–69.

Pan, W.H., L.B. Cedres, K. Liu, A. Dyer, J.A. Schoenberger, R.B. Shekelle, R. Stamler, D. Smith, P. Collette, and J. Stamler. 1986. Relationship of Clinical Diabetes and Asymptomatic Hyperglycemia to Risk of Coronary Heart Disease Mortality in Men and Women. *Am J Epidemiol* 123:504–16.

Rose G. 1992. *The Strategy of Preventive Medicine.* Oxford, England: Oxford University Press.

Schlosser E. 2002. *Fast Food Nation. The Dark Side of the All American Meal.* New York: Perennial-Harper Collins.

Sherwin, R., C.T. Kaelber, P. Kezdi, M.O. Kjelsberg, and H.E. Thomas, Jr. 1981. The Multiple Risk Factor Intervention Trial (MRFIT). II. The Development of the Protocol. *Prev Med* 10:405–25.

Stamler J. 1967. *Lectures on Preventive Cardiology.* New York: Grune and Stratton.

Stamler J. 1992. Established Major Coronary Risk Factors. Edited by M. Marmot and P. Elliott, *Coronary Heart Disease Epidemiology: From Aetiology to Public Health.* New York: Oxford University Press, pp. 35–66.

Stamler, J. 1997. The INTERSALT Study: Background, Methods, Findings, and Implications. *Am J Clin Nutr* 65(2 Suppl):626S–42S.

Stamler, J., D.M. Berkson, A. Dyer, M.H. Lepper, H.A. Lindberg, O. Paul, H. McKean, P. Rhomberg, J.A. Schoenberger, R.B. Shekelle, and R. Stamler. 1975. Relationship of Multiple Variables to Blood Pressure—Findings from Four Chicago Epidemiologic Studies. Edited by O. Paul, *Epidemiology and Control of Hypertension.* Miami: Symposia Specialists, pp. 307–356.

Stamler, J., A.R. Dyer, R.B. Shekelle, J. Neaton, and R. Stamler. 1993. Relationship of Baseline Major Risk Factors to Coronary and All-Cause Mortality, and to Longevity: Findings from Long-Term Follow-Up of Chicago Cohorts. *Cardiology* 82:191–222.

Stamler, J. and H.P. Hazuda. 1996. Executive Summary. *Report of the Conference on Socioeconomic Status and Cardiovascular Health and Disease;* Nov 6–7 1995; National Institutes of Health; National Heart, Lung, and Blood Institute, pp. 3–10. Also reprinted in *Circulation* 1996 94:2041–4 with an introduction by C. Lenfant.

Stamler, J., J.D. Neaton, D. Garside, and M.L. Daviglus. 2005. Current Status: Six Established Major Risk Factors and Low Risk. In: *Coronary Heart Disease Epidemiology,* 2nd ed. Edited by M.G. Marmot and P. Elliot. New York: Oxford University Press, pp. 32–70.

Stamler, J., R. Stamler, D. Garside, K. Greenlund, S. Archer, J.D. Neaton, and D.N. Wentworth. 1996. Socioeconomic Status, Cardiovascular Risk Factors, and Cardiovascular Disease: Findings on U.S. Working Populations. *Report of the Conference on Socioeconomic Status and Cardiovascular Health and Disease;* Nov 6–7 1995; National Institutes of Health; National Heart, Lung, and Blood Institute, pp. 109–118.

Stamler, J., R. Stamler, J.D. Neaton, D. Wentworth, M.L. Daviglus, D. Garside, A.R. Dyer, P. Greenland, and K. Liu. 1999. Low Risk Factor Profile and Long-Term Cardiovascular and Non-Cardiovascular Mortality and Life Expectancy: Findings for Five Large Cohorts of Young Adult and Middle-Aged Men and Women. *JAMA* 282:2012–8.

Stamler, J., D. Wentworth, and J.D. Neaton. 1986. Is Relationship Between Serum Cholesterol and Risk of Premature Death from Coronary Heart Disease Continuous and Graded? Findings in 356,222 Primary Screenees of the Multiple Risk Factor Intervention Trial (MRFIT). *JAMA* 256:2823–8.

Stamler, R., J. Stamler, J.A. Schoenberger, R.B. Shekelle, P. Collette, S. Shekelle, A. Dyer, D. Garside, and J. Wannamaker. 1979. Relationship of Glucose Tolerance to Prevalence of ECG Abnormalities and to 5-Year Mortality from Cardiovascular Disease: Findings of the Chicago Heart Association Detection Project in Industry. *J Chron Dis* 32:817–28.

Stampfer, M.J., F.B. Hu, J.R. Manson, E.B. Rimm, and W.C. Willett. 2000. Primary Prevention of Coronary Heart Disease in Women through Diet and Lifestyle. *N Engl J Med* 343:16–22.

PART II

Measures of the Atherosclerotic Process in Children and Young Adults

Relationship between Cardiovascular Risk Factors and Coronary Artery Calcification

Larry T. Mahoney, Trudy L. Burns, Lawrence F. Bielak, and Patricia A. Peyser

From examination of pathologic specimens, it is well known that calcium eventually becomes incorporated into the developing advanced atherosclerotic lesion. Early attempts to identify calcific lesions used the plain chest radiograph; however, the lesions had to be quite extensive to be seen as a radiopaque lesion using this technique. Advances in rapid acquisition computed tomography (CT) have led to a reliable, noninvasive technique for identifying, locating, and quantifying even small calcific lesions. This chapter provides background information on coronary artery calcification (CAC), a marker of subclinical atherosclerosis, and describes the results from investigations focused on validation of a noninvasive method to detect and quantify CAC. The chapter summarizes the results from epidemiologic investigations of the association between CAC and current and previously measured coronary risk factor (CRF) levels, including childhood measures, genetic studies, and studies of the progression of CAC. In adolescents and young adults, assessment of CAC may provide a measure of the early atherosclerotic process before occlusive cardiovascular disease becomes evident. Very little is known about the detection of CAC during childhood. There is a need to study its utility in high-risk children, such as those with markedly elevated cholesterol levels. Clearly, from a clinical perspective, CT measurement of CAC should not be recommended for general pediatric practice.

■ CORONARY ARTERY CALCIFICATION AND ATHEROSCLEROSIS

Atherosclerosis begins in childhood with the accumulation of lipid in the intima of arteries to form fatty streaks (McGill, 1989). Nearly all children have at least some degree of aortic fatty streaks by 3 years of age and the prevalence of fatty streaks increases rapidly after 8 years of age (Strong and McGill, 1962). Calcium uptake occurs during the development of atherosclerosis with deposition of insoluble calcium apatite crystals within the fibrous plaque by a mechanism similar to that found in active bone formation and remodeling (Anderson, 1983). The presence of calcified lesions, detected in vivo, accurately predicts the presence of atherosclerotic plaque and occurs almost exclusively when coronary atherosclerosis is present. In an early X-ray study of 89 randomly selected postmortem hearts, Blankenhorn (1961) found no radiopaque lesions without concomitant atherosclerosis. Small deposits close to the internal elastic lamina were not associated with arterial narrowing, but larger deposits were associated with more pronounced vessel narrowing. While CAC has been found in preatheromas, it occurs most often in fibroatheromas that usually develop during the third or the fourth decade of life (Stary, 1990).

At autopsy, Eggen et al. (1965) concluded that (1) white males have the highest prevalence of CAC in all examined coronary branches, followed by black males, white females, and black females in descending rank order; (2) the calcified lesions are most frequently located about 2 cm from the orifice; and (3) the value of information concerning CAC in the differential diagnosis of clinically significant coronary artery disease (CAD) is greatest in the fourth decade of life compared to that in later years. Extensive CAC appears to stabilize the arterial wall, rendering it less vulnerable to rupture, whereas the early or intermediate stages of calcification may actually enhance plaque vulnerability (Wexler et al., 1996). Mineralization of plaque is associated with a compensatory enlargement of the coronary artery, which may explain why coronary angiography frequently underestimates the severity of CAD compared to that from histologic studies (Clarkson et al., 1994).

■ DETECTION AND QUANTIFICATION OF CORNARY ARTERY CALCIFICATION BY ELECTRON-BEAM COMPUTED TOMOGRAPHY

Numerous techniques have been employed in an attempt to accurately identify calcium deposition in blood vessels. Standard radiography and CT do not acquire images with sufficient speed to image the coronary arteries of a beating heart. With the development of ultrafast CT scanners, images are acquired very rapidly. The speed of image acquisition reduces the distorting effects of cardiac motion and limits artifact. Accurate CAC detection and quantification is achieved without contrast medium by using the high-resolution mode of an electron-beam CT (EBCT) scanner in conjunction with a 100-ms scan time, 3-mm slice thickness and electrocardiographic triggering during held inspiration. A typical scan run obtains 40 contiguous images of the heart to examine the coronary arteries from their origins to the most distal distributions. Each image in a scan run is evaluated sequentially by a radiologist or trained technician.

While there is no universally accepted definition for the presence of CAC, the more widely used definition is at least one focus with three contiguous pixels, each with a pixel density ≥ 130 Hounsfield units (HU) (Fig. 4.1). Such a focus is at least 1 mm^2 when using a 30 cm^2 field of view and a 512 $\times$ 512 reconstruction matrix. From the acquired scan data, a three-dimensional reconstruction can also be made to identify the precise location of calcium deposits within the distribution of the coronary arteries (Fig. 4.2).

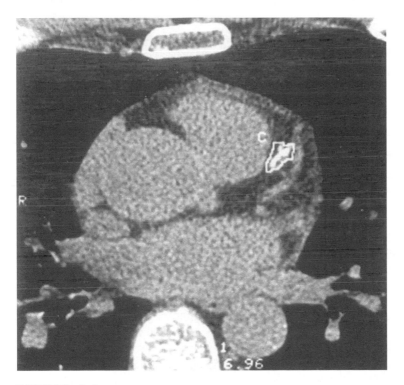

FIGURE 4.1
Electron-beam computed tomography scan of an asymptomatic male participant in the community-based Epidemiology of Coronary Artery Calcification Study. A focus of coronary artery calcification is outlined in the left anterior descending artery. The area of the focus was 20.6 mm^2 and the peak density in the focus was 385 HU; the Agatston score of the focus was 61.8. This participant's total area and score in his whole heart were 41.5 mm^2 and 120.9, respectively.

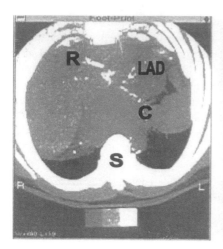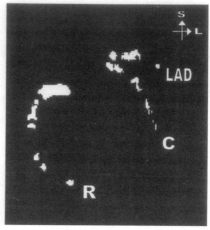

FIGURE 4.2
Volumetric calcium measurement. In the left panel, individual electron-beam computed tomography slices have been converted to a fast footprint composite image reconstruction display. Increasing pixel density ranges from subthreshold values in gray or speckled to ≥130 HU in white. The spine (S) and ribs are readily identified. Multiple calcific lesions are seen in the distribution of the right (R), left anterior descending (LAD), and circumflex (C) coronary arteries. In the right panel, a three-dimensional reconstruction shows the same distribution of calcium (orientation is superior [S] and leftward [L]). The image can be rotated in all directions. This would allow a more precise localization of each calcific deposit, which is very important for serial studies of regression or progression in the same subject.

Many investigators prefer to record the quantity of CAC as the area (in mm^2) of the hyperattenuating foci, rather than the originally described Agatston score (Agatston et al., 1990), in which an arbitrary weighting coefficient is used to multiply the area of each focus by a coefficient that is based on the highest pixel density in the focus. The total area (or Agatston score) is calculated by summing the areas (or scores) of all foci across all coronary segments. A volumetric calcium measure has also been described that requires a postprocessing regression approach of isotropic interpolation to derive a volume from the two-dimensional scan data (Callister et al., 1998a).

Inter- and intraobserver reliability of EBCT scoring for quantitative measures of CAC was studied in 25 adults with CAC (Kaufmann et al., 1994). The reliability among three observers (two radiologic technologists and one radiologist) was 0.997 for the quantity of CAC in all arteries combined. Intraobserver agreement was equally high when the EBCT scans were again scored after 6 months. Neither inter- nor intraobserver reliability was affected by the quantity of CAC.

EBCT is viewed as the standard method for quantification of CAC and most epidemiologic studies investigating CAC have used this technology. Unfortunately, access to this technology is somewhat limited. Since its introduction in the early 1990s, multislice helical CT has become the predominate technology for obtaining CT images for medical applications. The temporal resolution of the multislice CT has improved to the subsecond range, cardiac gating methods have been described and calcium scoring is comparable to that of EBCT. In one study Pearson and Spearman correlation coefficients both for Agatston (0.98 and 0.96, respectively) and volumetric (0.97 and 0.95, respectively) scores were nearly identical (Carr et al., 2000). A recent study also showed excellent correlation between techniques for volume scoring ($r = 0.994$, $p - 0.01$) and comparison of low (1–100), moderate (101–400), high (401–1000), and very high (>1000) scores showed no differences (Knez et al., 2002). CAC was measured with EBCT and multislice helical CT in 6814 participants in the Multi-Ethnic Study of Atherosclerosis with two consecutive scan runs of the heart (Detrano et al., 2005). Three study centers used EBCT, and three used multislice helical CT. Concordance for presence of CAC between dual scans was high and similar for both EBCT and multislice helical CT (96%, kappa = 0.92). EBCT and multislice helical CT scanners had equivalent reproducibility for measuring CAC (Detrano et al., 2005). Since data on the applicability of multislice techniques to epidemiologic studies are just unfolding, this chapter will focus primarily on evidence generated through EBCT detection of CAC.

■ HISTOPATHOLOGIC AND ANGIOGRAPHIC CORRELATIVE STUDIES OF EBCT-MEASURED CORONARY ARTERY CALCIFICATION

Studies examining the relationship between CAC detected by EBCT and histopathologic atheromatous plaque (Mautner et al., 1994; Rumburger et al., 1995) concluded that (1) while the CAC burden was positively associated with the histomorphometric analysis of calcified area and quantitative extent of coronary artery atheromatous plaque, the variation in the corresponding plaque areas at a given quantity of CAC was substantial; (2) the quantity of CAC measured by EBCT was significantly associated with the percent of lumen area stenosis; (3) the total absence of CAC did not confirm the absence of atheromatous plaque; however, in such instances, the extent of stenosis was minimal; and (4) when predicting the presence of any plaque within a given coronary artery segment using CAC from EBCT, the sensitivity and specificity in these studies ranged from 59% to 94%, and from 76% to 90%, respectively.

The diagnostic accuracy of EBCT measured CAC for CAD on angiography has varied widely in published reports. A meta-analysis of data from nine studies was performed to estimate the accuracy of EBCT in diagnosing obstructive

(≥50% diameter stenosis) CAD (Nallamothu et al., 2001). Using the definition of ≥130 HU and minimal areas to define a focus of CAC ranging from 0.5 to 2.0 mm², the pooled sensitivity of EBCT was 92% and the pooled specificity was 51%, that is, 92% of the subjects who were diagnosed with obstructive CAD had CAC on EBCT, and 51% of the subjects who were diagnosed without obstructive CAD did not have CAC on EBCT. As the threshold for defining an abnormal test based on CAC area was increased, the sensitivity decreased and specificity increased. For example, for a CAC threshold area that resulted in a sensitivity of 90%, the specificity was 54%. By increasing the CAC threshold area to one that resulted in a decrease of sensitivity to 80%, the specificity increased to 71%. The overall conclusion was that the performance of EBCT as a diagnostic test for obstructive disease is reasonably accurate, and is comparable to the accuracy of traditional exercise stress testing.

It should be noted that these estimates of sensitivity and specificity are biased since most information regarding the ability of EBCT to predict CAD is based on samples of symptomatic patients whose CAD status has been verified with angiography. As a result of this bias, the sensitivity will be overestimated and the specificity will be underestimated for the general population. In a study of 213 patients (examined with angiography and EBCT) and 765 asymptomatic research participants (examined with only EBCT), the estimated debiased sensitivity and specificity of EBCT for ≥50% stenosis were 97% and 72%, respectively (Bielak et al., 2000a). When only the 213 patients with angiography were considered, the sensitivity and specificity were 99% and 39%, respectively. Thus, after adjusting for verification bias, specificity was considerably higher than when estimated with patients only undergoing angiography (Bielak et al., 2000a).

▪ CARDIOVASCULAR DISEASE END POINTS RELATED TO CORONARY ARTERY CALCIFICATION

In a study of 800 patients followed over a 5-year period after they had undergone angiography, 40% of the 250 patients with CAC detected by fluoroscopy compared to 10% of the 550 without CAC died from CAD. This study suggested a prognostic significance of CAC that was independent of the information obtained from cardiac catheterization (Margolis et al., 1980). The quantity of CAC measured by EBCT appears to be associated with the risk of coronary events in both asymptomatic and symptomatic individuals (Arad et al., 2000; Wong et al., 2000; Keelan et al., 2001; Greenland et al., 2004; La Monte et al., 2005). EBCT has also been shown to be an effective triage tool for screening patients with angina-like chest pain in the emergency room setting. Laudon et al. (1999) found that patients with chest pain but normal cardiac enzyme concentrations, normal or indeterminate ECG findings, and no detectable CAC on EBCT may be safely discharged from the emergency room without further testing or observation. Measurement of CAC in patients can help guide initiation of prevention programs aimed at improving outcomes in patients felt to be at high risk for CAD.

■ CORONARY RISK FACTOR LEVELS RELATED TO CORONARY ARTERY CALCIFICATION

A number of studies have examined the association between known CRF levels and CAC. In a study of 675 males and 190 females, 22 to 85 years of age, Wong et al. (1994) examined the association between the presence and quantity of CAC and self-reported CRF information. A significantly greater prevalence of CAC was demonstrated in both the males and females who reported a history of hypertension or hypercholesterolemia, as well as in males with a history of diabetes, previous smoking, infrequent exercise, or obesity.

In another study of asymptomatic females, those 55 years of age or younger with CAC had significantly higher total cholesterol, low-density lipoprotein cholesterol (LDL-C), and triglyceride levels compared to those without detectable CAC; however, among females >55 years of age, there were no observed CRF differences between the two CAC groups (Hecht and Superko, 2001). Among hypertensive males, there was an association of CAC with age and hypertension duration, but not with blood pressure level (Megnien et al., 1996). Other risk factors such as smoking history, family history of CAD, and levels of fibrinogen, lipoprotein(a) [Lp(a)], C-reactive protein, homocysteine, and insulin either showed no association with CAC or the findings were inconsistent, perhaps because of the marked age differences among participants in different studies (Bielak et al., 2000b; Nishino et al., 2000; Mahoney et al., 2001; Taylor et al., 2001; Kullo et al., 2003). Since recognized CRFs have been shown to account for less than 40% of the variability in the quantity of CAC, it has been suggested that future studies of new risk factors for CAC and its progression could provide new insights into the etiology of the atherosclerotic process (Maher et al., 1996).

■ CORONARY ARTERY CALCIFICATION IN HETEROZYGOUS FAMILIAL HYPERCHOLESTEROLEMIA

Gidding et al. (1998) used EBCT to examine the presence of CAC in individuals 11 to 23 years of age with heterozygous familial hypercholesterolemia (FH). Of the 29 individuals examined, seven showed evidence of CAC, but the foci were small. Of the large number of risk factors examined, only an increased body mass index (BMI) was significantly associated with the presence of CAC (25.3 vs. 20.6 kg/m^2 in those with and without detectable CAC, respectively, $p < 0.05$). The authors suggested that the presence of increased BMI in individuals with FH is an additional and potent risk factor for acceleration of atherosclerosis.

■ CHILDHOOD AND YOUNG ADULT PREDICTORS OF CORONARY ARTERY CALCIFICATION: THE MUSCATINE STUDY

The association of childhood and young adult CRF levels with CAC was examined in participants of the Muscatine Study (Mahoney et al., 1996, 2001). This is the largest study to date of CRFs and CAC in young adults in a community-based study. Subjects were eligible for study if they had previously participated in at least one of the biennial school surveys during childhood conducted in Muscatine, Iowa, between 1971 and 1981 and at least one of the Young Adult Follow-up Surveys conducted between the ages of 20 and 38 years. Standardized methods were used to obtain body size and blood pressure measurements and blood samples were obtained from all participants contemporaneously with the EBCT examination. Initially, 385 males and 384 females, aged 29 to 37 years, completed all components of the study protocol. Because the prevalence of CAC was substantially lower in females (13%) than in males (30%) in this age group, the female population was enriched with 88 additional older subjects who were 40 to 43 years of age. The prevalence of CAC in the final sample was 30% for males and 16% for females. CAC was identified in 29 year old females (2 of 11) and males (2 of 16) in the Muscatine cohort.

Tables 4.1 and 4.2 describe the CRF levels, measured during childhood (males 15.2 ± 1.9; females 15.4 ± 1.8 years of age) and twice during young adult life (males 26.8 ± 3.6 and 34.1 ± 2.3; females 27.7 ± 4.2 and 35.2 ± 3.5 years of age), by CAC status in the 385 males and 472 females. Because of the age and sex associations with CRFs, all of the mean comparisons were made using age-, sex-, and survey-specific Z scores.

In young adult males, the mean childhood measures of body habitus (weight, BMI and triceps skinfold thickness) were significantly higher in those with than in those without detectable CAC (Table 4.1). In young adult females, the mean childhood measures of body habitus (weight, BMI, and triceps skinfold thickness) and blood pressure (systolic [SBP] and diastolic [DBP]) were significantly higher in those with CAC (Table 4.2). Measures of body habitus, including the waist-to-hip circumference ratio, SBP, and DBP from the third and fourth decades of life (young adult and most recent measurements) were consistently higher for young adult males and females with CAC. In addition, mean levels of high-density lipoprotein cholesterol (HDL-C), the total cholesterol/HDL-C ratio, triglycerides, and apolipoproteins A1 (apo A1) and B (apo B) were consistently different in males and females with CAC compared to those without detectable CAC. No differences were observed between groups for cholesterol, LDL-C, or Lp(a).

TABLE 4.1

Serial measurements (mean ± SD) during childhood and two young adult Muscatine Study examinations in males with (n = 116) and without (n = 265) detectable coronary artery calcification

Variable	Childhood Ages 8 to 18 years		Young Adult Ages 20 to 34 years		Most Recent Ages 29 to 37 years	
	+CAC	−CAC	+CAC	−CAC	+CAC	−CAC
Height (cm)	169.6 ± 11.3	169.3 ± 11.6	177.0 ± 6.2	177.8 ± 6.8	177.4 ± 6.2	178.3 ± 6.7
Weight (kg)	67.0 ± 14.9	62.7 ± 14.0**	86.3 ± 15.0	79.6 ± 12.8***	92.0 ± 16.5	85.1 ± 14.8***
BMI (kg/m^2)	23.1 ± 3.6	21.7 ± 3.4***	27.5 ± 4.5	25.2 ± 3.7***	29.2 ± 4.9	26.8 ± 4.5***
TSF (cm)	9.7 ± 5.0	8.1 ± 4.9**	14.2 ± 7.1	11.5 ± 6.3***	20.7 ± 7.7	17.4 ± 7.3***
Waist/hip					0.92 ± 0.07	0.89 ± 0.07***
Systolic BP (mmHg)	122.4 ± 12.7	119.8 ± 11.9	123.0 ± 12.4	118.0 ± 11.7***	121.9 ± 12.4	118.8 ± 11.0*
Diastolic BP (mmHg)	77.3 ± 9.4	76.5 ± 8.8	76.5 ± 9.3	70.4 ± 10.1***	79.5 ± 9.3	77.2 ± 8.7*
Total cholesterol (mg/dL)	151.6 ± 28.9	147.9 ± 25.8	181.9 ± 39.7	173.7 ± 33.5	191.3 ± 38.1	184.6 ± 40.5
Triglycerides (mg/dL)	79.8 ± 33.1	77.2 ± 40.5	117.6 ± 73.6	99.4 ± 60.3*	149.7 ± 91.2	127.9 ± 83.3*
HDL-C (mg/dL)			41.6 ± 10.7	44.6 ± 11.0*	40.4 ± 10.9	43.9 ± 11.5**
LDL-C (mg/dL)			115.2 ± 32.3	109.1 ± 29.6	119.1 ± 32.1	114.1 ± 33.9
LDL-C/HDL-C			3.0 ± 1.2	2.6 ± 0.9**	3.1 ± 1.1	2.7 ± 1.1**
Cholesterol/HDL-C			4.7 ± 2.2	4.1 ± 1.2**	5.1 ± 1.8	4.5 ± 1.9**
ApoA1 (mg/dL)					113.4 ± 24.4	117.8 ± 24.3*
ApoB (mg/dL)					81.4 ± 36.3	72.0 ± 34.5**
Lipoprotein(a) (mg/dL)					13.9 ± 17.5	13.2 ± 18.1
Homocysteine (nmol/mL)				9.4 ± 3.0	9.6 ± 4.9	

p values reflect analyses of age-survey standardized data; * p < 0.05; ** p < 0.01; *** p < 0.001. Apo, apolipoprotein; BMI, body mass index; BP, blood pressure; HDL, high-density lipoprotein; LDL, low-density lipoprotein; TSF, triceps skinfold thickness; +CAC, with coronary artery calcification, detected as a minimum of three contiguous pixels ≥130 HU; −CAC, without coronary artery calcification.

TABLE 4.2

Serial measurements (mean ± SD) during childhood and two young adult Muscatine Study examinations in females with (n = 75) and without (n = 397) detectable coronary artery calcification

Variable	Childhood Ages 8 to 18 years		Young Adult Ages 20 to 38 years		Most Recent Ages 29 to 43 years	
	+CAC	−CAC	+CAC	−CAC	+CAC	−CAC
Height (cm)	162.1 ± 6.9	161.5 ± 7.1	164.7 ± 5.5	164.2 ± 6.0	165.0 ± 5.6	164.7 ± 6.2
Weight (kg)	61.5 ± 14.5	56.1 ± 9.3*	77.4 ± 17.4	64.5 ± 12.3***	85.3 ± 18.6	70.0 ± 14.7***
BMI (kg/m^2)	23.3 ± 4.7	21.4 ± 3.0*	28.6 ± 6.3	23.9 ± 4.4***	31.4 ± 6.8	25.8 ± 5.3***
TSF (mm)	15.7 ± 6.6	13.7 ± 5.2*	25.0 ± 9.7	20.7 ± 7.9***	35.3 ± 9.2	28.6 ± 9.3***
Waist/hip					0.80 ± 0.07	0.75 ± 0.07***
Systolic BP (mmHg)	119.2 ± 12.3	113.8 ± 10.9***	113.8 ± 11.9	108.8 ± 9.5***	119.1 ± 14.8	111.8 ± 11.8***
Diastolic BP (mmHg)	78.5 ± 8.6	75.6 ± 8.9*	71.6 ± 10.0	67.4 ± 8.3**	76.4 ± 11.8	69.6 ± 10.0***
Total cholesterol (mg/dL)	152.2 ± 25.6	158.2 ± 28.0*	175.9 ± 35.0	172.6 ± 33.3	178.3 ± 36.3	174.9 ± 31.8
Triglycerides (mg/dL)	73.9 ± 32.3	75.8 ± 31.3	104.4 ± 58.3	88.5 ± 48.2*	125.0 ± 60.7	103.4 ± 68.6*
HDL-C (mg/dL)			44.7 ± 9.1	50.2 ± 12.5***	45.4 ± 11.6	51.8 ± 14.6***
LDL-C (mg/dL)			111.0 ± 31.9	104.7 ± 31.0	107.9 ± 33.3	102.7 ± 29.2
LDL-C/HDL-C			2.6 ± 1.0	2.3 ± 1.0**	2.6 ± 1.1	2.2 ± 1.0*
Cholesterol/HDL-C			4.1 ± 1.3	3.7 ± 1.2**	4.2 ± 1.3	3.7 ± 1.3**
ApoA1 (mg/dL)					125.6 ± 24.2	136.3 ± 27.0*
ApoB (mg/dL)					64.0 ± 26.7	56.2 ± 19.1*
Lipoprotein(a) (mg/dL)					13.2 ± 17.2	14.1 ± 19.2
Homocysteine (nmol/mL)					9.0 ± 5.1	8.1 ± 3.3

See Table 4.1 for abbreviations. *p < 0.05; **p < 0.01; ***p < 0.001.

Table 4.3 presents univariate age-adjusted risk odds ratios for CAC associated with having a CRF level in the upper decile of the age-, sex-, and survey-specific distribution relative to having a CRF level in the lower nine deciles. For HDL-C and apo A1, the odds ratios reflect a CRF level that is in the lower decile relative to a CRF level in the upper nine deciles. Upper-decile values of childhood weight, BMI, and SBP in females were associated with significantly increased odds of CAC. In both sexes, upper-decile values for young adult body habitus, blood pressure, and triglyceride measurements were associated with significantly increased odds of CAC. In young adult males, lower-decile values of HDL-C and upper-decile values of LDL-C/HDL-C and total cholesterol/HDL-C were associated with significantly increased odds of CAC. For females, upper decile values for the most recent measurements of body habitus, SBP and DBP showed very significant associations with CAC; the association with these measures was weaker in males. Upper-decile values for the most recent measurements of triglycerides, LDL-C, and apo B were also associated with significantly increased odds of CAC in females; lower-decile values of HDL-C were associated with significantly increased odds of CAC in males.

Table 4.4 presents the age-adjusted odds ratios and 95% confidence intervals for CAC from multiple logistic regression analysis for upper decile (lower for HDL-C) vs. the lower (upper) nine deciles of age-, sex-, and survey-specific CRF Z scores in males and females. Analysis of childhood CRF information in males did not identify any variable as a significant predictor of CAC in young adults. Childhood BMI in females was a significant independent predictor of CAC. The model resulting from the analysis of young adult CRF information in males identified DBP as a significant independent predictor. In females, BMI and triglycerides were significant predictors. Finally, the model resulting from the analysis of the most recent CRF information included HDL-C as a significant independent predictor in males, and BMI, DBP, and LDL-C as significant independent predictors in females.

The greater the number of aberrant CRF levels (blood pressure ≥140/90 mmHg, total cholesterol ≥200 mg/dL, HDL-C ≤35 mg/dL, or BMI ≥30), the more likely it was for CAC to be detected in these young adults (Mahoney et al., 2001). The percent of females positive for CAC increased from 10% in those with no aberrant CRF levels, to 16% in those with one, 37% in those with two, and 42% in those with three of these CRFs. The percent of males positive for CAC was 20% in those with no aberrant CRF levels, 34% in those with one, 41% in those with two, and 56% in those with three of these CRFs. However, only 12 of the 472 females and 25 of the 385 males had three aberrant CRF levels.

A simplified algorithm to predict multivariate CAD risk in persons without overt disease was developed using CRF data from the Framingham Heart Study (Wilson et al., 1998). We applied the model to participants in the Muscatine Study to determine its association with CAC in young adults (Mahoney et al., 2001). For every 2-point increase in the Framingham Score, the odds of CAC increased by 30% in females and by 20% in males.

TABLE 4.3
Univariate age-adjusted odds ratios† (95% confidence intervals) for presence of coronary artery calcification according to measured coronary risk factors from childhood, young adult, and most recent Muscatine Study examinations

Variable	Childhood Ages 8 to 18 years		Young Adult Ages 20 to 34 years		Most Recent Ages 29 to 43 years	
	Males	Females	Males	Females	Males	Females
Height	0.9 (0.4–1.9)	0.6 (0.2–1.5)	0.4 (0.2–1.1)	0.3 (0.1–1.0)	0.6 (0.3–1.3)	0.6 (0.2–1.5)
Weight	2.0 (1.0–3.8)	2.5 (1.2–5.2)**	2.1 (1.0–4.1)*	7.9 (4.0–15.5)***	2.0 (1.0–4.0)*	6.8 (3.5–13.1)***
BMI	1.3 (0.7–2.7)	2.5 (1.2–5.2)**	2.9 (1.5–5.8)**	6.9 (3.6–13.4)***	2.0 (1.0–4.0)*	8.2 (4.2–16.0)***
Waist/hip					1.4 (0.7–2.9)	3.1 (1.6–6.2)***
TSF	1.6 (0.8–3.1)	1.6 (0.8–3.5)	2.5 (1.2–4.9)*	3.0 (1.5–5.8)**	1.7 (0.8–3.4)	2.9 (1.4–5.8)**
Systolic BP	1.2 (0.6–2.4)	2.3 (1.2–4.7)*	3.2 (1.6–6.4)***	3.3 (1.7–6.5)***	2.3 (1.2–4.6)*	4.0 (2.0–7.8)***
Diastolic BP	1.5 (0.7–2.9)	2.0 (1.0–4.1)	3.7 (1.9–7.4)***	3.1 (1.6–6.2)**	2.2 (1.1–4.3)*	4.4 (2.3–8.7)***
Total cholesterol	1.2 (0.6–2.4)	0.5 (0.2–1.4)	1.5 (0.7–2.9)	1.3 (0.6–2.8)	1.8 (0.9–3.7)	1.7 (0.8–3.5)
Triglycerides	0.7 (0.3–1.6)	0.4 (0.1–1.2)	2.3 (1.2–4.5)*	3.6 (1.8–7.1)***	1.6 (0.8–3.3)	2.8 (1.4–5.6)**
HDL-C			2.0 (1.0–3.9)*	1.5 (0.7–3.2)	2.2 (1.1–4.4)*	1.6 (0.8–3.5)
LDL-C			1.5 (0.8–3.1)	1.2 (0.5–2.7)	1.7 (0.8–3.4)	2.7 (1.3–5.4)**
LDL-C/HDL-C			2.1 (1.1–4.1)*	1.8 (0.8–3.7)	1.6 (0.8–3.2)	1.8 (0.8–3.8)
Cholesterol/HDL-C			2.5 (1.3–5.0)**	1.8 (0.8–3.7)	1.9 (0.9–3.8)	1.8 (0.9–3.8)
ApoA1					1.9 (0.9–3.8)	1.2 (0.5–2.6)
ApoB					1.6 (0.8–3.3)	2.3 (1.1–4.7)*
Lipoprotein(a)					1.2 (0.6–2.5)	1.2 (0.6–2.7)
Homocysteine					0.8 (0.4–1.8)	1.3 (0.5–3.1)

See Table 4.1 for abbreviations. †Upper decile of coronary risk factor vs. lower nine deciles (lower decile of HDL-C and Apo A1 vs. upper nine deciles). * $p < 0.05$; ** $p < 0.01$; *** $p < 0.001$.

TABLE 4.4

Multivariate age-adjusted odds ratios† (95% confidence intervals) for presence of coronary artery calcification in males and females from multiple logistic regression analysis of Muscatine Study coronary risk factors

Variable	Males	Females
Childhood		
BMI	1.5 (0.7–3.3)	2.2 (1.0–4.7)*
Systolic BP	1.1 (0.5–2.3)	1.8 (0.8–4.0)
Diastolic BP	1.5 (0.7–3.0)	1.2 (0.5–2.8)
Cholesterol	1.2 (0.6–2.5)	0.5 (0.2–1.6)
Triglycerides	0.6 (0.2–1.4)	0.4 (0.1–1.5)
Young Adult		
BMI	2.1 (1.0–4.5)	4.4 (2.1–9.2)***
Systolic BP	2.0 (0.9–4.4)	1.4 (0.6–3.4)
Diastolic BP	2.5 (1.1–5.5)*	2.2 (0.9–5.1)
HDL-C	1.8 (0.8–3.8)	1.0 (0.4–2.3)
LDL-C	1.3 (0.6–2.7)	0.9 (0.4–2.3)
Triglycerides	1.4 (0.6–3.1)	2.6 (1.2–5.7)*
Most Recent		
BMI	1.7 (0.7–3.9)	5.7 (2.7–12.1)***
Waist/hip	0.8 (0.3–1.8)	2.2 (1.0–4.8)*
Systolic BP	1.8 (0.8–4.1)	1.6 (0.6–3.9)
Diastolic BP	1.6 (0.7–3.7)	2.9 (1.2–7.0)*
HDL-C	2.4 (1.1–5.3)*	1.5 (0.6–3.5)
LDL-C	1.5 (0.7–3.3)	2.8 (1.3–6.0)**
Triglycerides	1.2 (0.5–2.8)	1.8 (0.8–4.2)

See Table 4.1 for abbreviations. †Upper decile of coronary risk factor vs. lower nine deciles (lower decile of HDL-C vs. upper nine deciles).*$p < 0.05$; **$p < 0.01$; ***$p < 0.001$.

▓ PREDICTORS OF QUANTITY OF CORONARY ARTERY CALCIFICATION IN ADULTS: THE EPIDEMIOLOGY OF CORONARY ARTERY CALCIFICATION STUDY

The Rochester Family Heart Study (Turner et al., 1989; Kottke et al., 1991) is a community-based study of the genetic epidemiology of CAD and essential hypertension that included 3974 individuals, 5 to 90 years of age, between 1984 and 1991 in Rochester, Minnesota. The community-based Epidemiology of

Coronary Artery Calcification (ECAC) Study (Kaufmann et al., 1995; Maher et al., 1996), conducted between 1991 and 1998, examined 1151 participants (558 males and 593 females), ages 20 to 79 years, from the Rochester Family Heart Study. Participants in the ECAC Study never had coronary or noncoronary heart surgery. Standardized body size measurements, blood pressure measurements, and blood samples were obtained from all participants contemporaneous with the EBCT examination. The associations between traditional CRF levels and the quantity of CAC (defined as the Agatston score) were examined among participants. The prevalence of CAC was 54% and 25% among males and females, respectively. The quantity of CAC ranged from 0 to 3036.7 among males and from 0 to 2488.5 among females, with medians of 2.2 and 0, respectively. The youngest male with CAC was 21 years old and the youngest female with CAC was 28 years old. Sex-specific linear regression models were used to identify the traditional CRF levels that were associated with the quantity of CAC after adjusting for age. Separate models were fit for each CRF. Participants were considered hypertensive if their systolic blood pressure was ≥140 mmHg or their diastolic blood pressure was ≥90 mmHg, or if they reported a prior diagnosis and treatment of hypertension and were currently using blood pressure lowering medications. The quantity of CAC (score) was natural log transformed to reduce skewness [log(score + 1).] The estimated sex-specific age-adjusted regression coefficients and their corresponding p values are presented in Table 4.5. Stepwise linear regression models were also used to determine the "best" set of CRFs associated with log(score + 1) for males and females separately. For males, age, total cholesterol/HDL-C ratio, hypertension and a history of cigarette smoking were positively and significantly associated with log(score + 1). Height and having a college education (≥4 years of college/university education) were negatively and significantly associated with log(score + 1). The model R^2 was 0.45. For females, age, waist/hip ratio, pulse pressure, hypertension, and a history of cigarette smoking were positively and significantly associated with log(score + 1). The model R^2 was 0.36. In both males and females, the direction and strength of the coefficients in the stepwise models were very similar to those in the age-adjusted models.

▪ GENETIC FACTORS AND CORONARY ARTERY CALCIFICATION

Differences in the occurrence of CAC among genetically distinct inbred mouse strains provide evidence for a genetic component in the calcification process (Qiao et al., 1994). In the ECAC Study, the relative contributions of measured CRFs and genetic influences on CAC quantity measured by EBCT were quantified. Before adjusting for any CRFs, 43.5% of the variation in CAC quantity was attributable to genetic factors ($p < 0.001$). This estimate was obtained using a variance components approach that included the genetic relatedness among individuals in the

TABLE 4.5

Association of coronary risk factors with quantity of coronary artery calcification in asymptomatic participants in the Epidemiology of Coronary Artery Calcification Study

Variable	Males (n = 569)			Females (n = 596)		
	Beta	p value		Beta	p value	
Age (years)	1.50	<0.0001	I†	0.96	<0.0001	I
Height (cm)	−0.25	0.0030	I	−0.09	0.1825	
Weight (kg)	0.15	0.0581		0.06	0.3462	
BMI	0.27	0.0008		0.10	0.1305	
Waist/hip	0.34	0.0005		0.33	<0.0001	I
Systolic BP (mmHg)	0.28	0.0013		0.43	<0.0001	
Diastolic BP (mmHg)	0.11	0.1576		0.01	0.8180	
Pulse pressure (mmHg)	0.25	0.0036		0.53	<0.0001	I
Hypertension	0.79	0.0001	I	0.99	<0.0001	I
Cholesterol (md/dL)	0.20	0.0194		0.12	0.1004	
Cholesterol/HDL-C	0.27	0.0010	I	0.12	0.0750	
Triglycerides (mg/dL)	0.36	0.0005		0.22	0.0025	
HDL-C (mg/dL)	−0.13	0.1088		−0.08	0.2451	
LDL-C (mg/dL)	0.14	0.0915		0.08	0.2393	
Ever smoked cigarettes	0.64	<0.0001	I	0.37	0.0049	I
College education	−0.59	0.0002	I	−0.49	0.0005	

Abbreviations as in Table 4.1. Beta coefficients and *p* values are from linear regression models predicting log(CAC score + 1). All models were adjusted for age except the model with just age. Participants were considered hypertensive if their systolic BP was ≥140 mmHg or diastolic BP ≥90 mmHg, or if they reported a prior diagnosis and treatment of hypertension and were currently using blood pressure lowering medications. College education was defined as ≥4 years of college/university education. †Variables denoted with *I* are significant independent predictors of quantity of CAC in stepwise linear regression models.

model (Almasy et al., 1998). After adjusting for age, sex, fasting glucose, SBP, pack-years of smoking, and LDL-C, 41.8% of the residual variation in CAC quantity was attributable to genetic factors ($p < 0.0005$) (Peyser et al., 2002).

Investigations of specific candidate genes for CAC in humans are limited, and none of the findings have been replicated. Pfohl et al. (1998) reported an association between the insertion/deletion polymorphism of the angiotensin I-converting enzyme gene and CAC detected by intravascular ultrasound in patients with angiographically proven CAD. The apolipoprotein E genotype was found to influence the relationship between CRFs and EBCT measured CAC presence in both males and females from the ECAC Study (Kardia et al., 1999). Ellsworth et al. (2001) reported a significant association between the S128R polymorphism of the E-selectin gene and presence and quantity of EBCT measured

CAC in females ≤50 years of age from the ECAC Study, after adjusting for CRFs. In the Helsinki Sudden Death Study, a polymorphism within the tumor necrosis factor locus was associated with the extent of CAC (Keso et al., 2001). The hepatic lipase gene promoter polymorphism (*LIPC*-480C>T) was associated with CAC in type 1 diabetic patients after adjusting for duration of diabetes and CRFs (Hokanson et al., 2002). In first-degree relatives of persons with premature CAD, the Val64Ile polymorphism in the C-C chemokine receptor 2 gene was associated with CAC (Valdes et al., 2002).

A genome-wide linkage analysis was performed using affected sib-pairs, defined as being greater than or equal to the age- and sex-specific 70th percentile for CAC quantity, in a sample of 29 families enriched for hypertension from the ECAC Study (Lange et al., 2002). The results provided evidence that chromosomal regions 6p21.3 (maximum LOD score = 2.22, $p < 0.001$) and 10q21.3 (maximum LOD score = 3.24, $p < 0.0001$) may harbor genes associated with subclinical coronary atherosclerosis.

Taken together, all of these studies demonstrate the importance of genetic factors in subclinical coronary atherosclerosis variation as measured by CAC and indicate that unknown genes influencing CAC quantity are yet to be identified. Identification of genes that contribute to the CAC process will provide a better understanding of the origin of CAC and could ultimately establish a basis for improved prevention and treatment of asymptomatic coronary atherosclerosis.

■ PROGRESSION AND REGRESSION OF QUANTITY OF CORONARY ARTERY CALCIFICATION

Several studies have investigated the rate of progression of CAC and the variability in the rate of progression among different patient groups. Asymptomatic hypertensive patients with prominent atherosclerotic risk had progression rates, expressed as percent change in total calcium score after 3 years, that were similar to those for patients with hypertension and stable CAD (124% and 118%, respectively) when CAC was measured with dual-section spiral CT (Shemesh et al., 2001). However, the rates of progression for both of these groups were significantly less than the rate of progression for a group who experienced a coronary event during the 3-year period (180%, $p < 0.05$).

Baseline and follow-up examinations for CAC with EBCT were obtained a mean of 3.5 ± 0.4 years apart in 81 ECAC participants (Bielak et al., 2001). At follow-up, 59 participants had no apparent change in the quantity of CAC (46 had no CAC at either examination and 13 had similar quantities at both baseline and follow-up), 21 had large increases in the quantity of CAC, and 1 participant had a large decrease in the quantity suggesting regression. In another study, 246 patients with hypertension underwent baseline scanning and follow-up scanning 3 years later with dual-section spiral CT (Shemesh et al., 2000). Of the 152 patients with CAC at baseline, 106 (70%) showed progression (defined as absolute change in total calcium score from baseline); however, of the 94 with no CAC at baseline, only 26 (28%) showed progression ($p < 0.01$). The association of obesity with progression of CAC was examined among 443 asymptomatic participants (243 men) in the ECAC Study with baseline and follow-up CAC measurements an average of 8.9 years apart (Cassidy et al., 2005). In those at <10% 10-year coronary heart disease risk based on the Framingham Score, waist circumference ($p < 0.025$), waist-to-hip ratio ($p < 0.001$), body mass index ($p < 0.05$), and being overweight compared with being underweight or of normal weight ($p < 0.01$) were each significantly positively associated with progression of CAC (Cassidy et al., 2005).

The impact of lipid-lowering medications on CAC measured using EBCT was examined retrospectively in 149 subjects, ages 32 to 75 years, who underwent EBCT studies at baseline and 12 to 15 months later (Callister et al., 1998b). Three groups were identified: no therapy and LDL-C ≥120 mg/dL; therapy but LDL-C remaining above 120 mg/dL; and therapy with reduction of LDL-C to <120 mg/dL during the follow-up period. The first two groups showed a measurable increase in CAC expressed as the percent of baseline (mean ± SD of 52% + 36% and 24% ± 22%, respectively; $p < 0.001$ for both). The third group, however, showed a decrease (-7% + 23%; $p < 0.01$). The magnitude of the reduction in CAC quantity was directly related to treatment-induced reduction in LDL-C.

Patients with hypertension, hypercholesterolemia, and/or diabetes (ages 36 to 77 years) underwent two EBCT scans a mean of 2.2 ± 1.1 years apart (Budhoff et al., 2000). Of the 131 patients with hypercholesterolemia, those on therapy showed an increase in CAC of 15% ± 8% per year compared to 39% ± 12% per year for untreated participants ($p < 0.001$). Among the 60 patients on statin monotherapy, 37% exhibited a decrease in CAC from baseline to follow-up scan and 18% had no significant change. Conversely, of the 71 patients not on statin therapy, only 4% showed a decrease in CAC. This rate of regression is significantly less than that in patients receiving statin therapy ($p < 0.001$).

An efficacy study, comparing treatment with a calcium channel blocker (nifedipine) to treatment with a diuretic (co-amilozide), examined serial double-helix computerized tomographic scans for progression of CAC (Motro and Shemesh, 2001). Inhibition of CAC progression was significant in the nifedipine vs. co-amilozide group during the first (3.2% vs. 27%, respectively, $p < 0.025$) and third (40% vs. 78%, respectively, $p < 0.025$) but not the second ($p > 0.10$) years of study. While the authors acknowledged that the number of patients was not large enough in comparison to an evidenced-based controlled trial, the data suggest a slower progression of CAC with use of a calcium channel blocker.

▦ SUMMARY

• The deposition of calcium in the atherosclerotic plaque occurs as the plaque becomes more complex.

- Identification of calcium by a noninvasive technique, such as EBCT, indicates that the atherosclerotic process is present in the coronary arteries of an individual.
- An increasing quantity of CAC indicates narrowing somewhere in the coronary arteries and high levels predict subsequent CAD.
- The prevalence of CAC is associated with known CRF levels, even levels obtained in childhood.
- The quantity and distribution of CAC increase with increasing age, with the prevalence approaching 100% in the elderly. Thus, the specificity of presence of CAC for significant CAD diminishes in older individuals.
- Concentration on CRF associations with EBCT detection of CAC in younger individuals may provide more specific identification of at-risk individuals who would benefit most from early intervention strategies.
- Many ongoing studies should provide valuable information on both environmental and genetic factors that play a role in variation in quantity of CAC.
- Finally, EBCT may also be used in serial studies to measure change in quantity of CAC over time and to monitor the effectiveness of interventions designed to alter the atherosclerotic process.

■ REFERENCES

Agatston, A.S., W.R. Janowitz, F.J. Hildner, N.R. Zusmer, M. Viamonte, Jr., and R. Detrano. 1990. Quantification of Coronary Artery Calcium Using Ultrafast Computed Tomography. *J Am Coll Cardiol* 15:827–32.

Almasy, L., and J. Blangero. 1998. Multipoint Quantitative Linkage Analysis in General Pedigrees. *Am J Hum Genet* 62:1198–211.

Anderson, H.C. 1983. Calcific Diseases. *Arch Pathol Lab Med* 107:341–8.

Arad, Y., L.A. Spadaro, K. Goodman, D. Newstein, and A.D. Guerci. 2000. Prediction of Coronary Events with Electron Beam Computed Tomography. *J Am Coll Cardiol* 36:1253–60.

Bielak, L.F., J.A. Rumberger, P.F. Sheedy, R.S. Schwartz, and P.A. Peyser. 2000a. Probabilistic Model for Prediction of Angiographically Defined Obstructive Coronary Artery Disease Using Electron Beam Computed Tomography Calcium Score Strata. *Circulation* 102:380–5.

Bielak, L.F., G.G. Klee, P.F. Sheedy, S.T. Turner, R.S. Schwartz, and P.A. Peyser. 2000b. Association of Fibrinogen with Quantity of Coronary Artery Calcification Measured by Electron Beam Computed Tomography. *Arterioscler Thromb Vasc Biol* 20:2167–71.

Bielak, L.F., P.F. Sheedy, II, and P.A. Peyser. 2001. Coronary Artery Calcification Measured at Electron-Beam CT: Agreement in Dual Scan Runs and Change Over Time. *Radiology* 218: 224–9.

Blankenhorn, D. 1961. Coronary Arterial Calcification, a Review. *Am J Med Sci.* 242:1–10.

Budoff, M.J., K.L. Lane, H. Bakhsheshi, S. Mao, B.O. Grassmann, B.C. Friedman, and B.H. Brundage. 2000. Rates of Progression of Coronary Calcium by Electron Beam Tomography. *Am J Cardiol* 86:8–11.

Callister, T.Q., B. Cooil, S.P. Raya, N.J. Lippolis, D.J. Russo, and P. Raggi. 1998a. Coronary Artery Disease: Improved Reproducibility of Calcium Scoring with an Electron-Beam CT Volumetric Method. *Radiology* 208:807–14.

Callister, T.Q., P. Raggi, B. Cooil, N.J. Lippolis, and D.J. Russo. 1998b. Effect of HMG-CoA Reductase Inhibitors on Coronary Artery Disease as Assessed by Electron-Beam Computed Tomography. *N Engl J Med* 339:1972–8.

Carr, J.J., J.R. Crouse, III, D.C. Goff, R.B. D'Agostino, Jr., N.P. Peterson, and G.L. Burke. 2000. Evaluation of Subsecond Gated Helical CT for Quantification of Coronary Artery Calcium and Comparison with Electron Beam CT. *AJR Am J Roentgenol* 174:915–21.

Cassidy, A.E., L.F. Bielak, Y. Zhou, P.F. Sheedy II, S.T. Turner, J.F. Breen, P.A. Araoz, I.J. Kullo, X.Lin, and P.A. Peyser. 2005. Progression of Subclinical Coronary Atherosclerosis. Does Obesity Make a Difference? *Circulation* 111:1877–82.

Clarkson, T.B., R.W. Prichard, T.M. Morgan, G.S. Petrick, and K.P. Klein. 1994. Remodeling of Coronary Arteries in Human and Nonhuman Primates. *JAMA* 271:289–94.

Detrano R.C., M. Anderson, J. Nelson, N.D. Wong, J.J. Carr, M. McNitt-Gray, and D.E. Bild. 2005. Coronary Calcium Measurements: Effect of CT Scanner Type and Calcium Measure on Rescan Reproducibility—MESA Study. *Radiology* 236:477–84.

Eggen, D.A., J.P. Strong, and H.C. McGill, Jr. 1965. Coronary Calcification: Relationship to Clinically Significant Coronary Lesions and Race, Sex, and Topographic Distribution. *Circulation* 32:948–55.

Ellsworth, D.L., L.F. Bielak, S.T. Turner, P.F. Sheedy, II, F. Boerwinkle and P.A. Peyser. 2001. Gender- and Age-Dependent Relationships between the E-Selectin S128R Polymorphism and Coronary Artery Calcification. *J Mol Med* 79:390–8.

Gidding, S.S., L.C. Bookstein, and E.V. Chomka. 1998. Usefulness of Electron Beam Tomography in Adolescents and Young Adults with Heterozygous Familial Hypercholesterolemia. *Circulation* 98:2580–3.

Greenland, P., L. LaBree, S.P. Azen, T.M. Doherty, and R.C. Detrano. 2004. Coronary Artery Calcium Score Combined with Framingham Score for Risk Prediction in Asymptomatic Individuals. *JAMA* 291:210–5.

Hecht, H.S., and R. Superko. 2001. Electron Beam Tomography and National Cholesterol Education Program Guidelines in Asymptomatic Women. *J Am Coll Cardiol* 37:1506–11.

Hokanson, J.E., S. Cheng, J.K. Snell Bergeon, D.A. Fijal, M.A. Grow, C. Hung, H.A. Erlich, J. Ehrlich, R.H. Eckel, and M. Rewers. 2002. A Common Promoter Polymorphism in the Hepatic Lipase Gene (LIPC-480C>T) Is Associated with an Increase in Coronary Calcification in Type 1 Diabetes. *Diabetes* 51:1208–13.

Kardia, S.L.R., M.B. Haviland, R.E. Ferrell, and C.F. Sing. 1999. The Relationship between Risk Factor Levels and Presence of Coronary Artery Calcification Is Dependent on Apolipoprotein E Genotype. *Arterioscler Thromb Vasc Biol* 19:427–35.

Kaufmann, R.B., P.F. Sheedy, II, J.F. Breen, J.R. Kelzenberg, B.L. Kruger, R.S. Schwartz and P.P. Moll. 1994. Detection of Heart Calcification with Electron Beam CT: Interobserver and Intraobserver Reliability for Scoring Quantification. *Radiology* 190:347–52.

Kaufmann, R.B., P.F. Sheedy, J.F. Maher, L.F. Bielak, J.F. Breen, R.S. Schwartz, and P.A. Peyser. 1995. Quantity of Coronary Artery Calcium Detected by Electron Beam Computed Tomography in Asymptomatic Subjects and Angiographically Studied Patients. *Mayo Clin Proc* 70:223–32.

Keelan, P.C., L.F. Bielak, K. Ashai, L.S. Jamjoum, A.E. Denktas, J.A. Rumberger, P.F. Sheedy, P.A. Peyser, and R.S. Schwartz. 2001. Long-Term Prognostic Value of Coronary Calcification Detected by Electron-Beam Computed Tomography in Patients Undergoing Coronary Angiography. *Circulation* 104:412–7.

Keso, T., M. Perola, P. Laippala, E. Ilveskoski, T.A. Kunnas, J. Mikkelsson, A. Penttila, M. Hurme, and P.J. Karhunen. 2001. Polymorphisms within the Tumor Necrosis Factor Locus and Prevalence of Coronary Artery Disease in Middle-Aged Men. *Atherosclerosis* 154:691–7.

Knez, A., C. Becker, A. Becker, A. Leber, C. White, M. Reiser, and G. Steinbeck. 2002. Determination of Coronary Calcium with Multi-Slice Spiral Computed Tomography: a Comparative Study with Electron-Beam CT. *Int J Cardiovasc Imag* 18:295–303.

Kottke, B.A., P.P. Moll, V.V. Michels, and W.H. Weidman. 1991. Levels of Lipids, Lipoproteins, and Apolipoproteins in a Defined Population. *Mayo Clin Proc* 66:1198–208.

Kullo, I.J., J.P. McConnell, K.R. Bailey, S.L. Kardia, L.F. Bielak, P.A. Peyser, P.F. Sheedy, II, E. Boerwinkle, and S.T. Turner. 2003. Relation of C-Reactive Protein and Fibrinogen to Coronary Artery Calcium in Subjects with Systemic Hypertension. *Am J Cardiol* 92:56–8.

LaMonte, M.J., S.J. FitzGerald, T.S. Church, C.E. Barlow, N.B. Radford, B.D. Levine, J.J. Pippin, L.W. Gibbons, S.N. Blair, and M.Z. Nichaman. 2005. Coronary Artery Calcium Score and Coronary Heart Disease Events in a Large Cohort of Asymptomatic Men and Women. *Am J Epidemiol* 162:421–9.

Lange, L.A., E.M. Lange, L.F. Bielak, C.D. Langefeld, S.L. Kardia, P. Royston, S.T. Turner, P.F. Sheedy, II, E. Boerwinkle, and P.A. Peyser. 2002. Autosomal Genome-Wide Scan for Coronary Artery Calcification Loci in Sibships at High Risk for Hypertension. *Arterioscler Thromb Vasc Biol* 22:418–23.

Laudon, D.A., L.F. Vukov, J.F. Breen, J.A. Rumberger, P.C. Wollan, and P.F. Sheedy. II. 1999. Use of Electron-Beam Computed Tomography in the Evaluation of Chest Pain Patients in the Emergency Department. *Ann Emerg Med* 33:15–21.

Maher, J.E., J.A. Raz, L.F. Bielak, P.F. Sheedy, R.S. Schwartz, and P.A. Peyser. 1996. Potential of Quantity of Coronary Artery Calcification to Identify New Risk Factors for Asymptomatic Atherosclerosis. *Am J Epidemiol* 144:943–53.

Mahoney, L.T., T.L. Burns, W. Stanford, B.H. Thompson, J.D. Witt, C.A. Rost, and R.M. Lauer. 1996. Coronary Risk Factors Measured in Childhood and Young Adult Life are Associated with Coronary Artery Calcification in Young Adults: The Muscatine Study. *J Am Coll Cardiol* 27:277–84.

Mahoney, L.T., T.L. Burns, W. Stanford, B.H. Thompson, J.D. Witt, C.A. Rost, and R.M. Lauer. 2001. Usefulness of the Framingham Risk Score and Body Mass Index to Predict Early Coronary Artery Calcium in Young Adults (Muscatine Study). *Am J Cardiol* 88:509–15.

Margolis, J.R., J.T.T. Chen, Y. Kong, R.H. Peter, V.S. Behar, and J.A. Kisslo. 1980. The Diagnostic and Prognostic Significance of Coronary Artery Calcification. *Radiology* 137:609–16.

Mautner, G.C., S.L. Mautner, J. Froehlich, I.M. Feuerstein, M.A. Proschan, W.C. Roberts, and J.L. Doppman. 1994. Coronary Artery Calcification: Assessment with Electron Beam CT and Histomorphometric Correlation. *Radiology* 192:619–23.

McGill, H.C. 1989. The Pathogenesis of Atherosclerosis. *Clin Chem* 34:B33–B39.

Megnien, J.L., A. Simon, M. Lemariey, M.C. Plainfosse, and J. Levenson. 1996. Hypertension Promotes Coronary Calcium Deposit in Asymptomatic Men. *Hypertension* 27:949–54.

Motro, M., and J. Shemesh. 2001. Calcium Channel Blocker Nifedipine Slows Down Progression of Coronary Calcification in Hypertensive Patients Compared with Diuretics. *Hypertension* 37:1410–3.

Nallamothu, B.K., S. Saint, L.F. Bielak, S.S. Sonnad, P.A. Peyser, M. Rubenfire, and A.M. Fendrich. 2001. Electron-Beam Computed Tomography in the Diagnosis of Coronary Artery Disease. *Arch Intern Med* 161:833–8.

Nishino, M., M.J. Malloy, J. Naya-Vigne, J. Russell, J.P. Kane, and R.F. Redberg. 2000. Lack of Association of Lipoprotein(a) Levels with Coronary Calclium Deposits in Asymptomatic Postmenopausal Women. *J Am Coll Cardiol* 35:314–20.

Peyser, P.A., L.F. Bielak, J.S. Chu, S.T. Turner, D.L. Ellsworth, E. Boerwinkle, and P.F. Sheedy, II. 2002. Heritability of Coronary Artery Calcium Quantity Measured by Electron Beam Computed Tomography in Asymptomatic Adults. *Circulation* 106:304–8.

Pfohl, M., A. Athanasiadis, M. Koch, P. Clemens, N. Benda, H.U. Haring, and K.R. Karsch. 1998. Insertion/Deletion Polymorphism of the Angiotensin I Converting Enzyme Gene Is Associated with Coronary Artery Plaque Calcification as Assessed by Intravascular Ultrasound. *J Am Coll Cardiol* 31:987–91.

Qiao, J.-H., P.-Z. Xie, M.C. Fishbein, J. Kreuzer, T. Drake, L. Demer, and A. Lusis. 1994. Pathology of Atheromatous Lesions in Inbred and Genetically Engineered Mice. *Arterioscler Thromb* 14:1480–97.

Rumberger, J.A., D.B. Simons, L.A. Fitzpatrick, P.F. Sheedy, and R.S. Schwartz. 1995. Coronary Artery Calcium Area by Electron-Beam Computed Tomography and Coronary Atherosclerotic Plaque Area. A Histopathologic Correlative Study. *Circulation* 92:2157–62.

Shemesh, J., S. Apter, D. Stolero, Y. Itzchak, and M. Motro. 2001. Annual Progression of Coronary Artery Calcium by Spiral Computed Tomography in Hypertensive Patients without Myocardial Ischemia but with Prominent Atherosclerotic Risk Factors, in Patients with Previous Angina Pectoris or Healed Acute Myocardial Infarction, and in Patients with Coronary Events During Follow-Up. *Am J Cardiol* 87:1395–7.

Shemesh, J., S. Apter, C.I. Stroh, Y. Itzchak, and M. Motro. 2000. Tracking Coronary Calcification by Using Dual-Section Spiral CT: A 3-Year Follow-Up. *Radiology* 217:461–5.

Stary, H.C. 1990. The Sequence of Cell and Matrix Changes in Atherosclerotic Lesions of Coronary Arteries in the First Forty Years of Life. *Eur Heart J* 11:3–19.

Strong, J.P., and H.C. McGill. 1962. The Natural History of Coronary Atherosclerosis. *Am J Pathol* 40:37–49.

Taylor, A.J., I. Feuerstein, H. Wong, W. Barko, M. Brazaitis, and P.G. O'Malley. 2001. Do Conventional Risk Factors Predict Subclinical Coronary Artery Disease? Results from the Prospective Army Coronary Calcium Project. *Am Heart J* 141:463–8.

Turner, S.T., W.H. Weidman, V.V. Michels, T.J. Reed, C.L. Ormson, T. Fuller, and C.F. Sing. 1989. Distribution of Sodium-Lithium Countertransport and Blood Pressure in Caucasians Five to Eighty-Nine Years of Age. *Hypertension* 13:379–91.

Valdes, A.M., M.L. Wolfe, E.J. O'Brien, N.K. Spurr, W. Gefter, A. Rut, P.H. Groot, and D.J. Rader. 2002. Val64Ile polymorphism in the C-C chemokine receptor 2 Is associated with reduced coronary artery calcification. *Arterioscler Thromb Vasc Biol* 22:1924–8.

Wexler, L., B. Brundage, J. Crouse, R. Detrano, V. Fuster, J. Maddahi, J. Rumberger, W. Stanford, R. White, and K. Taubert. 1996. Coronary Artery Calcification: Pathophysiology, Epidemiology, Imaging Methods and Clinical Implications. A Statement for Health Professionals from the American Heart Association. *Circulation* 94:1175–92.

Wilson, P.W.F., R.B. D'Agostino, D. Levy, A.M. Belanger, H. Silbershatz, and W.B. Kannel. 1998. Prediction of Coronary Heart Disease Using Risk Factor Categories. *Circulation* 97:1837–47.

Wong, N.D., J.C Hsu, R.C. Detrano, G. Diamond, H. Eisenberg, and J.M. Gardin. 2000. Coronary Artery Calcium Evaluation by Electron Beam Computed Tomography and Its Relation to New Cardiovascular Events. *Am J Cardiol* 86:495–8.

Wong, N.D., D. Kouwabunpat, A.N. Vo, R.C. Detrano, H. Eisenberg, M. Goel, and J.M. Tobis. 1994. Coronary Calcium and Atherosclerosis by Ultrafast Computed Tomography in Asymptomatic Men and Women: Relation to Age and Risk Factors. *Am Heart J* 127:422–30.

CHAPTER 5

Relationship between Cardiovascular Risk Factors and Carotid Artery Intimal-Medial Thickness

Patricia H. Davis and Jeffrey D. Dawson

In older adults, measurement of carotid artery intimal-medial thickness (IMT) has gained acceptance as a noninvasive, inexpensive method to assess the extent of atherosclerosis. Several pieces of evidence support the validity of this method. Measurements of carotid IMT with ultrasonography in vivo (Fig. 5.1) correlate well with pathologic measurements (Schulte-Altedorneburg et al., 2001) and are reproducible (Riley et al., 1992). Increased carotid IMT and the rate of change of carotid IMT over time are significantly related to known cardiovascular risk factors (Chambless et al., 2002). Carotid IMT is positively associated with incident myocardial infarction (MI) (Salonen and Salonen, 1993; Bots et al., 1997; Chambless et al., 1997; O'Leary et al., 1999), and stroke (Chambless et al., 2000) and this association persists after adjustment for known cardiovascular risk factors. Similarly, increased carotid IMT has been associated with a reduction in the ankle-arm index, a marker of peripheral vascular disease (Bots et al., 1994). The Writing Group II of the American Heart Association Prevention Conference V concluded that measurement of carotid IMT in asymptomatic persons over 45 years of age adds incremental information to traditional risk factor assessment (Greenland et al., 2000). In addition, progression of the atherosclerotic lesion by serial measurements of carotid IMT is used as an end point in clinical trials of therapies to retard the atherosclerotic process (Mukherjee and Yadav, 2002).

Identification of children and adolescents with premature atherosclerosis based on increased carotid IMT, long before they develop morbidity and mor-

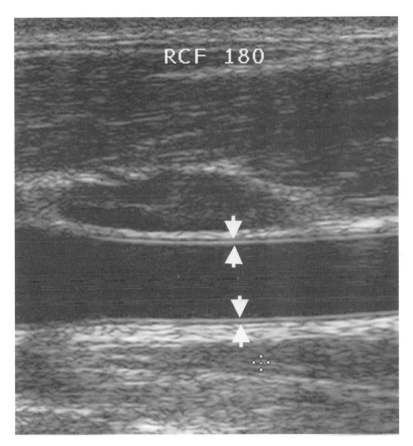

FIGURE 5.1

Ultrasound frame demonstrating measurement of the carotid intimal-medial thickness between the arrows, which indicate the intimal surface and the interface between the media and adventitia.

tality, would be useful in selecting those at highest risk. In young adults, the predictability of cardiovascular risk factors for clinical events in later life has not been established; however, the association of these risk factors with carotid IMT would lend support to measuring risk factors at a young age.

■ METHOD OF MEASURING INTIMAL-MEDIAL THICKNESS

Carotid IMT can be measured in both the near and far walls of the common carotid artery (CCA), bifurcation, and internal carotid artery (ICA) (Fig. 5.2)

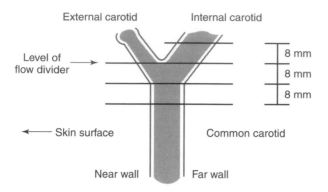

FIGURE 5.2
Schematic diagram illustrating the method of measuring the near and far wall intimal-medial thickness at the level of the common carotid artery, carotid bifurcation, and internal carotid artery with B-mode ultrasound. (Reproduced from Riley et al., 1992, with the permission of the American Heart Association.)

giving a total of 12 measurements when both sides are imaged. There are differing opinions about the optimal method of measurement (O'Leary et al., 1996; Raitakari, 1999; Dwyer et al., 2001). Raitakari (1999) recommends the measurement of only the far wall of the CCA in young adults because there are more missing data for measurements of the ICA and the near wall is technically more difficult to measure. Other studies have used the average of 12 measurements of maximal IMT. Stronger risk factor associations have been observed using the composite of 12 measurements compared to measuring the far wall of the CCA alone (O'Leary et al., 1996; Davis et al., 2001; Schillaci et al., 2002). In the Cardiovascular Health Study, risk factors accounted for 25% of the variability for a composite of CCA and ICA IMT but only 17% of the variability in the CCA IMT (O'Leary et al., 1996).

■ RISK FACTORS FOR INCREASED CAROTID INTIMAL-MEDIAL THICKNESS IN CHILDREN AND ADOLESCENTS

There are limited data concerning measurement of carotid IMT in children and adolescents. In a study of 85 boys and 108 girls who ranged in age from 10 to 24 years from the Stanislas cohort, the mean carotid IMT was 0.50 ± 0.04 mm for boys and 0.48 ± 0.03 mm for girls. Carotid IMT was not related to age or sex before 18 years of age. In those over 18 years of age, males had thicker IMTs. There were no risk factor associations with carotid IMT except for systolic blood pressure (SBP) in the males (Sass et al., 1998). In a study of 141 healthy 17- to 18-year-old males, carotid (CCA, ICA and bifurcation) and femoral IMT were measured and considered to be high if at least one vessel segment exceeded the 90th percentile. High IMT was positively associated with cigarette smoking, diastolic blood pressure (DBP), and immunoreactivity to heat shock protein (a marker of chronic infection or an autoimmune response), and negatively associated with high-density lipoprotein cholesterol (HDL-C) and alcohol intake (Knoflach et al., 2003). Another study of 249 healthy high school students demonstrated small but significant univariate associations between CCA IMT and low-density lipoprotein cholesterol (LDL-C), HDL-C, SBP, DBP, and body mass index (BMI); multivariate analysis was not performed (Sanchez et al., 2000).

Children with hypercholesterolemia have significantly higher carotid IMT when compared to controls (Pauciullo et al., 1994; Tonstad et al., 1996). In a study from Finland, a group of 88 children with either type 1 diabetes or hypercholesterolemia had increased carotid IMT compared to controls, and carotid IMT was positively associated with aortic IMT (Jarvisalo et al., 2001). In these high-risk children, DBP was also associated with carotid IMT. In a case-control study of children with type 1 diabetes, independent correlates with carotid IMT included the diabetic state, LDL-C, and SBP (Jarvisalo et al., 2002b). In another case-control study, carotid IMT was not increased in diabetic teenagers compared to healthy controls (Singh et al., 2003). In a study of 32 hypertensive children, carotid IMT was measured in the far wall of the CCA. Carotid IMT was significantly associated with left ventricular mass even after adjustment for age, sex and BMI. In those with increased carotid IMT ($\geq$0.80 mm which defined the top quartile), the prevalence of left ventricular hypertrophy was 89% as compared to 25% in those with normal carotid IMT (Sorof et al., 2003).

Elevated high sensitivity C-reactive protein (hsCRP) has been established as an independent predictor of subsequent myocardial infarction and stroke in older, asymptomatic adults even after adjustment for conventional risk factors (Ridker et al., 1998). In the Framingham Offspring Study, hsCRP was significantly higher in those in the top quartile of carotid IMT, but this association remained significant ($p = 0.01$) only in men after multivariate adjustment (O'Donell et al., 1999). However, a large cross-sectional study of older adults did not demonstrate an association of carotid IMT with hsCRP after multivariate adjustment (Folsom et al., 2001). In 70 healthy children, hsCRP was significantly associated with greater CCA far wall IMT as well as impaired brachial artery flow-mediated dilatation (a marker of disturbed endothelial function) (Jarvisalo et al., 2002a). This finding would suggest that elevated hsCRP may have a role in early atherosclerosis.

These studies demonstrate that carotid IMT can be measured in children and adolescents and that significantly increased carotid IMT is associated with hypercholesterolemia, hypertension and diabetes, and possibly hsCRP, even at a young age. It is not known whether increased carotid IMT measured in childhood will predict future cardiovascular risk as an adult.

■ PREDICTORS OF CAROTID INTIMAL-MEDIAL THICKNESS IN YOUNG AND MIDDLE-AGED ADULTS

A large population-based study of carotid IMT in young and middle-aged adults was conducted in Muscatine, Iowa. Subjects were eligible for this study if they had participated during childhood in at least one of the biennial school surveys conducted in Muscatine between 1971 and 1981, at least one of the Young Adult Follow-up surveys between ages 20 and 34 years, and had coronary artery calcification (CAC) measured at ages 29 to 37 years. Between 1996 and 1999, carotid ultrasound studies were performed in 346 men and 379 women aged 33 to 42 years who met these criteria and who were representative of the entire childhood cohort. The mean of the maximal carotid IMTs measured in 12 segments was 0.79 mm (SD 0.12) for men and 0.72 mm (SD 0.10) for women (Davis et al., 2001). The sex-specific distributions of the carotid IMT in this cohort are shown in Figure 5.3.

Tables 5.1 and 5.2 describe the cardiovascular risk factor levels measured during childhood (ages 8 to 18 years), young adulthood (ages 20 to 34 years), and concurrent with the measurement of carotid IMT (ages 33 to 42 years) for those with carotid IMT in the upper quartile (high carotid IMT) compared to those in the lower three quartiles. All mean comparisons were made using age-, sex-, and survey–specific Z scores.

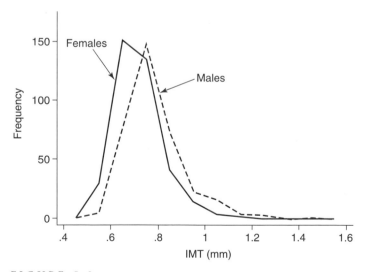

FIGURE 5.3
Sex-specific distribution of carotid intimal-medial thickness (IMT) in the Muscatine cohort, aged 33 to 42 years. The mean IMT for males was 0.79 mm (SD 0.12) and for females it was 0.72 mm (SD 0.10). The median IMT was 0.77 mm (interquartile range 0.12) for males and 0.71 mm (IQR 0.12) for females.

TABLE 5.1

Serial measurements (mean ± SD) during childhood and two young adult Muscatine Study examinations in males with high (upper quartile; $n = 86$) or low (lower three quartiles; $n = 260$) carotid IMT.

Variable	Childhood Ages 8 to 18 years		Young Adult Ages 20 to 34 years		Most Recent Ages 33 to 42 years	
	High IMT	Low IMT	High IMT	Low IMT	High IMT	Low IMT
Height (cm)	167.6 ± 13.3	170.3 ± 10.7	177.5 ± 6.4	177.7 ± 6.5	177.7 ± 6.5	177.9 ± 6.2
Weight (kg)	63.9 ± 6.5	64.6 ± 13.7	82.9 ± 15.1	81.7 ± 13.4	93.4 ± 17.2	89.5 ± 16.3
BMI (kg/m²)	22.4 ± 3.9	22.1 ± 3.4	26.3 ± 4.6	25.8 ± 3.9	29.6 ± 5.2	28.2 ± 4.8*
TSF (cm)	9.2 ± 5.6	8.4 ± 4.9	12.7 ± 6.8	12.3 ± 6.7	19.6 ± 8.5	17.8 ± 7.1
Waist/hip ratio					0.93 ± 0.07	0.91 ± 0.10*
Systolic BP (mmHg)	121.7 ± 11.0	120.5 ± 12.7	122.3 ± 11.5	113.5 ± 12.3*	121.0 ± 13.2	115.7 ± 10.6**
Diastolic 3P (mmHg)	77.4 ± 7.9	76.9 ± 9.4	74.4 ± 10.8	71.4 ± 10.1	79.9 ± 9.9	76.4 ± 8.2**
Total cholesterol (mg/dL)	156.7 ± 24.8	146.4 ± 26.5*	185.0 ± 39.5	173.6 ± 34.1*	200.3 ± 31.9	184.8 ± 37.7***
Triglycerides (mg/dL)	119.7 ± 81.1	100.2 ± 61.8*	119.7 ± 81.1	100.2 ± 61.8*	167.7 ± 134.5	141.8 ± 108.2*
HDL-C (mg/dL)			41.2 ± 9.2	44.8 ± 11.4**	39.3 ± 10.0	42.7 ± 14.4*
LDL-C (mg/dL)			119.8 ± 34.1	108.0 ± 28.2**	131.2 ± 29.2	112.9 ± 29.9***
LDL-C/HDL-C			3.0 ± 1.0	2.6 ± 1.0***	3.5 ± 1.3	2.9 ± 1.5***
Cholesterol/HDL-C			4.7 ± 1.4	4.2 ± 1.7***	5.4 ± 1.7	5.3 ± 7.2***
ApoA1 (mg/dL)					119.3 ± 17.3	125.6 ± 25.6
ApoB (mg/dL)					86.6 ± 31.6	78.9 ± 30.8*
Lipoprotein(a) (mg/dL)					13.2 ± 18.0	14.4 ± 18.2
Homocysteine (nmol/mL)					9.4 ± 3.1	9.7 ± 3.0

Apo, apolipoprotein; BMI, body mass index; BP, blood pressure; HDL, high-density lipoprotein; IMT, intimal-medial thickness; LDL, low-density lipoprotein; TSF, triceps skinfold thickness. P values based on Wilcoxon rank-sum test statistics; $p < 0.05$; $**p < 0.01$; $***p < 0.001$.

TABLE 5.2

Serial measurements (mean ± SD) during childhood and two young adult Muscatine Study examinations in females with high (upper quartile; $n = 94$) or low (lower three quartiles; $n = 285$) carotid IMT

Variable	Childhood Ages 8 to 18 years		Young Adult Ages 20 to 38 years		Most Recent Ages 33 to 46 years	
	High IMT	Low IMT	High IMT	Low IMT	High IMT	Low IMT
Height (cm)	161.3 ± 6.8	161.9 ± 7.3	164.0 ± 5.6	164.5 ± 6.1	164.3 ± 5.3	164.8 ± 6.1
Weight (kg)	58.9 ± 10.9	56.3 ± 10.1*	70.0 ± 14.4	65.6 ± 13.6**	79.0 ± 18.6	74.3 ± 16.9*
BMI (kg/m²)	22.6 ± 3.6	21.4 ± 3.3**	26.0 ± 5.2	24.3 ± 5.0**	29.2 ± 6.6	27.4 ± 6.2*
TSF (mm)	14.5 ± 5.7	13.7 ± 5.4	22.5 ± 8.9	21.2 ± 8.0	31.1 ± 10.0	29.2 ± 8.1
Waist/hip ratio					0.80 ± 0.07	0.77 ± 0.07**
Systolic BP (mmHg)	116.2 ± 12.0	114.2 ± 10.8	111.1 ± 10.4	109.2 ± 9.5	114.2 ± 11.3	110.5 ± 11.3**
Diastolic BP (mmHg)	75.9 ± 8.9	75.8 ± 9.3	69.0 ± 9.2	67.9 ± 8.7	73.5 ± 10.1	70.1 ± 9.3**
Total cholesterol (mg/dL)	164.5 ± 28.5	154.3 ± 26.5**	184.5 ± 34.2	169.2 ± 32.4***	195.2 ± 35.6	176.8 ± 31.6***
Triglycerides (mg/dL)	104.6 ± 53.2	85.9 ± 46.3*	104.6 ± 53.2	85.9 ± 46.3**	140.1 ± 100.3	117.5 ± 130.0*
HDL-C (mg/dL)			46.8 ± 11.4	50.5 ± 12.2*	46.4 ± 14.3	48.9 ± 13.3
LDL-C (mg/dL)			116.9 ± 33.1	101.5 ± 29.9***	121.7 ± 34.4	105.4 ± 27.3***
LDL-C/HDL-C			2.7 ± 1.2	2.2 ± 0.9***	2.9 ± 1.3	2.3 ± 1.0***
Cholesterol/HDL-C			4.2 ± 1.5	3.5 ± 1.1***	4.6 ± 1.7	3.9 ± 1.4***
ApoA1 (mg/dL)					129.3 ± 25.0	132.7 ± 23.7
ApoB (mg/dL)					88.5 ± 30.5	80.4 ± 31.1*
Lipoprotein(a) (mg/dL)					11.7 ± 13.0	14.0 ± 20.3
Homocysteine (nmol/mL)					7.7 ± 2.5	7.9 ± 3.0

See Table 5.1 for abbreviations. *$p < 0.05$, **$p < 0.01$, ***$p < 0.001$.

In males, childhood total cholesterol and triglycerides were higher in those with high carotid IMT (Table 5.1) while in females, childhood weight, BMI, total cholesterol and triglycerides were elevated in those with high carotid IMT (Table 5.2). In males, young adult SBP, total cholesterol, triglycerides, and LDL-C were significantly higher in those with upper-quartile carotid IMT, whereas HDL-C was significantly lower. In females weight and BMI were also significantly higher and SBP was not significant. Concurrent BMI, waist/hip ratio, SBP, DBP, total cholesterol, triglycerides, LDL-C, and apolipoprotein B (apo B) were significantly elevated and HDL-C was significantly lower in both males and females with upper-quartile carotid IMT. Triceps skinfold thickness, apolipoprotein A1 (apo A1), lipoprotein(a) and homocysteine were not different between the two groups (Tables 5.1 and 5.2).

Pack-years of smoking and prevalence of diabetes mellitus were not different between those with and those without upper-quartile carotid IMT, but the prevalence of diabetes was low in this cohort (1.2% in males and 6.4% in females); the mean number of pack-years of smoking was also low (5.7 ± 9.3 in females and 9.8 ± 12.1 in males). This lack of association may be due to an insufficient number of years of exposure to these risk factors.

Table 5.3 presents the age-adjusted odds of upper-quartile IMT relative to IMT in the lower three quartiles (odds ratios, OR) for childhood, young adult and concurrent risk factors. Each OR corresponds to a 1 SD increase in the risk factor. Increased childhood cholesterol was associated with a significantly increased risk of upper-quartile carotid IMT in both males and females, while childhood weight and BMI were significant only in females. Increased young adult total cholesterol, triglycerides, and LDL-C were associated with a significantly increased risk, while HDL-C was associated with a significantly decreased risk of upper-quartile carotid IMT in males and females. In addition, in males, elevated SBP and DBP were associated with an increased risk, whereas in females, high weight and BMI were associated with a significantly increased risk of upper-quartile IMT. Concurrent increased BMI, waist/hip ratio, SBP, DBP, total cholesterol, LDL-C, and apo B were all associated with a significantly increased risk in males and females. Elevated Apo A1 and HDL-C levels were associated with a significantly decreased risk of upper-quartile carotid IMT only in males, while there was no association with triglycerides, lipoprotein(a), or homocysteine.

Table 5.4 presents the age-adjusted ORs for upper-quartile carotid IMT in males and females from a multiple logistic regression analysis of risk factors. Elevated childhood cholesterol measured at a mean age of 15.2 years in males and 15.5 years in females was significantly associated with upper-quartile adult carotid IMT in both males and females. When this multivariate analysis was repeated with only measurements obtained between 8 and 11 years of age, total cholesterol remained significant with an OR of 1.5 (95% CI 1.0–2.1) in males and 1.7 (95% CI 1.2–2.5) in females. Childhood BMI was also significantly associated with upper-quartile adult carotid IMT in females. Higher young adult

T A B L E 5 . 3
Univariate age-adjusted odds ratios† (95% confidence intervals) for having high IMT according to measured coronary risk factors from childhood and two young adult Muscatine Study examinations

	Childhood Ages 8 to 18 years		Young Adult Ages 20 to 38 years		Most Recent Ages 33 to 46 years	
Variable	Males	Females	Males	Females	Males	Females
Height (cm)	0.9 (0.7–1.1)	1.0 (0.7–1.2)	0.9 (0.7–1.2)	0.9 (0.7–1.2)	0.9 (0.7–1.2)	0.9 (0.7, 1.2)
Weight (kg)	1.1 (0.8–1.4)	1.4 (1.1–1.8)**	1.1 (0.8–1.4)	1.4 (1.1–1.8)**	1.3 (1.0–1.6)	1.3 (1.0, 1.6)*
BMI (kg/m²)	1.2 (0.9–1.5)	1.5 (1.2–1.9)**	1.1 (0.9–1.5)	1.4 (1.1–1.8)**	1.3 (1.0–1.7)*	1.3 (1.0, 1.6)*
TSF (mm)	1.1 (0.9–1.4)	1.2 (0.9–1.5)	1.0 (0.8–1.3)	1.2 (0.9–1.5)	1.3 (1.0–1.6)	1.2 (1.0, 1.5)
Waist/Hip			1.3 (1.0–1.7)*		1.3 (1.0–1.7)*	1.4 (1.1, 1.8)**
Systolic BP (mmHg)	1.2 (0.9–1.5)	1.2 (0.9–1.6)	1.4 (1.1–1.8)**	1.3 (1.0–1.6)	1.6 (1.2–2.0)***	1.4 (1.1, 1.8)**
Diastolic BP (mmHg)	1.2 (0.9–1.6)	1.0 (0.8–1.3)	1.4 (1.1–1.7)*	1.1 (0.9–1.5)	1.5 (1.2–1.9)**	1.5 (1.2, 1.9)**
Total cholesterol (mg/dL)	1.5 (1.2–2.0)***	1.5 (1.2–1.9)**	1.3 (1.1–1.7)*	1.5 (1.2–1.9)***	1.6 (1.2–2.0)***	1.8 (1.4, 2.2)***
Triglycerides (mg/dL)	1.2 (0.9–1.5)	1.2 (1.0–1.6)	1.3 (1.0–1.7)*	1.4 (1.1–1.8)**	1.3 (1.0–1.6)	1.2 (1.0, 1.5)
HDL-C (mg/dL)			0.7 (0.5–0.9)**	0.7 (0.5–0.9)*	0.7 (0.5–0.9)*	0.8 (0.6, 1.0)
LDL-C (mg/dL)			1.4 (1.1–1.8)**	1.6 (1.3–2.0)***	2.0 (1.5–2.7)***	1.8 (1.4, 2.2)***
LDL-C/HDL-C			1.5 (1.2–1.9)***	1.6 (1.3–2.0)***	1.6 (1.2–2.2)***	1.6 (1.3, 2.1)***
Cholesterol/HDL-C			1.4 (1.1–1.7)**	1.7 (1.3–2.1)***	1.2 (1.0–1.5)	1.6 (1.3, 2.0)***
ApoA1 (mg/dL)					0.7 (0.6–1.0)*	0.9 (0.7, 1.1)
ApoB (mg/dL)					1.6 (1.2–2.0)***	1.5 (1.2, 2.0)**
Lipoprotein(a) (mg/dL)					0.9 (0.7–1.1)	0.9 (0.7, 1.1)
Homocysteine (nmol/mL)					0.9 (0.7–1.2)	0.9 (0.7, 1.2)

See Table 5.1 for abbreviations. †Odds ratios correspond to a 1 SD increase in the cardiovascular risk factor level. $*p < 0.05$, $**p < 0.01$, $***p < 0.001$.

TABLE 5.4

Multivariate age-adjusted odds ratios† (95% confidence intervals) for having high IMT in males and females, based on multiple logistic regression analysis of Muscatine Study coronary risk factors

Variable	Males	Females
Childhood		
BMI	1.1 (0.8–1.4)	1.5 (1.1–1.9)**
Systolic BP	1.1 (0.8–1.5)	1.1 (0.8–1.6)
Diastolic BP	1.1 (0.8–1.5)	0.9 (0.7–1.1)
Total cholesterol	1.5 (1.1–2.0)**	1.4 (1.1–1.8)*
Triglycerides	1.0 (0.7–1.3)	1.1 (0.9–1.5)
Young Adult		
BMI	0.8 (0.6 1.2)	1.2 (0.9–1.6)
Systolic BP	1.3 (0.9–1.8)	1.1 (0.8–1.6)
Diastolic BP	1.1 (0.8–1.5)	1.0 (0.7–1.3)
HDL-C	0.7 (0.5–0.9)*	0.9 (0.7–1.2)
LDL-C	1.3 (1.0–1.7)*	1.4 (1.1–1.8)**
Triglycerides	1.0 (0.8–1.4)	1.2 (0.9–1.5)
Most Recent		
BMI	1.0 (0.7–1.4)	1.0 (0,7–1,3)
Waist/hip ratio	1.1 (0.8–1.5)	1.2 (0.8–1.6)
Systolic BP	1.3 (0.9–1.9)	1.1 (0.8–1.6)
Diastolic BP	1.1 (0.7–1.6)	1.3 (0.9–1.8)
HDL-C	0.7 (0.5–1.1)	1.1 (0.8–1.6)
LDL-C	1.8 (1.3–2.4)***	1.7 (1.3–2.2)***
Triglycerides	1.0 (0.6–1.5)	1.3 (0.9–2.0)

See Table 5.1 for abbreviations. †Odds ratios correspond to a 1SD increase in the cardiovascular risk factor level. *$p < 0.05$; **$p < 0.01$; ***$p < 0.001$.

LDL-C in both males and females and lower HDL-C in males were significant predictors of upper-quartile adult carotid IMT. Concurrent LDL-C was also significantly associated with upper-quartile adult carotid IMT.

Two other longitudinal studies have also shown an association between cardiovascular risk factors measured during childhood and adolescence and carotid IMT measured as a young adult. In the Young Finns Study, 2229 young adults aged 24 to 39 years had risk factors measured at ages 3 to 18 years, an average of 21 years before measurement of carotid IMT. Childhood LDL-C, SBP, BMI and smoking were predictive of young adult IMT after adjustment for age and sex with multivariate models. Concurrent SBP, BMI, and smoking also showed a significant association. Childhood LDL-C and SBP remained significant predictors of carotid IMT even after adjustment for concurrent risk factors. The number of risk factors present measured at ages 12 to 18 years was significantly associated with adult carotid IMT in both males and females whereas the number of risk factors present at ages 3 to 9 years was only weakly associated with IMT and only in men. These results suggest that risk factors measured after puberty play a significant role in determining adult risk of cardiovascular disease. Multiple measures of risk factors over time were used to calculate a cumulative risk load, but this produced only marginally stronger correlations with IMT compared to a single measurement (Raitakari et al., 2003).

In the Bogalusa Heart Study, 486 young adults aged 25 to 37 years underwent carotid ultrasound to measure IMT. All subjects had had cardiovascular risk factors measured at least three times an average of 22 years earlier. Childhood LDL-C and BMI were predictive of adult carotid IMT in the top quartile compared to the lower three quartiles in multivariate analysis. Adult predictors included LDL-C, HDL-C, and SBP. The cumulative loads for LDL-C and HDL-C were also associated with adult carotid IMT. Similar to the Muscatine Study and the Young Finns Study, use of the cumulative burden or risk factor load did not improve the predictive value for carotid IMT over that of a single childhood or adult measurement (Li et al., 2003).

In the Muscatine cohort, childhood total cholesterol level measured as early as ages 8 to 11 years was a significant risk factor for carotid IMT measured in young adulthood. In women, childhood BMI was also a risk factor (Davis et al., 2001). Similar results were found in the other two longitudinal cohort studies: childhood LDL-C and BMI were both significant risk factors for adult IMT (Li et al., 2003; Raitakari et al., 2003). In the Young Finns Study, childhood smoking and SBP were also significant predictors of IMT (Raitakari et al., 2003). These findings support the initiation of preventive measures at an early age in childhood and adolescence and are relevant in a time when the incidence of childhood obesity is increasing (Sorof and Daniels, 2002). All three studies also suggest that a single measurement during childhood or adolescence may be adequate to predict long-term risk of subsequent cardiovascular disease.

Further confirmation that cardiovascular risk factors are associated with carotid IMT measured in young adults is provided by a cross-sectional study of 750 healthy young adults aged 27 to 30 years living in the Netherlands. In this study, age, male sex, pulse pressure, BMI, and LDL-C were independent predictors of CCA IMT and explained 36% of the variation in IMT. In addition, the total pack-years of smoking showed a linear trend with increased CCA IMT ($p = 0.02$). Carotid IMT increased significantly with the number of risk factors present (Oren et al., 2003).

Case–control studies of young adults with familial hypercholesterolemia have demonstrated increased carotid IMT compared to that in controls (Wendelhag et al., 1992; Rubba et al., 1994; Lavrencic et al., 1996; Raal et al., 1999).

Emerging evidence supports the hypothesis that subclasses of LDL may be important in the atherosclerotic process. Small, dense LDL particles are frequently observed in conjunction with other lipid abnormalities and have been associated with increased carotid IMT (Hulthe et al., 2000). There is also evidence for an important role of oxidative modification in mediating the atherogenicity of LDL-C. In a study of 55 healthy men less than 45 years of age, oxidized LDL-C was significantly associated with carotid IMT (Raitakari et al., 2001). Oxidized LDL-C was also significantly associated with carotid IMT in a small case-control study of men less than 45 years of age with borderline hypertension (Toikka et al., 2000).

Two case-control studies showed increased carotid IMT in type 1 diabetics under the age of 40 years compared to controls (Yamasaki et al., 1994; Frost and Beischer, 1998). In one of the studies which included 105 insulin-dependent diabetics aged 4 to 25 years, age and duration of diabetes were the only significant risk factors for increased carotid IMT (Yamasaki et al., 1994). At baseline, the mean carotid IMT of type 1 diabetics aged 19 to 51 years (mean of 35 years) was not significantly increased compared to controls in the Epidemiology of Diabetes Interventions and Complications (EDIC) Study. However, age, smoking, and LDL-C were significantly associated with carotid IMT after multivariate adjustment (Epidemiology of Diabetes Interventions and Complications [EDIC] Research Group, 1999).

Three case-control studies of young adults with borderline hypertension showed increased carotid IMT in cases even after multivariate adjustment for other cardiovascular risk factors (Lonati et al., 1993; Lemne et al., 1995; Pauletto et al., 1999).

Elevated plasma homocysteine has been shown to be a significant risk factor for increased carotid IMT in older adults (McQuillan et al., 1999; Tsai et al., 2000). In the National Heart, Lung and Blood Institute's (NHLBI) Family Heart Study, the association between plasma homocysteine and increased carotid IMT was significant in those participants 55 years of age or older but not in participants under 55 years of age (Tsai et al., 2000). Elevated homocysteine levels may be a less important risk factor for increased carotid IMT at a younger age.

■ RELATIONSHIP OF CAROTID INTIMAL-MEDIAL THICKNESS AND CORONARY ARTERY CALCIFICATION

Carotid IMT may also be used as a surrogate measure of coronary artery atherosclerosis. Several studies have shown an association between carotid IMT and the degree of coronary artery disease (CAD) measured angiographically (Wexler et al., 1996; Greenland et al., 2000). In older adults carotid IMT is predictive of incident MI, in studies from Finland (Salonen and Salonen, 1993), the United States (Chambless et al., 1997), and the Netherlands (Bots et al., 1997). All of these studies demonstrated that the association between carotid IMT and incident MI persisted after adjustment for known cardiovascular risk factors although the effect was attenuated. Long-term follow-up in a clinical trial has shown that measurement of carotid IMT predicted coronary events beyond that predicted by angiographic measurement of coronary atherosclerosis and lipid measurements (Hodis et al., 1998). Thus the link between carotid IMT and CAD appears to have been established.

Detection of the presence of CAC through electron-beam computed tomography (EBCT) (see Chapter 4) is another method used to noninvasively evaluate the early atherosclerotic process in asymptomatic individuals (Wexler et al., 1996; Greenland et al., 2000). Since both carotid IMT and the presence of CAC are associated with the early atherosclerotic process and the presence of CAD, an association between increased carotid IMT and CAC would not be unexpected. In a subset of the Muscatine cohort who underwent carotid ultrasound studies, 182 men and 136 women had concurrent EBCT to measure CAC. CAC was present ($\geq$3 contiguous pixels, $\geq$130 HU) in 27% of the men and 14% of the women, and was significantly associated with a higher mean carotid IMT in men ($p < 0.025$) and women ($p < 0.005$). Presence of proximal CAC was a significant predictor of high carotid IMT (upper quartile) even after adjustment for known cardiovascular risk factors as shown in Table 5.5 (Davis et al., 1999). This finding suggests that the association of carotid IMT and CAC is not solely due to shared risk factors and lends further weight to the assumption that both CAC and carotid IMT are measures of early atherosclerosis.

Studies in older adults have also examined the association between CAC and carotid IMT. In a study of 102 subjects with a mean age of 78 years, the coronary calcification score was highly correlated with subclinical atherosclerosis in the carotid arteries (Kuller and Sutton-Tyrell, 1999). In 2013 participants in the Rotterdam Coronary Calcification Study, a graded association between CAC and common carotid IMT was seen ($p < 0.001$) after adjustment for known cardiovascular risk factors (Oei et al., 2002). A similar association of CAC was seen with a carotid plaque score. In the Cardiovascular Health Study, the ICA IMT was most strongly correlated with the presence of CAC ($r = 0.30$; $p < 0.0001$) when different measures of subclinical disease were evaluated as predictors of CAC (Newman et al., 2002). However, in a small study of 111 asymptomatic middle-aged men with hypercholesterolemia, presence of CAC was significantly associated with plaque in the aorta and femoral arteries but not in the carotid arteries (Megnien et al., 1992). Megnien et al. (1998) evaluated 94 men with an age range of 30 to 65 years who were asymptomatic but had multiple cardiovascular risk factors. While carotid IMT was associated with the presence of CAC, this association did not persist after adjustment for age (Megnien et al., 1998).

It remains unclear whether CAC or increased carotid IMT or the combination of both will be predictive of subsequent clinical events in young and middle-aged, asymptomatic subjects. Long-term follow-up of the Muscatine cohort may provide an answer to this question.

TABLE 5.5
Coronary artery calcification and cardiovascular risk factors as predictors of high carotid IMT*

Predictor Variable	Adjusting for Age and Sex Only		Also adjusting for BMI, HDL-C, Triglycerides, SBP, and Triceps Skinfold Thickness	
	OR (95% CI)	p	OR (95% CI)	p
CAC†	2.10 (1.14–3.87)	0.02	2.34 (1.20–4.55)	0.01
LDL-C	1.74 (1.33–2.28)	<0.001	1.77 (1.34–2.35)	<0.001
DBP	1.39 (1.05–1.84)	0.02	1.38 (0.91–2.08)	0.13

BMI, body mass index; CAC, coronary artery calcification; CI, confidence interval; DBP, diastolic blood presure; HDL-C, high-density lipoprotein cholesterol; IMT, intimal–medial thickness; LDL, low-density lipoprotein; OR, odds ratio; SBP, systolic blood pressure.
*Results of multiple logistic regression models to predict high carotid IMT (upper quartile) as a function of risk factors and the presence of proximal CAC in 182 males and 136 females. With the exception of CAC, all reported ORs represent a 1 SD increase in the predictor variable. Adjustments were made for age and sex by computing age- and sex-specific Z scores for IMT and risk factors.
†Presence of CAC, ≥3 contiguous pixels ≥130 HU.

▪ FAMILIAL AND GENETIC FACTORS

The adult relatives of children with adverse cardiovascular risk factor levels more frequently have a history of premature death due to cardiovascular disease (Burns et al., 1992; Bao et al., 1997). Intimal thickening was detected more commonly in autopsy specimens of the coronary arteries of infants who had a grandparent with CAD than in infants without a family history (Kaprio et al., 1993). Three studies (Riley et al., 1986; Gaeta et al., 2000; Wang et al., 2003) have investigated the association between carotid wall abnormalities in subjects with a parental history of MI. Increased carotid stiffness was significantly associated with a positive parental history of MI in a sample of participants aged 10 to 17 years from the Bogalusa Heart Study (Riley et al., 1986). A case–control study compared 40 young adults ("cases") with a mean age of 19.0 years (SD 5.2) who had a parent hospitalized for acute MI that occurred before 60 years of age, matched by age and sex to 40 "control" subjects who were the offspring of patients hospitalized at the same institution for diagnoses other than CVD or diabetes. The mean IMT of the far wall of the CCA was significantly greater ($p < 0.005$) in the cases, and this association persisted after multivariate risk factor adjustment (Gaeta et al., 2000). Framingham Offspring Study participants (mean age 57 years) with a parental history of premature cardiovascular disease (occurring before age 60 years) had significantly increased ICA IMT (men, $p < 0.01$; women, $p < 0.05$). This association was not found for CCA IMT or when no restriction was placed on the parental age at CHD diagnosis (Wang et al., 2003).

In Muscatine, Iowa, carotid IMT was determined in 725 individuals aged 33 to 42 years representing 579 families. Vital status was known for 512 fathers and 546 mothers. Death certificates were obtained for all of the 165 deceased fathers (32%) and 91 deceased mothers (17%). There was no significant difference in the mean maximal carotid IMT in those whose fathers died from CVD at any age, age <60 years, or age <50 years compared to those without this family history. Similar results were found for mothers and for both parents combined (P. Davis and J. Dawson, unpublished results).

Estimates of the heritability of carotid IMT have been obtained from multiple studies (Duggirala et al., 1996; Zannad et al., 1998; Wagenknecht et al., 2001; Hunt et al., 2002; Lange et al., 2002; Fox et al., 2003). Duggirala et al. (1996) reported heritability estimates of 0.92 ± 0.05 for the CCA IMT and 0.86 ± 0.13 for the ICA IMT, based on sibship data from a small epidemiologic survey in Mexico where the study population had a 33% prevalence of diabetes. In a study of 252 individuals with type 2 diabetes belonging to 122 families, the heritability of CCA IMT was 0.41 (SE 0.16) after adjustment for other cardiovascular risk factors (Lange et al., 2002). In populations with a lower prevalence of diabetes, the heritability estimates are lower. Genetic factors explained 30% of IMT variation in 76 healthy families in France with family members ranging in age from 10 to 54 years (Zannad et al., 1998). In the NHLBI Family Heart Study, the heritability of CCA IMT was estimated to be 0.23 (Wagenknecht et al., 2001) whereas it was 0.13 in the San Antonio Family Heart Study (Hunt et al., 2002). When carotid artery plaque rather than IMT was used as a marker of subclinical atherosclerosis in the latter study, the heritability was 0.23 ± 0.15 ($p < 0.05$) after adjustment for known cardiovascular risk factors. In the Framingham Heart Study, 1630 sibling pairs from 586 families underwent carotid ultrasound studies to measure mean CCA and ICA IMT (Fox et al., 2003). For CCA IMT, 27% of the overall variance was due to measured cardiovascular risk factors while 38% was due to heritable factors. The multivariate-adjusted heritability for ICA IMT was similar at 0.35 ($p < 0.001$). These studies suggest that subclinical atherosclerosis of the carotid arteries has a significant familial component.

To date, very few genetic factors that appear to be involved in the determination of carotid IMT have been identified. Several population-based studies have examined the association of apolipoprotein E (*APOE*) genotype and carotid IMT, with the largest studies showing either no effect of *APOE* (Beilby et al., 2003) or a small protective effect of the *E2E3* genotype (Slooter et al., 2001). Several other genetic polymorphisms have been investigated for their possible association with carotid IMT. The insertion/deletion polymorphism of the angiotensin-converting enzyme (*ACE*) gene (Hung et al., 1999) and a polymorphism in the angiotensinogen gene (Arnett et al., 1998) were not associated with mean carotid IMT. The factor V Leiden mutation (Garg et al., 1998), the C677T polymorphism in the methylenetetrahydrofolate reductase gene (McQuillan et al., 1999), and the C282Y polymorphism in the hemochromatosis gene (Rossi et al., 2000) also do not appear to be associated with carotid IMT. However, several small studies have shown a positive association between carotid IMT and the glu298asp polymorphism in the endothelial nitric oxide synthase (*eNOS*) gene (Lembo et al., 2001), the signal peptide of neuropeptide Y (Karvonen et al., 2001), the PON1 polymorphism of the paraoxonase gene (Schmidt et al., 1998), and mutations of the gene for ATP-binding cassette A1 transporter (*ABCA1*), which plays an important role in mediating cholesterol efflux from cells, the rate-limiting step in producing HDL particles (van Dam et al., 2002). Further studies to identify genetic factors involved in the determination of carotid artery IMT are warranted.

■ LONGITUDINAL MEASUREMENTS OF CAROTID INTIMAL-MEDIAL THICKNESS

Serial measurements of carotid IMT have been used in older adults to evaluate the efficacy of interventions to slow the atherosclerotic process. The use of progression of carotid IMT as an end point in a clinical trial has the advantage of decreasing the sample size and reducing the time of follow-up as compared to the end points of cardiovascular morbidity and mortality (Bots et al., 2003). Treatment with statins, other lipid-lowering medications, angiotensin-converting enzyme inhibitors, calcium channel blockers, and insulin sensitizers has been associated with a decrease in the rate of progression of carotid IMT or in some studies with regression of carotid IMT (Mukherjee et al., 2002; Bots et al., 2003). In a pooled analysis of the placebo groups from clinical trials, the annual progression rate of mean CCA IMT was 0.0147 mm (95% CI 0.0122–0.0173) and for mean maximal CCA IMT was 0.0176 mm (95% CI 0.0149–0.0203) (Bots et al., 2003). Results of a 3-year clinical trial of lovastatin compared to placebo demonstrated that serial measurements of carotid IMT were reproducible and reliable when there was careful monitoring and training of sonographers and the readers of the IMT studies. Only 11% of the total variance of IMT was attributable to systematic difference among readers and less than 7% was due to nonvisualization of carotid walls (missing data). Little if any temporal drift was detected. On the basis of these data, a follow-up time of 6 years was felt to be the minimum to detect progression within individuals (Espeland et al., 1996). In the Atherosclerosis Risk in Communities Study (ARIC), which enrolled subjects aged 45 to 64 years, the degree of progression of carotid IMT over 6 years was associated with baseline diabetes, current smoking, HDL-C, pulse pressure, white blood cell count, and fibrinogen as well as changes in LDL-C and triglycerides or the onset of diabetes and hypertension during the follow-up period (Chambless et al., 2002). As expected, because of limited precision when measuring IMT change, the associations with risk factors were less significant than those found on cross-sectional analysis but were still statistically significant. No data are available concerning rate of progression of carotid IMT in children and adolescents. The increase in IMT was estimated to be 0.006 mm/ year according to cross-sectional data from the Bogalusa Study of young adults aged 25 to 37 years. This finding suggests that studies of progression in children will require long-term follow-up. Since measurement error related to the resolution of the ultrasound equipment is the same in children as that in adults but the carotid IMT is thinner, reproducibility may also be lower. The effects of puberty and growth during childhood on carotid IMT are also unknown. Data from the Young Finns Study suggest that associations between cardiovascular risk factors and carotid IMT are not seen until after puberty (Raitakari et al., 2003). Clearly a number of methodologic problems need to be addressed to determine whether measurement of progression of IMT in children is feasible. However, controlled clinical trials of interventions in children with an end point of cardiovascular morbidity would take 30 to 40 years to complete and are clearly impractical, thus noninvasive measures of atherosclerosis such as serial measurements of carotid or aortic IMT are attractive. While lifestyle modifications such as regular exercise, maintaining an appropriate weight, and avoiding cigarette smoking are safe measures to implement in children and adolescents, the safety and efficacy of long-term pharmacologic therapy to reduce risk factors are unknown in childhood. For this reason, an objective measure of subclinical progression of atherosclerosis in children and adolescents would be invaluable.

■ SUMMARY

- In older adults, measurement of carotid IMT is a well-established method to evaluate subclinical atherosclerosis and provides additional information in predicting which asymptomatic subjects are at the highest risk for subsequent clinical events.
- In older adults, measurement of carotid IMT is a research tool used to identify novel risk factors for atherosclerosis, as a gold standard for new noninvasive methods to measure atherosclerosis, and as a surrogate end point for clinical events in clinical trials of therapies to retard the atherosclerotic process.
- While much less information is available about the use of carotid IMT as a marker of atherosclerosis in children, elevated lipids, hypertension, and type 1 diabetes have been shown to be associated with increased carotid IMT in this age group.
- In young and middle-aged adults, increased carotid IMT is associated with hypertension, elevated LDL-C, decreased HDL-C, diabetes, obesity, and smoking, although the link to subsequent clinical cardiovascular events has not yet been proven.

- The association between carotid IMT and CAC further supports the use of carotid ultrasound to identify young adults and middle-aged adults at risk for premature atherosclerosis.
- Childhood risk factors measured as early as ages 8 to 11 years predict carotid IMT measured in young adulthood. Thus early preventive measures to retard progression of atherosclerosis prior to the development of symptomatic disease should be applied.

▓ REFERENCES

Arnett, D.K., I.B. Borecki, E.H. Ludwig, J.S. Pankow, R. Myers, G. Evans, A.R. Folsom, G. Heiss, and M. Higgins. 1998. Angiotensinogen and Angiotensin Converting Enzyme Genotypes and Carotid Atherosclerosis: Atherosclerosis Risk in Communities and the NHLBI Family Heart Studies. *Atherosclerosis* 138:111–6.

Bao, W., S.R. Srinivasan, R. Valdez, K.J. Greenland, W.A. Wattigney, and G.S. Berenson. 1997. Longitudinal Changes in Cardiovascular Risk from Childhood to Young Adulthood in Offspring of Parents with Coronary Artery Disease: The Bogalusa Heart Study. *JAMA* 278:1749–54.

Beilby, J.P., C.C.J. Hunt, L.J. Palmer, C.M.L. Chapman, J.P. Burley, B.M. McQuillan, P.L. Thompson, and J. Hung. 2003. Apolipoprotein E Gene Polymorphisms are Associated with Carotid Plaque Formation but not with Intima Media Wall Thickening. Results for the Perth Carotid Ultrasound Disease Assessment Study (CUDAS). *Stroke* 34:869–74.

Bots, M.L., G.W. Evans, W.A. Riley, and D.E. Grobbee. 2003. Carotid Intima-Media Thickness Measurements in Intervention Studies: Design Options, Progression Rates, and Sample Size Considerations: A Point of View. *Stroke* 34:2985–94.

Bots, M.L., A.W. Hoes, P.J. Koudstaal, A. Hofman, and D.E. Grobbee. 1997. Common Carotid Intima-Media Thickness and Risk of Stroke and Myocardial Infarction. The Rotterdam Study. *Circulation* 96:1432–7.

Bots, M.L., A. Hofman, and D.E. Grobbe. 1994. Common Carotid Intima-Media Thickness and Lower Extremity Arterial Atherosclerosis. *Arterioscler Thromb* 14:1885–91.

Burns, T.L., P.P. Moll, and R.M. Lauer. 1992. Increased Familial Cardiovascular Mortality in Obese Schoolchildren: The Muscatine Ponderosity Family Study. *Pediatrics* 89:262–8.

Chambless, L.E., A.R. Folsom, L.X. Clegg, A.R. Sharrett, E. Shahar, F.J. Nieto, W.D. Rosamond, and G. Evans. 2000. Carotid Wall Thickness Is Predictive of Incident Clinical Stroke. *Am J Epidemiol* 151:478–87.

Chambless, L.E., A.R. Folsom, and G.W. Evans. 2002. Risk Factors for Progression of Common Carotid Atherosclerosis: The Atherosclerosis Risk in Communities Study, 1987–1998. *Am J Epidemiol* 155:38–47.

Chambless, L.E., G. Heiss, A.R. Folsom, W. Rosamond, M. Szklo, A.R. Sharrett, and L.X. Clegg. 1997. Association of Coronary Heart Disease Incidence with Carotid Arterial Wall Thickness and Major Risk Factors: The Atherosclerosis Risk in Communities (ARIC) Study, 1987–1993. *Am J Epidemiol* 146:483–94.

Davis, P.H., J.D. Dawson, L.T. Mahoney, and R.M. Lauer. 1999. Increased Carotid Intimal-Medial Thickness and Coronary Calcification are Related in Young and Middle-Aged Adults: The Muscatine Study. *Circulation* 100:838–42.

Davis, P.H., J.D. Dawson, W.A. Riley, and R.M. Lauer. 2001. Carotid Intimal-Medial Thickness Is Related to Cardiovascular Risk Factors Measured from Childhood Through Middle Age. *Circulation* 104:2815–9.

Duggirala, R., C.G. Villalpando, D.H. O'Leary, M.P. Stern, and J. Blangero. 1996. Genetic Basis of Variation in Carotid Artery Wall Thickness. *Stroke* 27:833–7.

Dwyer, J.H., M. Navab, K.M. Dwyer, K. Hassan, P. Sun, A. Shircore, S. Hama-Levy, G. Hough, X. Wang, T. Drake, C.N. Bairey, and A.M. Fogelman. 2001. Oxygenated Carotenoid Lutein and Progression of Early Atherosclerosis. *Circulation* 103:2922–7.

Epidemiology of Diabetes Interventions and Complications (EDIC) Research Group. 1999. Effect of Intensive Diabetes Treatment on Carotid Artery Wall Thickness in the Epidemiology of Diabetes Interventions and Complications. *Diabetes* 48:383–90.

Espeland, M.A., T.E. Craven, W.A. Riley, J. Corson, A. Romomt, and C.D. Furberg, for the Asymptomatic Carotid Artery Progression Study Research Group. 1996. Reliability of Longitudinal Ultrasonographic Measurements of Carotid Intimal-Medial Thickness. *Stroke* 27:480–5.

Folsom, A.R., J.S. Pankow, R.P. Tracy, D.K. Arnett, J.M. Peacock, Y. Hong, L. Djousse, and J.H. Eckfeldt. 2001. Association of C-Reactive Protein with Markers of Prevalent Atherosclerotic Disease. *Am J Cardiol* 88:112–7.

Fox, C.S., J.F. Polak, I. Chazaro, A. Cupples, P.A. Wolf, R.A. D'Agostino, and C.J. O'Donnell. 2003. Genetic and Environmental Contributions to Atherosclerosis Phenotypes in Men and Women: Heritability of Carotid Intima-Media Thickness in the Framingham Heart Study. *Stroke* 34:397–401.

Frost, D., and W. Beischer. 1998. Determinants of Carotid Artery Wall Thickening in Young Patients with Type-1 Diabetes Mellitus. *Diabet Med* 15:841–57.

Gaeta, G., M. De Michele, S. Cuomo, P. Guarini, M.C. Foglia, G. Bond, and M. Trevisan. 2000. Arterial Abnormalities in the Offspring of Patients with Premature Myocardial Infarction. *N Engl J Med* 343:840–6.

Garg, U.C., D.K. Arnett, G. Evens, and J.H. Eckfeldt. 1998. No Association between Factor V Leiden Mutation and Coronary Heart Disease or Carotid Intima Media Thickness: The NHLBI Family Heart Study. *Thromb Res* 89:289–93.

Greenland, P.G., J. Abrams, G.P. Aurigemma, M.G. Bond, L.T. Clark, M.H. Criqui, J.R. Crouse, III, L. Friedman, V. Fuster, D. Herrington, L.H. Kuller, P.M. Ridker, W.C. Roberts, W. Standford, N. Stone, J. Swan, and K.A. Taubert. 2000. Prevention Conference V: Beyond Secondary Prevention: Identifying the High-Risk Patient for Primary Prevention. Noninvasive Tests of Atherosclerotic Burden. *Circulation* 101:e16–e22.

Hodis, H.N., W.J. Mack, L. LaBree, R.H. Selzer, C.R. Liu, C.H. Liu, and S.P. Azen, 1998. The Role of Carotid Intima-Media Thickness in Predicting Clinical Coronary Events. *Ann Intern Med* 128:262–9.

Hulthe, J., L. Bokemark, J. Wikstrand, and B. Fagerberg. 2000. The Metabolic Syndrome, LDL Particle Size, and Atherosclerosis. *Arterioscler Thromb Vasc Biol* 20:2140–7.

Hung, J., B.M. McQuillan, M. Nidorf, P.L. Thompson, and J.P. Beilby. 1999. Angiotensin-Converting Enzyme Gene Polymorphism and Carotid Wall Thickening in a Community Population. *Arterioscler Thromb Vasc Biol* 19:1969–74.

Hunt, K.J., R. Duggirala, H.H. Goring, J.T. Williams, L. Almasy, J., Blangero, D.H. O'Leary, and M.P. Stern. 2002. Genetic Basis of Variation in Carotid Artery Plaque in the San Antonio Family Heart Study. *Stroke* 33:2775–80.

Jarvisalo, M.J., A. Harmoinen, M. Hakanen, U. Paakkunainen, J. Viikari, J. Hartiala, T. Lehtimaki, O. Simell, and O.T. Raitakari. 2002a. Elevated Serum C-Reactive Protein Levels and Early Arterial Changes in Healthy Children. *Arterioscler Thromb Vasc Biol* 22:1323–8.

Jarvisalo, M.J., L. Jartti, K. Nanto-Salonen, K. Irjala, T. Ronnemaa, J.J. Hartiala, D.S. Celermajer, and O.T. Raitakari. 2001. Increased Aortic Intima-Media Thickness. A Marker of Preclinical Atherosclerosis in High-Risk Children. *Circulation* 104:2943–7.

Jarvisalo, M.J., A. Putto-Laurila, L. Jartti, T. Lehtimaki, T. Solakivi, T. Ronnemaa, and O.T. Raitakari. 2002b. Carotid Artery Intima-Media Thickness in Children with Type 1 Diabetes. *Diabetes* 51:493–8.

Kaprio, J., R. Norio, E. Pesonen, and S. Sarna. 1993. Intimal Thickening of the Coronary Arteries in Infants in Relation to Family History of Coronary Artery Disease. *Circulation* 87:1960–8.

Karvonen, M.K., V.P. Valkonen, T.A. Lakka, R. Salonen, M. Koulu, U. Pesonen, T.P. Tuomainen, J. Kauhanen, K. Nyyssonen, H.M. Lakka, M.I.J. Uusitupa, and J.T. Salonen. 2001. Leucine7 to Proline7 Polymorphism in the Preproneuropeptide Y Is Associated with the Progression of Carotid Atherosclerosis, Blood Pressure and Serum Lipids in Finnish Men. *Atherosclerosis* 159:145–51.

Knoflach, M., S. Kiechl, M. Kind, M. Said, R. Sief, M. Gisinger, R. van der Zee, H. Gaston, E. Jarosch, J. Willeit, and G. Wick. 2003. Cardiovascular Risk Factors and Atherosclerosis in Young Males. ARMY Study (Atherosclerotic Risk-Factors in Male Youngsters). *Circulation* 108:1064–9.

Kuller, L.H., and K. Sutton-Tyrell. 1999. Aging and Cardiovascular Disease. *Cardiol Clinics* 17:51–65.

Lange, L.A., D.W. Bowden, C.D. Langefeld, L.E. Wagenknecht, J.J. Carr, S.S. Rich, W.A. Riley, and B.I. Freedman. 2002. Heritability of Carotid Artery Intima-Medial Thickness in Type 2 Diabetes. *Stroke* 33:1876–81.

Lavrencic, A., B. Kosmina, I. Keber, V. Videcnik, and D. Keber. 1996. Carotid Intima-Media Thickness in Young Patients with Familial Hypercholesterolaemia. *Heart* 76:321–5.

Lembo, G., N. De Luca, C. Battagli, G. Iovino, A.Aretini, M. Musicco, G. Frati, F. Pompeo, C. Vecchione, and B. Trimarco. 2001. A Common Variant of Endothelial Nitric Oxide Synthase (glu298asp) Is an Independent Risk Factor for Carotid Atherosclerosis. *Stroke* 32:735–40.

Lemne, C., T. Jogestrand, and U. de Faire. 1995. Carotid Intima-Media Thickness and Plaque in Borderline Hypertension. *Stroke* 26:34–9.

Li, S., W. Chen, S.R. Srinivasan, M.G. Bond, R. Tang, E.M. Urbina, and G.S. Berenson. 2003. Childhood Cardiovascular Risk Factors and Carotid Vascular Changes in Adulthood: The Bogalusa Heart Study. *JAMA* 290:2271–6.

Lonati, L., C. Cuspidi, L. Sampieri, L. Boselli, M. Bocciolone, G. Leonetti, and A. Zanchetti. 1993. Ultrasonographic Evaluation of Cardiac and Vascular Changes in Young Borderline Hypertensives. *Cardiology* 83:298–303.

McQuillan, B.M., J.P. Beilby, M. Nidorf, P.L. Thompson, and J. Hung. 1999. Hyperhomocysteinemia but not the C677T Mutation of Methylenetetrahydrofolate Reductase Is an Independent Risk Determinant of Carotid Wall Thickening. *Circulation* 99:2383–8.

Megnien, J.L., V. Sene, S. Jeannin, A. Hernigou, M.C. Plainfosse, I. Merli, V. Atger, N. Moatti, J. Levenson, and A. Simon, and the PCV METRA Group. 1992. Coronary Calcification and its Relation to Extracoronary Atherosclerosis in Asymptomatic Hypercholesterolemic Men. *Circulation* 85:1799–807.

Megnien, J.L., A. Simon, J. Gariepy, N. Denaire, M. Cocaul, A. Linhart, and J. Levenson. 1998. Preclinical Changes of Extracoronary Arterial Structures as Indicators of Coronary Atherosclerosis in Men. *J Hypertens* 16:157–63.

Mukherjee, D., and J.S. Yadav. 2002. Carotid Artery Intimal-Medial Thickness: Indicator of Atherosclerotic Burden and Response to Risk Factor Modification. *Am Heart J* 144:753–9.

Newman, A.B., B.L. Naydeck, K. Sutton-Tyrell, D. Edmundowicz, D. O'Leary, R. Kronmal, G.L. Burke, and L.H. Kuller. 2002. Relationship between Coronary Artery Calcification and Other Measures of Subclinical Cardiovascular Disease in Older Adults. *Arterioscler Thromb Vasc Biol* 22:1674–9.

O'Donell, C.J., H. Sibershatz, and R.B. D'Agostino. 1999. Relationship of C-Reactive Protein to Carotid Stenosis and Intimal Medial Thickness in the Framingham Heart Study. *Circulation* 100:I-477.

Oei, H.H., R. Vliegenthart, A.E. Hak, D.S. Iglesias, A. Hofman, M. Oudkerk, and J.C. Witteman. 2002. The Association Between Coronary Calcification Assessed by Electron Beam

Computed Tomography and Measures of Extracoronary Atherosclerosis: The Rotterdam Coronary Calcification Study. *J Am Coll Cardiol* 39:1745–51.

O'Leary, D.H., J.F. Polak, R.A. Kronmal, T.A. Manolio, G.L. Burke, and S.K. Wolfeson. 1999. Carotid-Artery Intima and Media Thickness as a Risk Factor for Myocardial Infarction and Stroke in Older Adults. *N Engl J Med* 340:14–22.

O'Leary, D.H., J.F. Polak, R.A. Kronmal, P.J. Savage, N.O. Borhani, S.J. Kittner, R. Tracey, J.M. Gardin, T.R. Price, and C.D. Furberg, and CHS Collaborative Research Group. 1996. Thickening of the Carotid Wall. A Marker for Atherosclerosis in the Elderly? *Stroke* 27:224–31.

Oren, A., L.E. Vos, C.S.P.M. Uiterwaal, D.E. Grobbee, and M.L. Bots. 2003. Cardiovascular Risk Factors and Increased Carotid Intima-Media Thickness in Healthy Young Adults: The Atherosclerosis Risk in Young Adults (ARYA) Study. *Arch Intern Med* 163:1787–92.

Pauciullo, P., A. Iannuzzi, R. Sartorio, C. Irace, G. Covetti, A.D. Costanzo, and P. Rubba. 1994. Increased Intima-Media Thickness of the Common Carotid Artery in Hypercholesterolemic Children. *Arterioscler Thromb* 14:1075–9.

Pauletto, P., P. Palatini, S. DaRos, V. Pagliara, N. Santipolo, E. Baccillieri, E. Casiglia, P. Mormino, and A.C. Pessina. 1999. Factors Underlying the Increase in Carotid Intima-Media Thickness in Borderline Hypertensives. *Arterioscler Thromb Vasc Biol* 19:1231–7.

Raal, F., G.J. Pilcher, R. Waisberg, E.P. Buthelezi, M.G. Veller, and B.I. Joffe. 1999. Low-Density Lipoprotein Cholesterol Bulk Is the Pivotal Determinant of Atherosclerosis in Familial Hypercholesterolemia. *Am J Cardiol* 83:1330–3.

Raitakari, O. 1999. Imaging of Subclinical Atherosclerosis in Children and Young Adults. *Ann Med* 31:33–40.

Raitakari, O.T., M. Juonala, M. Kahonen, L. Taittonen, T. Laitinen, N. Maki-Torkko, M.J. Jarvisalo, M. Uhari, E. Jokinen, T. Ronnemaa, H.K. Akerblom, and J.S.A. Viikari. 2003. Cardiovascular Risk Factors in Childhood and Carotid Artery Intima-Media Thickness in Adulthood: The Cardiovascular Risk in Young Finns Study. *JAMA* 290:2277–83.

Raitakari, O.T., J.O. Toikka, H. Laine, M. Ahotupa, H. Iida, J.S.A. Viikari, J. Hartiala, and J. Knuuti. 2001. Reduced Myocardial Flow Reserve Relates to Increased Carotid Intima-Media Thickness in Healthy Young Men. *Atherosclerosis* 156:469–75.

Ridker, P.M., R.J. Glynn, and C.H. Hennekens. 1998. C-Reactive Protein Adds to the Predictive Value of Total and HDL Cholesterol in Determining Risk of First Myocardial Infarction. *Circulation* 97:2007–11.

Riley, W.A., R.W. Barnes, W.B. Applegate, R. Dempsey, T. Hartwell, V.G. Davis, M.G. Bond, and C.D. Furberg. 1992. Reproducibility of Noninvasive Ultrasonic Measurement of Carotid Artherosclerosis. The Asymptomatic Carotid Artery Plaque Study. *Stroke* 23:1062–8.

Riley, W.A., D.S. Freedman, N.A. Higgs, R.W. Barnes, S.A. Zinkgraf, and G.S. Berenson. 1986. Decreased Arterial Elasticity Associated with Cardiovascular Disease Risk Factors in the Young. *Arteriosclerosis* 6:378–86.

Rossi, E., B.M. McQuillan, J. Hung, K. Thompson, C. Kuek, and J.P. Beilby. 2000. Serum Ferritin and C282Y Mutation of the Hemochromatosis Gene as Predictors of Asymptomatic Carotid Atherosclerosis in a Community Population. *Stroke* 31:3015–20.

Rubba, P., M. Mercuri, F. Faccenda, A. Iannuzzi, C. Irace, S P. Trisciuglio, A. Gnasso, R. Tang, G. Andria, G. Bond, and M. Mancini. 1994. Premature Carotid Atherosclerosis: Does it Occur in both Familial Hypercholesterolemia and Homocystinuria? *Stroke* 25:943–50.

Salonen, J.T., and R. Salonen. 1993. Ultrasound B-Mode Imaging in Observational Studies of Atherosclerotic Progression. *Circulation* 87[Suppl II]:II-56–II-65.

Sanchez, A., J.D. Barth, and L. Zhang. 2000. The Carotid Artery Wall Thickness in Teenagers Is Related to Their Diet and the Typical Risk Factors of Heart Disease Among Adults. *Atherosclerosis* 152:265–6.

Sass, C., B. Herbeth, O. Chapet, G. Siset, S. Visvikis, and F. Zannad. 1998. Intima-Media Thickness and Diameter of Carotid and Femoral Arteries in Children, Adolescents and Adults from the Stanislas Cohort. *J Hypertens* 16:1593–603.

Schillaci, G., G. Vaudo, S. Marchesi, G. Lupattelli, G. Reboldi, P. Verdecchia, L. Pasqualini, and E. Mannarino. 2002. Optimizing Assessment of Carotid and Femoral Intima-Media Thickness in Essential Hypertension. *Am J Hypertens* 14:1025–31.

Schmidt, H., R. Schmidt, K. Niederkorn, A. Gradert, M. Schumacher, N. Watzinger, H.P. Hartung, and G.M. Kostner. 1998. Paraoxanase PON1 Polymorphism Leu-Met54 Is Associated with Carotid Atherosclerosis: Results of the Austrian Stroke Prevention Study. *Stroke* 29:2043–8.

Schulte-Altedorneburg, G., D.W. Droste, S. Felszeghy, M. Kellermann, V. Popa, K. Hegedus, C. Hegedus, M. Schmid, L. Modis, E.B.Ringelstein, and L. Csiba. 2001. Accuracy of in vivo Carotid B-Mode Ultrasound Compared with Pathological Analysis. *Stroke* 32:1520–4.

Singh, T.P., H. Groehn, and A. Kazmers. 2003. Vascular Function and Carotid Intimal-Medial Thickness in Children with Insulin-Dependent Diabetes Mellitus. *J Am Coll Cardiol* 41:661–5.

Slooter, A.J.C., M.L. Bots, L.M. Havekes, A. Iglesias del Sol, M. Cruts, D.E. Grobbee, A. Hofman, C. Van Broeckhoven, J.C.M. Witteman, and C.M. van Duijn. 2001. Apolipoprotein E and Carotid Artery Atherosclerosis. *Stroke* 32:1947–52.

Sorof, J., and S. Daniels. 2002. Obesity Hypertension in Children: A Problem of Epidemic Proportions. *Hypertension* 40:441–7.

Sorof, J.M., A.V. Alexandrov, G. Cardwell, and R.J. Portman. 2003. Carotid Artery Intimal-Medial Thickness and Left Ventricular Hypertrophy in Children with Elevated Blood Pressure. *Pediatrics* 111:61–6.

Toikka, J.O., H. Laine, M. Ahotupa, A. Haapanen, J.S.A. Viikari, J. Hartiala, and O.T. Raitakari. 2000. Increased Arterial Intima-Media Thickness and in vivo LDL Oxidation in Young Men with Borderline Hypertension. *Hypertension* 36:929–33.

Tonstad, S., O. Joakimsen, E. Stensland-Bugge, T.P. Leren, L. Ose, D. Russell, and K.H. Bonaa. 1996. Risk Factors Related to Carotid Intima-Media Thickness and Plaque in Children with Familial Hypercholesterolemia and Control Subjects. *Arterioscler Thromb Vasc Biol* 16:984–91.

Tsai, M.Y., D.K. Arnett, J.H. Eckfeldt, R.R. Williams, and R.C. Ellison. 2000. Plasma Homocysteine and its Association with Carotid Intimal-Medial Wall Thickness and Prevalent Coronary Heart Disease. *Atherosclerosis* 151:519–24.

van Dam, M.J., E. de Groot, S.M. Clee, G.K. Hovingh, R. Roelants, A. Dorks-Wilsaon, A.H. Zwinderman, A.J. Smir, H.M. Smelt, A.K.Groen, M.R. Hayden, and J.J.P. Kastelein. 2002. Association between Increased Arterial-Wall Thickness and Impairment in ABCA1–driven Cholesterol Efflux: An Observational Study. *Lancet* 359:37–42.

Wagenknecht, L.E., D.W. Bowden, J.J. Carr, C.D. Langefeld, B.I. Freedman, and S.S. Rich. 2001. Familial Aggregation of Coronary Artery Calcium in Families with Type 2 Diabetes. *Diabetes* 50:861–6.

Wang, T.J., B. Nam, R.B. D'Agostino, P.A. Wolf, D.M. Lloyd-Jones, C.A. MacRae, P.W. Wilson, J.F. Polak, and C.J. O'Donnell. 2003. Carotid Intima-Media Thickness Is Associated with Premature Parental Coronary Heart Disease. The Framingham Heart Study. *Circulation* 108:572–6.

Wendelhag, I., O. Wiklund, and J. Wikstrand. 1992. Arterial Wall Thickness in Familial Hypercholesterolemia. *Arterioscler Thromb* 12:70–7.

Wexler, L., B. Brundage, J. Crouse, R. Detrano, V. Fuster, J. Maddahi, J. Rumberger, W. Stanford, R. White, and K. Taubert. 1996. Coronary Artery Calcification: Pathophysiology, Epidemiology, Imaging Methods, and Clinical Implications. *Circulation* 94:1175–92.

Yamasaki, Y., R. Kawamori, H. Matsushima, H. Nishizawa, M. Kodama, Y. Kajimoto, T. Morishima, and T. Kamada. 1994. Atherosclerosis in Carotid Artery of Young IDDM Patients Monitored by Ultrasound High-Resolution B-Mode Imaging. *Diabetes* 43:634–9.

Zannad, F., S. Visvikis, R. Gueguen, C. Sass, O. Chapet, B. Herbeth, and G. Siest. 1998. Genetics Strongly Determines the Wall Thickness of the Left and Right Carotid Arteries. *Hum Genet* 103:183–8.

PART III

Cholesterol in Childhood
and Adolescence

CHAPTER 6

The Epidemiology
of Childhood Cholesterol

Laura E. Beane Freeman, Ronald M. Lauer, and William R. Clarke

Elevated cholesterol levels in adults are predictive of cardiovascular disease (CVD). In addition, drug trials to lower cholesterol levels in adults have demonstrated a reduction in the risk of morbidity and mortality from CVD. While children with elevated cholesterol levels have been shown to be at increased risk for elevated cholesterol levels as adults, long-term studies of children and adolescents with elevated cholesterol levels have not been conducted to show that elevated childhood cholesterol levels are predictive of adult CVD.

■ LIPIDS AND LIPOPROTEINS

Cholesterol and triglycerides are water-insoluble lipids that are transported in the blood by lipoproteins. Lipoproteins can be classified into four categories: low-density lipoprotein (LDL) cholesterol, very-low-density lipoprotein (VLDL) cholesterol, high-density lipoprotein (HDL) cholesterol, and chylomicrons. Apolipoproteins are large lipid complexes and the ligands that react with receptor sites in cells. Apolipoproteins, together with phospholipids, serve to solubilize triglycerides and the proteins in different lipoproteins. The principal lipoprotein associated with LDL cholesterol is apolipoprotein (apo) B-100; apo A-I and apo A-II are associated with HDL cholesterol. The complex of apo B-100 and LDL cholesterol is the primary transporter of cholesterol. HDL cholesterol provides a reverse transport to remove cholesterol from the cells and deliver it to the liver for catabolism. VLDL cholesterol is the main carrier for triglycerides, which are the carrier or storage form of fatty acids in the tissues and plasma. Chylomicrons are the triglycerides of dietary origin and are lipid complexes consisting of three fatty acids linked to a glycerol molecule by an ester bond (Guyton, 1990). In many large epidemiologic studies of adults, elevated LDL cholesterol levels and low HDL cholesterol levels are associated with accelerated CVD (National Cholesterol Education Program, 1993).

■ EPIDEMIOLOGIC INVESTIGATIONS OF LIPIDS AND LIPOPROTEINS

Many epidemiologic studies have established elevated blood cholesterol levels, specifically LDL cholesterol levels, as one of several major risk factors for CVD in men and women. These investigations include case–control studies, comparisons of populations with low and high rates of CVD, migrant studies, and international studies of diet, atherosclerosis, cholesterol levels, and CVD (Stamler, 1967; LaRosa et al., 1990).

Noteworthy are the findings of many prospective, observational studies within populations, such as the Framingham Heart Study (Castelli et al., 1986) the Honolulu Heart Program (Kagan et al., 1981), the British Regional Heart Study (Pocock et al., 1986), and studies of men screened for the Multiple Risk Factor Intervention Trial (Kannel et al., 1986; Martin et al., 1986; Stamler et al., 1986; Multiple Risk Factor Intervention Trial Research Group, 1990). Such investigations have consistently shown the cholesterol level to be a powerful and independent predictor of CVD. On average, each 1% rise in cholesterol level is associated with an approximate 2% increase in the risk of CVD (Stamler et al., 1986). Davis and coworkers (1990) suggested that this relationship has been underestimated because of a failure to take into account intraindividual variation in cholesterol levels and each 1% rise in blood cholesterol level is actually associated with an approximate 3% increase in risk (see Chapter 2). The level of HDL cholesterol, in contrast, is inversely and independently associated with CVD in both men and women at all ages (Gordon and Rifkind, 1989).

■ DISTRIBUTION OF CHOLESTEROL AND TRIGLYCERIDE LEVELS IN CHILDREN AND ADOLESCENTS

The National Health and Nutrition Examination Survey (NHANES) is a nationally representative survey of diet and health conducted in the United States by the Centers for Disease Control and Prevention (CDC). Table 6.1 describes the total, LDL, and HDL cholesterol levels along with the triglyceride levels for children and adolescents by age group during the period from 1988 to 1994 (NHANES III). Total cholesterol levels appear to be marginally higher in females than in males, but do not vary much by age. HDL and LDL levels do not follow a particular pattern with respect to age or sex. Triglyceride levels are higher in adolescents.

■ DEFINITION OF ELEVATED CHOLESTEROL LEVELS IN CHILDREN AND ADOLESCENTS

In 1992, the National Cholesterol Education Program (NCEP) published the following guidelines for the classification of total cholesterol in children:

- Acceptable   ≤170 mg/dL (4.4 mmol/L)
- Borderline   >170 and ≤199 mg/dL (4.4 to 5.2 mmol/L)
- High   ≥200 mg/dL (5.2 mmol/L)

While the NCEP did not specifically recommend drug therapy for those children under the age of 10 with high cholesterol, it did urge that children with high cholesterol be further evaluated (see Chapters 7 and 8). As can be seen in Table 6.1, the 75th percentile for all age groups is similar to the guidelines set by this panel for borderline cholesterol levels, and the 90th percentile approximates the cut point for high cholesterol levels in children and adolescents.

■ INTERNATIONAL COMPARISONS OF CHOLESTEROL LEVELS

In children, the major nutritional determinant of differences in serum total cholesterol levels among countries appears to be the proportion of saturated fat in the diet (Blackburn 1983; Knuiman et al., 1983, 1987). For example, in countries such as the Philippines, Italy, and Ghana, saturated fat constitutes between 9.3% and 10.5% of the dietary energy intake, and the mean total cholesterol level of boys aged 7 to 9 years is ≤159 mg/dL (4.1 mmol/L) (Table 6.2) (National Health Survey, 1978; Knuiman et al., 1983; National Center for Health Statistics, 1983). These countries also often have lower dietary cholesterol intakes than countries such as the United States, the Netherlands, and Finland, where saturated fat intake has been shown to be between 13.5% and 17.7% of dietary energy intake, and mean cholesterol levels are ≥167 mg/dL (4.3 mmol/L).

Although cholesterol levels are lowest in countries in which nutrition is not optimal and growth is delayed, there are many industrialized countries (such as Portugal, Israel, and Italy) where children have lower cholesterol levels and where normal growth is maintained (Knuiman et al., 1980, 1987; Halfon et al., 1982). As shown in Table 6.2, higher serum cholesterol levels in boys are associated with higher levels in middle-aged men in the same country and with higher mortality rates of CVD in the adult population.

TABLE 6.1

Cholesterol and triglyceride levels in U.S. children and adolescents by age group and sex (NHANES III)

Age Category	Mean mg/dL (mmol/L)	Median mg/dL (mmol/L)	75th Percentile mg/dL (mmol/L)	90th Percentile mg/dL (mmol/L)
Ages 5 to 9				
Total				
Males	165 (4.3)	164 (4.3)	180 (4.7)	197 (5.1)
Females	169 (4.4)	168 (4.4)	184 (4.8)	201 (5.2)
LDL				
Males	95 (2.5)	93 (2.4)	106 (2.8)	121 (3.1)
Females	103 (2.7)	101 (2.6)	118 (3.1)	129 (3.4)
HDL				
Males	57 (1.5)	56 (1.5)	65 (1.7)	72 (1.9)
Females	55 (1.4)	54 (1.4)	63 (1.6)	69 (1.8)
Triglycerides				
Males	56 (1.5)	53 (0.60)	67 (0.76)	88 (0.99)
Females	60 (1.6)	57 (0.64)	73 (0.82)	93 (1.05)
Ages 10 to 14				
Total				
Males	162 (4.2)	160 (4.2)	178 (4.6)	196 (5.1)
Females	164 (4.3)	163 (4.2)	179 (4.7)	196 (5.1)
LDL				
Males	99 (2.6)	97 (2.5)	112 (2.9)	126 (3.3)
Females	100 (2.6)	97 (2.5)	113 (2.9)	130 (3.4)
HDL				
Males	57 (1.5)	57 (1.5)	63 (1.6)	73 (1.9)
Females	54 (1.4)	54 (1.4)	60 (1.6)	66 (1.7)
Triglycerides				
Males	68 (0.77)	61 (0.69)	80 (0.90)	105 (1.19)
Females	78 (0.88)	72 (0.81)	93 (1.05)	117 (1.32)
Ages 15 to 19				
Total				
Males	154 (4.0)	150 (3.9)	170 (4.4)	188 (4.9)
Females	162 (4.2)	160 (4.1)	177 (4.6)	197 (5.1)
LDL				
Males	97 (2.5)	96 (2.5)	112 (2.9)	127 (3.3)
Females	99 (2.6)	96 (2.5)	114 (3.0)	133 (3.4)
HDL				
Males	48 (1.2)	47 (1.2)	54 (1.4)	61 (1.6)
Females	54 (1.4)	53 (1.4)	63 (1.6)	70 (1.8)
Triglycerides				
Males	80 (0.90)	71 (0.80)	94 (1.06)	124 (1.40)
Females	78 (0.88)	70 (0.79)	90 (1.02)	117 (1.32)

HDL, high-density lipoprotein, LDL, low-density lipoprotein.
Source: National Health and Nutrition Examination Survey III (NHANES III).

TABLE 6.2
Dietary saturated fat and cholesterol intake and mean total cholesterol in boys 7 to
9 years of age, mean total cholesterol, and cardiovascular disease mortality in men from
six countries

| | Dietary Intake | | Mean Total Cholesterol mg/dL (mmol/L) | | CVD Mortality per 100,000 Men |
Country	Saturated Fat (% of energy)	Cholesterol (mg/1000 calories)	In Boys	In Adult Men	Ages 45 to 54
Philippines	9.3	97	147 (3.8)	186 (4.8)	—
Italy	10.4	159	159 (4.1)	200 (5.2)	91
Ghana	10.5	48	128 (3.3)	159 (4.1)	—
United States	13.5	151	167 (4.3)	217 (5.6)	170
Netherlands	15.1	142	174 (4.5)	221 (5.7)	134
Finland	17.7	157	190 (4.9)	240 (6.2)	264

Sources: Dietary intake data from National Health and Nutrition Examination Survey (NHANES) II (National Center for Health Statistics, 1983) for U.S. boys ages 7 to 9, and from Knuiman et al. (1983) for boys ages 8 to 9 from the other five countries. Serum cholesterol data from NHANES I (National Health Survey, 1978) for U.S. boys ages 5 to 9, and from Knuiman et al. (1983) for boys ages 8 to 9 from the other five countries, from NHANES II (NCHS-NHLBI Collaborative Lipid Group, 1987) for U.S. men ages 35 to 44, and from Knuiman et al. (1982) for men ages 33 to 48 from the other five countries. Mortality data for 1985 from the World Health Organization (1986, 1987, 1988). Data reproduced from Knuiman et al. (1982) by permission of Oxford University Press.

■ TRENDS IN TOTAL CHOLESTEROL LEVELS OF CHILDREN AND ADOLESCENTS

Comparing data from NHANES I (1971 to 1974) to that of NHANES III (1988 to 1994), it appears that total cholesterol levels have declined (Fig. 6.1). During this time period, intervention efforts were under way to reduce fat intake (NCEP, 1992; American Academy of Pediatrics, 1998). Indeed, total and saturated fat consumption decreased during this time interval (National Health Survey, 1978; Blackburn, 1983), which likely impacted cholesterol levels in the pediatric population.

■ CLASSIFICATION OF LDL, HDL, AND TOTAL CHOLESTEROL LEVELS IN ADULTS

In 2002, the NCEP established the third adult treatment panel (ATP III) guidelines with the intention of providing clinical guidance for the prevention of CVD through the management of serum cholesterol levels (NCEP, 2002). The panel was comprised of leading clinicians and experts from a variety of governmental agencies and academies. Using published results from clinical trials and observational studies, the panel objectively reviewed the literature to set guidelines

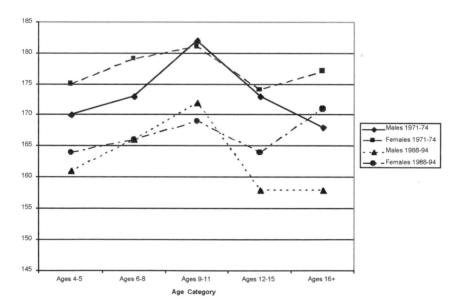

FIGURE 6.1
Comparison of mean childhood total serum cholesterol levels (mg/dL) from the National Health and Nutrition Examination Survey (NHANES) I (1971 to 1974) and NHANES III (1988 to 1994).

for treatment of elevated cholesterol for the prevention of CVD. These guidelines were updated from the ATP II guidelines, which were published in 1993. The new ATP III guidelines for cholesterol levels in adults are presented in Table 6.3. For total cholesterol, a desirable level is defined as being <200 mg/dL (5.2 mmol/L). Total cholesterol levels of 200 to 239 mg/dL (5.2 to 6.2 mmol/L) are defined as being borderline high, and levels ≥240 mg/dL (6.2 mmol/L) are considered to be high.

■ TRACKING OF TOTAL CHOLESTEROL LEVELS FROM CHILDHOOD AND ADOLESCENCE INTO ADULTHOOD

Tracking implies the maintenance of rank order. If cholesterol levels track well, then children in the highest percentiles of cholesterol would become adults with high cholesterol, and children in the lowest percentiles of cholesterol would become adults with low cholesterol. Two large cohort studies have shown that there is some utility of using childhood cholesterol levels to predict who will have high cholesterol levels later in life. Studies have shown that rank order of

TABLE 6.3

Adult treatment panel III classification
of LDL, HDL, and total cholesterol in
adults mg/dL (mmol/L)

Type	Classification
LDL Cholesterol	
<100 (2.6)	Optimal
100–129 (2.6–3.3)	Near optimal/above optimal
130–159 (3.4–4.1)	Borderline high
160–189 (4.1–4.9)	High
≥190 (4.9)	Very high
HDL Cholesterol	
<40 (1.0)	Low
≥60 (1.6)	High
Total Cholesterol	
<200 (5.2)	Desirable
200–239 (5.2–6.2)	Borderline high
≥240 (6.2)	High

Source: National Cholesterol Education Program, Adult Treatment Panel III.

cholesterol levels in childhood is maintained, but not as consistently as rank order of height and weight (Clarke et al., 1967, 1978; Laskarzewski et al., 1979; Freedman et al., 1985).

The Bogalusa Heart Study is a longitudinal epidemiologic study of the early history of CVD in children and young adults in a biracial population (Berenson, 1980). Using data from two cross-sectional surveys administered as part of this study, investigators tracked cholesterol levels of 1169 children in this cohort. Serum cholesterol measurements were obtained for children and adolescents who were 5–14 years of age in 1973–74 and again on the same participants in 1988–91. Among the children and adolescents with total cholesterol levels ≥80th percentile for their age and sex, more than 40% had elevated levels 15 years later (Nicklas et al., 2002). Correlation coefficients between baseline and 15-year follow-up were highest for LDL cholesterol, with correlation as high as 0.69 (Lenfant and Savage, 1995).

In another longitudinal cohort study, school children ages 5 to 18 years in Muscatine, Iowa were examined between 1971 and 1981. Established risk factors for adult CVD, including total cholesterol, triglycerides, triceps skinfold thickness, body mass index (BMI), and blood pressure, were measured during six biennial cross-sectional surveys. Individuals who participated in the childhood examinations were asked to participate in follow-up examinations as adults between the ages of 20 and 35. The follow-up examinations were designed to measure each adult in the years that they turned 23, 28, or 33 years of age. These longitudinal risk factor measurements in the Muscatine cohort were examined to characterize the association between the childhood measures and elevated (≥200 mg/dL or ≥240 mg/dL) cholesterol levels at the time of the adult examinations. Adults were classified into three age categories, 20 to 24, 25 to 29, and 30+ years of age. This study (Lauer and Clarke, 1990) showed that of children 5 to 18 years of age who had total cholesterol levels >90th percentile on two occasions, 75% had high levels (≥200 mg/dL, 5.2 mmol/L); 25% had desirable levels (<200 mg/dL, 5.2 mmol/L) at ages 20 to 24 years with no intervention. The 75th percentile of total cholesterol for adults in their 20s is approximately 200 mg/dL (5.2 mmol/L). Therefore, the percentage of individuals among those who were at the 90th percentile of total cholesterol as children who had levels ≥200 mg/dL (5.2 mmol/L) as adults is about three times the percentage expected for the general population.

The association of childhood (ages 5 to 18 years) risk factors with elevated adult cholesterol levels is presented in Table 6.4. The odds that a child with an age- and sex-specific cholesterol level 1 standard deviation above the mean will have high cholesterol when re-examined between 20 and 24 years of age are 3.6 times higher than the odds for a child whose age- and sex-specific cholesterol level is at the mean. The 95% confidence interval indicates that the odds ratio could be as low as 2.9 or as high as 4.5. Similarly, the odds ratio for cholesterol ≥240 mg/dL at 20 to 24 years of age is 4.2 with a 95% confidence interval of 2.9 to 6.0. Note that all the odds ratios for cholesterol are statistically significant (the

TABLE 6.4
Odds ratios and 95% confidence intervals for childhood predictors of adult cholesterol levels ≥200 mg/dL (5.2 mmol/L) and ≥240 mg/dL (6.2 mmol/L), Muscatine, Iowa*

Childhood Measurement†	Adult Cholesterol ≥200 mg/dL (5.2 mmol/L)			Adult Cholesterol ≥240 mg/dL (6.2 mmol/L)		
	Ages 20 to 24 OR (95% CI)	Ages 25 to 29 OR (95% CI)	Age 30+ OR (95% CI)	Ages 20 to 24 OR (95% CI)	Ages 25 to 29 OR (95% CI)	Age 30+ OR (95% CI)
Cholesterol	3.6 (2.9–4.5)	3.0 (2.4–3.7)	3.2 (2.5–4.0)	4.2 (2.9–6.0)	4.0 (2.8–5.9)	2.8 (2.1–3.8)
Triglycerides	1.4 (1.2–1.6)	1.4 (1.2–1.6)	1.3 (1.1–1.5)	1.0 (0.7–1.4)	1.1 (0.8–1.6)	1.4 (1.1–1.7)
Height	0.8 (0.7–1.0)	0.8 (0.7–0.9)	0.8 (0.7–1.0)	0.7 (0.5–1.0)	0.9 (0.5–1.3)	0.7 (0.5–0.9)
Weight	1.1 (1.0–1.3)	1.2 (1.0–1.4)	1.0 (0.8–1.2)	1.1 (0.8–1.5)	1.2 (0.9–1.7)	1.0 (0.8–1.4)
BMI	1.2 (1.1–1.5)	1.3 (1.1–1.5)	1.1 (0.9–1.3)	1.3 (0.9–1.7)	1.3 (0.9–1.7)	1.3 (1.0–1.7)
Triceps skinfold	1.2 (1.0–1.4)	1.3 (1.1–1.5)	1.1 (0.9–1.3)	1.4 (1.0–1.8)	1.3 (1.0–1.8)	1.3 (1.0–1.7)
Diastolic BP	1.1 (0.9–1.3)	1.1 (0.9–1.30)	1.1 (0.9–1.3)	0.9 (0.6–1.3)	1.7 (1.1–2.6)	0.8 (0.6–1.1)
Systolic BP	1.2 (1.0–1.4)	1.1 (0.9–1.3)	1.2 (1.0–1.4)	1.0 (0.7–1.4)	1.2 (0.8–1.7)	0.9 (0.7–1.2)

*For example, the odds ratio (OR) for cholesterol in adults 20 to 24 years of age is 3.6 with a 95% confidence interval (CI) of 2.9 to 4.5. This means the odds that a child with cholesterol level 1 standard deviation above the mean will become an adult 20 to 24 years of age with high cholesterol is 3.6 times higher than the odds for a child whose cholesterol level is at the mean. This could be as low as 2.9 or as high as 4.5. If the CI does not contain 1.0, then the OR is statistically significant at the 5% level.
†Mean of the last two age-, sex-, and survey-specific Z scores from school surveys conducted at ages 5 to 18. Results were comparable when the mean of the first two age-, sex-, and survey-specific Z scores were used.

95% confidence interval does not include 1.0), indicating that elevated childhood cholesterol levels are predictive of elevated adult cholesterol levels.

Table 6.4 also displays odds ratios for other childhood predictors of elevated cholesterol, including triglycerides, height, weight, BMI, triceps skinfold thickness, and diastolic and systolic blood pressures. Childhood total cholesterol, triglycerides, weight, BMI, and triceps skinfold thickness are statistically significant univariate predictors of high adult cholesterol. Note that these individual childhood risk factors may be acting jointly to affect adult cholesterol levels.

These data show that high levels of cholesterol in childhood are predictive of high cholesterol levels in adulthood (the positive predictive value) where such levels are known to be predictive of CVD. However, the positive predictive value column in Table 6.5 shows that, depending on age and sex, from 13% to 40% (1 − positive predictive value) of children with cholesterol levels ≥90th percentile on at least two occasions would not qualify for individual medical intervention, as defined by the NCEP, when they became adults (NCEP, 1992). Clearly, many children with high cholesterol levels do not become adults with high cholesterol. To provide appropriate early intervention for the treatment of elevated cholesterol levels in children and adolescents, it would be of benefit to identify those individuals who will become adults with high cholesterol levels at an age when primordial prevention could be initiated with high sensitivity, specificity, and predictive value.

■ PREDICTIVE VALUE OF HIGH CHILDHOOD CHOLESTEROL LEVELS

Tables 6.5 and 6.6, and Figures 6.2 and 6.3 illustrate the utility of using age- and sex-specific percentiles of childhood cholesterol as a screening test. These tables provide estimates from the Muscatine Study of the sensitivity, specificity, positive predictive value and negative predictive value of potential screening strategies for identifying children who are most likely to become adults with high cholesterol. For this analysis, two different definitions of an elevated childhood total cholesterol level were considered: ≥75th and ≥90th age- and sex-specific percentiles on two occasions. Two different definitions of an elevated adult total cholesterol level were also considered on the basis of ATP III: ≥200 and ≥240 mg/dL. In the context of predicting elevated cholesterol levels in adults based on classification of cholesterol levels measured when they were children and adolescents, *sensitivity* refers to the probability of an elevated adult cholesterol level given an elevated childhood cholesterol level. The *specificity* is the proportion of those adults who do not have elevated total cholesterol whose childhood cholesterol levels were not elevated. However, in this situation the positive predictive value and negative predictive value are the more important measures of the suitability of the screening test because they represent the probability that a

TABLE 6.5
Predictive value of childhood total cholesterol levels (≥75th and
≥90th percentiles on two occasions) for adult total cholesterol levels
≥200 mg/dL, Muscatine, Iowa

Childhood Percentile and Sex	Number of Participants	Sensitivity (%)	Specificity (%)	Positive Predictive Value (%)	Negative Predictive Value (%)
Adults 20 to 24 Years of Age					
≥75th					
Females	539	43.0	88.5	50.6	88.5
Males	479	49.2	93.3	52.5	92.4
≥90th					
Females	539	20.4	98.7	76.0	85.6
Males	479	20.6	99.3	81.3	89.2
Adults 25 to 29 Years of Age					
≥75th					
Females	510	41.0	92.9	58.6	86.6
Males	409	36.1	92.6	56.4	92.6
≥90th					
Females	510	13.0	98.5	68.4	82.3
Males	409	14.0	98.1	66.7	98.1
Adults 30+ Years of Age					
≥75th					
Females	650	33.3	93.5	61.9	81.6
Males	602	31.6	93.4	71.4	77.4
≥90th					
Females	650	9.6	98.0	60.0	77.4
Males	602	9.7	99.2	87.0	67.9

child with high cholesterol will become an adult with high cholesterol (positive predictive value) and the probability that a child with low cholesterol will become an adult with a cholesterol level that is not significantly elevated to be predictive of adult CVD (negative predictive value).

Positive Predictive Value

Table 6.5 shows that 50.6% of the females whose childhood total cholesterol level was ≥75th percentile on two occasions had total cholesterol levels above 200 mg/dL (5.2 mmol/L) when they were examined between the ages of 20 and 24 years; that

TABLE 6.6

Predictive value of childhood serum cholesterol levels (≥75th and ≥90th percentiles on two occasions) for adult total cholesterol levels ≥240 mg/dL, Muscatine, Iowa

Percentile and Sex	Number of Participants	Sensitivity (%)	Specificity (%)	Positive Predictive Value (%)	Negative Predictive Value (%)
Adults 20 to 24 Years of Age					
≥75th					
Females	539	56.5	87.2	16.5	97.8
Males	479	60.0	88.7	10.2	99.1
≥90th					
Females	539	34.8	96.7	32.0	97.1
Males	479	50.0	97.7	31.3	98.9
Adults 25 to 29 Years of Age					
≥75th					
Females	510	73.3	88.1	15.7	99.1
Males	409	66.7	88.6	18.2	98.6
≥90th					
Females	510	33.3	97.2	26.3	98.0
Males	409	46.7	97.2	38.9	98.0
Adults 30+ Years of Age					
≥75th					
Females	650	48.5	89.0	19.1	97.0
Males	602	40.7	87.4	24.2	93.7
≥90th					
Females	650	18.2	96.9	24.0	95.7
Males	602	18.5	97.6	43.5	97.6

is, the predictive value of a positive childhood test is 50.6%. In the same adult age category, 76.0% of females whose childhood total cholesterol level was ≥90th percentile on two occasions had elevated adult total cholesterol levels.

■ Negative Predictive Value

Generally, there is a trade-off between maximizing the positive predictive value and the negative predictive value of a screening test (Figs. 6.2 and 6.3). For example, among females 20 to 24 years of age (Table 6.5), the predictive value of a negative test was 88.5% and 85.6%, using childhood criteria of ≥75th and ≥90th percentiles, respectively. Because estimation of the negative predictive value fo-

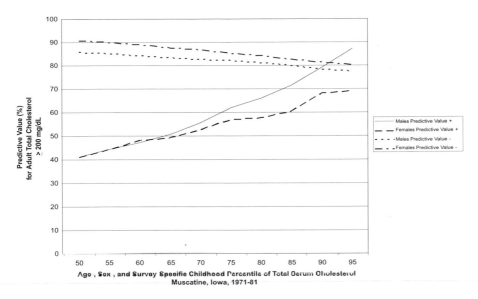

FIGURE 6.2
Predictive value of age-, sex-, and survey-specific percentiles of childhood total cholesterol level for adult total cholesterol level ≥200 mg/dL. Predictive Value + is the positive predictive value.

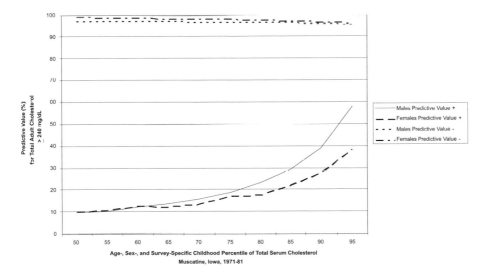

FIGURE 6.3
Predictive value of age-, sex-, and survey-specific percentiles of childhood total cholesterol level for adult total cholesterol level ≥240 mg/dL. Predictive Value + is the positive predictive value.

121

cuses on participants whose childhood total cholesterol levels were not elevated, this indicates that 88.5% of females whose childhood total cholesterol levels were <75th percentile on two occasions had total cholesterol <200 mg/dL (5.2 mmol/L) as adults 20 to 24 years of age.

■ WHY NOT CONDUCT POPULATION-WIDE SCREENING IN CHILDREN?

As described in the examples above, screening all children and following and possibly treating those whose total cholesterol levels are at the highest percentiles for their age and sex might reduce the risk of elevated cholesterol levels later in life, consequently reducing CVD risk. However, for a variety of reasons, the NCEP does not recommend a population-wide approach to childhood cholesterol screening, but rather a more measured approach, including screening for those children with a family history of premature CVD or at least one parent with high cholesterol (see Chapter 7). The reasons for this selective screening approach include the following:

- While childhood cholesterol levels predict adult cholesterol levels with some accuracy, many children with elevated cholesterol levels will not have elevated cholesterol levels as adults.
- The implementation of population-wide screening could lead to unnecessarily labeling children as patients with a "disease," which could cause anxiety for them and their families.
- There is sufficient time to initiate cholesterol-lowering therapies in adulthood for most children who are not members of high-risk families.
- The long-term safety and efficacy of cholesterol-lowering drugs have not been studied sufficiently to exclude the possibility of long-term toxicities.

■ REFERENCES

American Academy of Pediatrics: Committee on Nutrition. 1998. Cholesterol in Childhood. *Pediatrics* 101:1141–7.

Berenson, G.S. 1980. *Cardiovascular Risk Factors in Children.* New York, NY: Oxford University Press.

Blackburn, H. 1983. Diet and Atherosclerosis: Epidemiologic Evidence and Public Health Implications. *Prev Med* 12:2–10.

Castelli, W.P., R.J. Garrison, P.W.F. Wilson, R.D. Abbott, S. Kalousdian, and W.B. Kannel. 1986. Incidence of Coronary Heart Disease and Lipoprotein Cholesterol Levels. The Framingham Study. *JAMA* 256:2835–8.

Clarke, D.A., M.F. Allen, and F.H. Wilson, Jr. 1967. Longitudinal Study of Serum Lipids. 12-Year Report. *Am J Clin Nutr* 20:743–52.

Clarke, W.R., H.G. Schrott, P.E. Leaverton, W.E. Connor, and R.M. Lauer. 1978. Tracking of Blood Lipids and Blood Pressures in School Age Children: The Muscatine Study. *Circulation* 58:626–34.

Davis, C.E., B.M. Rifkind, H. Brenner, and D.J. Gordon. 1990. A Single Cholesterol Measurement Underestimates the Risk for Coronary Heart Disease. An Empirical Example from the Lipid Research Clinics Mortality Follow-up Study. *JAMA* 264:3044–6.

Freedman, D.S., C.L. Shear, S.R. Srinivasan, L.S. Webber, and G.S. Berenson. 1985. Tracking of Serum Lipids and Lipoproteins in Children over an 8–Year Period: The Bogalusa Heart Study. *Prev Med* 14:203–16.

Gordon, D.J., and B.M. Rifkind. 1989. High-Density Lipoprotein: The Clinical Implications of Recent Studies. *N Engl J Med* 321:1311–6.

Guyton, J.R. 1990. Lipid Metabolism and Atherosclerosis. In: *The Science and Practice of Pediatric Cardiology*. Edited by A. Garson, J.T. Bricker, and D.G. McNamara. Philadelphia: Lea & Febiger, pp. 475–91.

Halfon, S.T., B.M. Rifkind, S. Harlap, N.A. Kaufmann, M. Baras, P.E. Slater, G. Halperin, S. Eisenberg, A.M. Davis, and Y. Stein. 1982. Plasma Lipids and Lipoproteins in Adult Jews of Different Origins: The Jerusalem Lipid Research Clinic Prevalence Study. *Isr J Med Sci* 18:1113–20.

Kagan, A., D.L. McGee, K. Yano, G.G. Rhoads, and A. Nomura. 1981. Serum Cholesterol and Mortality in a Japanese-American Population: The Honolulu Heart Program. *Am J Epidemiol* 114:11–20.

Kannel, W.B., J.D. Neaton, D. Wentworth, H.E. Thomas, J. Stamler, S.B. Hulley, and M.O. Kjelsberg. 1986. Overall and Coronary Heart Disease Mortality Rates in Relation to Major Risk Factors in 325,348 Men Screened for the MRFIT. *Am Heart J* 112:825–36.

Knuiman, J.T., R.J.J. Hermus, and J.G. Hautvast. 1980. Serum Total and High Density Lipoprotein (HDL) Cholesterol Concentrations in Rural and Urban Boys from 16 Countries. *Atherosclerosis* 36:529–37.

Knuiman, J.T., C.E. West, J. Burema. 1982. Serum Total and High Density Lipoprotein Cholesterol Concentrations and Body Mass Index in Adult Men From 13 Countries. *Am J Epidemiol* 116:631–42.

Knuiman, J.T., C.E. West, M.B. Katan, and J.G. Hautvast. 1987. Total Cholesterol and High Density Lipoprotein Cholesterol Levels in Populations Differing in Fat and Carbohydrate Intake. *Arteriosclerosis* 7:612–9.

Knuiman, J.T., S. Westenbrink, L. van der Heyden, C.E. West, J. Burema, J. De Boer, J.G. Hautvast, L. Rasanen, L. Viikkunen, J. Vilkari, P. Lokko, J.O.M. Pobee, A. Ferro-Luzzi, A.M. Ferrini, C. Scaccini, S. Sette, G.M. Villavieja, and J. Bulatao-Jayme. 1983. Determinants of Total and High Density Lipoprotein Cholesterol in Boys from Finland, the Netherlands, Italy, the Philippines and Ghana with Special Reference to Diet. *Hum Nutr Clin Nutr* 37:237–54.

LaRosa, J.C., D. Hunninghake, D. Bush, M.H. Criqui, G.S. Getz, A.M. Gotto, Jr., S.M. Grundy, L. Rakita, R.M. Robertson, and M.L. Weisfeldt. 1990. The Cholesterol Facts. A Summary of the Evidence Relating Dietary Fats, Serum Cholesterol, and Coronary Heart Disease. A Joint Statement by the American Heart Association and the National Heart, Lung, and Blood Institute. *Circulation* 81:1721–33.

Laskarzewski, P.M., J.A. Morrison, I. deGroot, K.A. Kelly, M.J. Mellies, P. Khoury, and C.J. Glueck. 1979. Lipid and Lipoprotein Tracking in 108 Children over a Four-Year Period. *Pediatrics* 64:584–91.

Lauer, R.M., and W.R. Clarke. 1990: Use of Cholesterol Measurements in Childhood for the Prediction of Adult Hypercholesterolemia: The Muscatine Study. *JAMA* 264:3034–8.

Lenfant, C., and P.F. Savage. 1995. The Early Natural History of Atherosclerosis and Hypertension in the Young: National Institutes of Health Perspectives. *Am J Med Sci* 310:S3–7.

Martin, M.J., S.B. Hulley, W.S. Browner, L.H. Kuller, and D. Wentworth. 1986. Serum Cholesterol, Blood Pressure, and Mortality: Implications from a Cohort of 361,662 Men. *Lancet* 328:933–6.

Multiple Risk Factor Intervention Trial Research Group. 1990. Mortality Rates after 10.5

Years for Participants in the Multiple Risk Factor Intervention Trial: Findings Related to a priori Hypotheses of the Trial. *JAMA* 263:1795–801.

National Center for Health Statistics, Carroll, M.D., and S. Abraham. 1983. Dietary Intake Source Data: United States 1976–80. Vital and Health Statistics. Hyattsville, MD: U.S. Department of Health and Human Services, Public Health Service, National Center for Health Statistics. DHHS Publication PHS 83–1681. Series 11, No. 231.

[NCEP] National Cholesterol Education Program. 1992. Report of the Expert Panel on Blood Cholesterol Levels in Children and Adolescents. *Pediatrics* 89:495–501.

[NCEP] National Cholesterol Education Program. 1993. Report of the Expert Panel on Detection, Evaluation, and Treatment of High Blood Cholesterol in Adults (Adult Treatment Panel II). Bethesda, MD: U.S. Department of Health and Human Services, National Institutes of Health, National Heart, Lung and Blood Institute. NIH Publication 9-3095.

[NCEP] National Cholesterol Education Program. 2002. Report of the Expert Panel on Detection, Evaluation, and Treatment of High Blood Cholesterol in Adults (Adult Treatment Panel III). Bethesda, MD: U.S. Department of Health and Human Services, National Institutes of Health, National Heart, Lung and Blood Institute. NIH Publication 02–5215.

National Health Survey. 1978. Total Serum Cholesterol Levels in Children 4–17 Years, United States, 1971–1974. Data from the National Health Survey. Hyattsville, MD: U.S. Department of Health, Education, and Welfare, Public Health Service, National Center for Health Statistics. DHEW Publication PHS 78-1655.

NCHS-NHLBI Collaborative Lipid Group. 1987. Trends in Serum Cholesterol Levels among US Adults Aged 20 to 74 Years: Data from the National Health and Nutrition Examination Surveys, 1960 to 1980. *JAMA* 257:937–42.

Nicklas, T.A., S.P. von Duvillard, and G.S. Berenson. 2002. Tracking of Serum Lipids and Lipoproteins from Childhood to Dyslipidemia in Adults: The Bogalusa Heart Study. *Int J Sports Med* 23:S39–S43.

Pocock, S.J., A.G. Shaper, A.N. Phillips, M. Walker, and T.P. Whithead. 1986. High Density Lipoprotein Cholesterol Is not a Major Risk Factor for Ischaemic Heart Disease in British Men. *BMJ* 22:515–9.

Stamler, J. 1967. *Lectures on Preventive Cardiology.* New York: Grune & Stratton.

Stamler, J., D. Wentworth, and J.D. Neaton. 1986. Is the Relationship between Serum Cholesterol and Risk of Premature Death from Coronary Heart Disease Continuous and Graded? Findings in 356,222 Primary Screens of the Multiple Risk Factor Intervention Trial (MRFIT). *JAMA* 256:2823–8.

World Health Organization. 1986. *World Health Statistics Annual, 1986.* Geneva: World Health Organization.

World Health Organization. 1987. *World Health Statistics Annual, 1987.* Geneva: World Health Organization.

World Health Organization. 1988. *World Health Statistics Annual, 1988.* Geneva: World Health Organization.

CHAPTER 7

Identification and Treatment of Children and Adolescents with High Cholesterol

Ronald M. Lauer

There is convincing pathologic evidence (see Chapter 1) that the atherosclerotic process begins during childhood and adolescence (Newman et al., 1986; Davies, 1990; Haust, 1990; PDAY Research Group, 1990). The Bogalusa Heart Study has reported research relating cholesterol levels to the extent of early arterial lesions of atherosclerosis in children (Freedman et al., 1988; Berenson et al., 1998). In addition to cholesterol levels, other risk factors in children and adolescents require attention. Specifically, smoking should be discouraged, hypertension should be identified and treated, obesity should be avoided and reduced, exercise should be encouraged, and diabetes mellitus should be identified and treated (Kavey et al., 2003). This chapter discusses lipids and lipoproteins, their relationship to the atherosclerotic process, and their medical management in children and adolescents.

■ SIGNIFICANCE OF LIPIDS AND LIPOPROTEINS IN CHILDREN AND ADOLESCENTS

In adult population studies, elevated cholesterol levels are major predictors of cardiovascular disease (CVD). The link between lipid disorders and CVD is the atherosclerotic plaque, a cap of intimal, lipid-containing cells (macrophages and modified smooth muscle cells) with some collagen covering a deeper deposit of extracellular lipid and cell debris. Subsequently, there may be calcification, cell necrosis, and rupture of or hemorrhage into the plaque; these changes result in overlying thrombosis. These lesions may narrow or occlude coronary, renal, or cerebral arteries or the aorta and lead to embolism of cholesterol crystals or thrombi.

In adults, drug trials of cholesterol-lowering agents have shown major reductions in CVD rates (Brensike et al., 1984; Lipid Research Clinics Program, 1984a, 1984b). Follow-up studies of childhood populations have examined the predictive value of childhood cholesterol levels for adult cholesterol levels (see Chapter 6). The safety, efficacy, and acceptability of lower-fat diets and drugs used to lower cholesterol levels have been assessed in short-term studies in children and adolescents (DISC Collaborative Research Group, 1995; Lagstrom et al., 1998; Salo et al., 1999; also see Chapter 8); however, no long-term studies of drug therapy beginning in childhood have been conducted. Thus, the long-term CVD benefit of lowering cholesterol levels has been inferred from less direct evidence in children and adolescents.

▧ IDENTIFYING HIGH-RISK INDIVIDUALS: FAMILIAL DISORDERS AND DYSLIPIDEMIA ASSOCIATED WITH OBESITY

Several human dyslipidemias have in common raised concentrations of cholesterol and lipoproteins; many result from specific genetic mutations (Breslow, 2000; Kwiterovich, 2002). These disorders are characterized by severe atherosclerosis and the occurrence of CVD at a young age.

▧ Familial Hypercholesterolemia

Familial hypercholesterolemia (FH) is a dominantly inherited defect in the low-density lipoprotein (LDL) receptor that causes faulty LDL uptake and metabolism. The heterozygous form of FH is the most commonly encountered dyslipoproteinemia in children and adolescents, affecting 1 in 500 persons. In some countries where the population has been maintained with inbreeding, the rates of FH are higher; examples are the French-Canadians, Afrikaners, and Norwegians. Many different mutations of the LDL receptor gene have been reported (Leren et al., 1994; Goldstein et al., 2001; Ose, 2002).

To determine whether a child or adolescent with primary elevation of LDL cholesterol has heterozygous FH, an evaluation of family members is particularly helpful (Civeira et al., 2004). Because a parent, grandparent, or sibling of an FH child will often have elevated total and LDL cholesterol levels, they should have their lipid and lipoprotein levels evaluated. The triglyceride levels of individuals with FH are usually normal (<95th percentile). Children and adolescents with heterozygous FH often have LDL cholesterol levels >160 mg/dL (4.1 mmol/L), with average levels about 240 mg/dL (6.2 mmol/L) (Kwiterovich et al., 1974;

Kwiterovich, 1989, 1996). Adults with FH may have tendon xanthomas; however, tendon xanthomas are rarely found before 10 years of age, and only 10% to 15% of FH patients develop xanthomas in the second decade of life. Xanthomas most often appear in the Achilles tendon and the extensor tendons of the hands. The clinical manifestations of CVD are rare in children and adolescents with heterozygous FH (Kwiterovich et al., 1974). CVD develops in approximately one-half of heterozygous fathers by 55 years of age and in heterozygous mothers by 65 years of age. The premature CVD in relatives provides a strong rationale for the early detection and treatment of children and adolescents with FH (Goldstein et al., 2001).

The homozygous form of FH is rare, affecting 1 per million in the population. Affected children have cholesterol levels that average about 700 mg/dL (18.1 mmol/L), and may reach levels >1000 mg/dL (25.9 mmol/L) (Sprecher et al., 1984). The profoundly elevated LDL cholesterol levels in these children result in physical signs, such as planar xanthomas, that are present by 5 years of age. These occur in the webs of the hands, over the elbows, and over the buttocks. Tendon xanthomas, corneal arcus, and clinically significant CVD are often present by 10 years of age, and aortic stenosis due to atherosclerosis in the valve may also occur (Sprecher et al., 1984).

Familial Combined Hyperlipidemia

Familial combined hyperlipidemia, a more frequent lipid disorder than FH among the adult population, results in increased LDL production. Phenotypic expression is infrequent in children and adolescents, however, and results in mild dyslipoproteinemia. This disorder is thought to be transmitted as an autosomal dominant trait, but no specific genetic mutations have been identified.

Familial Hypertriglyceridemia

Familial hypertriglyceridemia with a normal LDL cholesterol level is a disorder of triglyceride-rich lipoproteins that results in the abnormal production of VLDL cholesterol. Familial hypertriglyceridemia does not predispose individuals to premature CVD. This disease is thought to be an autosomal dominant trait carried by approximately 1.8 in 10,000 persons. Triglyceride levels generally range between 200 mg/dL (2.3 mmol/L) and 500 mg/dL (5.6 mmol/L), and a low high-density lipoprotein (HDL) cholesterol level is often seen.

The hypertriglyceridemia may be due to a deficiency in lipoprotein lipase (Brunzell and Deeb, 2001) or the carrier apolipoprotein (apo) C-II (Cox et al., 1988); the decreased removal of VLDL particles results in the high triglyceride levels. Inherited deficiency of lipoprotein lipase, the enzyme responsible for catabolism of triglycerides in triglyceride-rich lipoproteins, results in a profound increase in chylomicrons. Deficiency of lipoprotein lipase or apo C-II manifests in the same manner clinically. A child or adolescent with this disorder may present with eruptive xanthomas over the mucous membranes or buttocks. Lipemia retinalis and hepatosplenomegaly may also be present. The lipid profile shows marked elevation of chylomicrons and triglycerides. Other disorders resulting in hypertriglyceridemia include hypothyroidism, alcoholism, and diabetes. In a less common form of triglyceride-rich lipoprotein abnormality both chylomicrons and VLDL are elevated. This disease can cause pancreatitis, abdominal pain, glucose intolerance, and hyperuricemia.

Familial Dysbetalipoproteinemia

Familial dysbetalipoproteinemia is due to an underlying defect in apolipoprotein E (Mahley and Rall, 2001) and results in an accumulation of remnants of VLDL and chylomicrons. Clinical manifestations include palmar and tuberous xanthomas. More than 90% of individuals with this disease are homozygous for apo E-2. Triglyceride and cholesterol levels are both elevated. This disorder is not usually seen in childhood.

Familial Decreased HDL

Other primary disorders of lipid and lipoprotein metabolism are associated with deficiencies of HDL cholesterol. Hypoalphalipoproteinemia involves a low HDL cholesterol level most often accompanied by normal triglyceride and LDL cholesterol levels. In families with low HDL cholesterol levels, some affected members may have elevated levels of triglycerides. When triglyceride levels are high (>150 mg/dL; 1.7 mmol/L), the low HDL cholesterol levels may not be a primary defect but rather a result of the hypertriglyceridemia (Deckelbaum et al., 1984). Abnormalities in the gene for the major lipoprotein of HDL, apo A-I, have been detected in some families with hypoalphalipoproteinemia (Schaefer, 1984; Breslow, 1989; Assman, 1990).

Atherogenic Dyslipidemia

A common form of dyslipidemia incorporates three lipid abnormalities: elevated triglycerides; small, dense LDL particles; and reduced HDL cholesterol (Austin et al., 1998; Grundy, 1998; Krauss, 1998). The measurement of small dense LDL particle size is not clinically available except where sophisticated research methods are used. The characteristics of subjects with atherogenic dyslipoproteinemia are abdominal obesity, insulin resistance, and physical inactivity. The high insulin levels found in such subjects have been shown to increase sympathetic nerve tone as well as renal retention of sodium, which may result in higher blood pressure levels (Dyer et al., 1999; Falkner et al., 1999).

Metabolic Syndrome

This syndrome (also referred to as syndrome X) has become more common not only in adults but also in children. Not unlike atherogenic dyslipoproteinemia, the metabolic syndrome is characterized by a constellation of metabolic risk factors in an individual patient (Reaven, 1995; Grundy, 1999). The various risk factors observed include (1) abdominal obesity; (2) atherogenic dyslipidemia; (3) raised blood pressure; (4) insulin resistance and/or glucose intolerance; (5) prothombotic state; and (6) proinflammatory state. This syndrome and its associated risk factors have become as important as other risk factors for premature CVD (U.S. Department of Health and Human Services, 1996; Eckel and Krauss, 1998; National Institutes of Health, 1998; Wilson et al., 1998). Children and adolescents who are obese and hypertensive and have elevated triglycerides and low HDL cholesterol levels may have insulin resistance (Sinaiko et al., 2001; also see Chapter 15).

■ FAMILIAL AGGREGATION OF CHOLESTEROL LEVELS

Cardiovascular disease occurs more frequently in adult members of families in which the children's levels of cholesterol, triglycerides, LDL cholesterol, and apo B or combinations thereof are elevated. The cholesterol levels in children and adolescents aggregate with those of their family members. The prevalence of CVD in adult relatives is significantly increased among children with high cholesterol levels compared to children with normal cholesterol levels (Hennekens et al., 1976; Schrott et al., 1982; Moll et al., 1983; Lee et al., 1986). In addition, when the progeny of young (<55 years of age) CVD victims are examined, more than one-half have dyslipoproteinemia. Familial aggregation of lipid and lipoprotein levels is the result of a shared environment and shared genetic factors.

■ CLINICAL TRIALS OF CHOLESTEROL-LOWERING AGENTS

Clinical trials in adult populations have provided convincing evidence that lowering cholesterol levels through the use of medication or diet reduces CVD risk

(Lipid Research Clinics Program, 1984a, 1984b; Canner et al., 1986; Frick et al., 1987; Carlson and Rosenhamer, 1988). Angiographic trials of cholesterol lowering have reported that progression of atherosclerotic lesions can definitely be slowed, and regression occurs in some patients after lipid lowering (Brensike et al., 1984; Blankenhorn et al., 1987; Brown et al., 1990; Buchwald et al., 1990; Kane et al., 1990; Ornish et al., 1990). No studies have provided direct evidence that lowering cholesterol levels in children and adolescents will reduce their risk of CVD in adulthood. Such studies may never be possible because they would involve following large numbers of children for several decades. The available evidence, however, strongly suggests that the benefit of reducing cholesterol levels in childhood will be realized in adulthood. A number of clinical studies of children and adolescents have shown significant lowering of cholesterol levels with diet (DISC Collaborative Research Group, 1995; Salo et al., 1999). Other studies have shown the safety, efficacy and acceptability of drugs in lowering cholesterol levels in children and adolescents. Such drugs include bile acid sequestrants and hydroxy methyglutaryl-CoA reductase inhibitors—the statins (Stein, 1989; Sinzinger et al., 1992; McCrindle et al., 1997; McCrindle et al., 2002, 2003; Gotto, 2004).

■ STRATEGIES FOR LOWERING CHOLESTEROL LEVELS IN CHILDREN AND ADOLESCENTS

Two strategies have been suggested for lowering cholesterol levels in children and adolescents to prevent or retard the atherosclerotic process: the population approach, and the individualized approach (National Cholesterol Education Program [NCEP], 1991).

■ The Population Approach

The aim of the population approach is to lower the average cholesterol level in all children and adolescents by encouraging their adoption of a diet lower in saturated fat, total fat, and cholesterol. Changes in diet are thus designed as the principal means of preventing CVD. These recommendations are directed to groups that influence the eating patterns of children and adolescents, including schools, health professionals, government agencies, the food industry, and the mass media. The advantage of this approach is that even a small reduction in mean total and LDL cholesterol levels in children and adolescents, if carried into adult life, could substantially decrease the incidence of CVD (Rose, 1985). The National Cholesterol Education Program Expert Panel on Blood Cholesterol Levels in Children and Adolescents (NCEP, 1991) recommended a diet low in saturated fat and cholesterol to lower cholesterol levels and promote primordial prevention in children over 2 years of age as well as in adolescents. There is evidence that such a diet will lower cholesterol levels in children without adversely affecting normal growth and development (DISC, 1995; Salo et al., 1999). The NCEP diet guidelines include the following:

- Adequate nutrition should be achieved by eating a wide variety of foods low in saturated fat and cholesterol.
- Total caloric intake should be sufficient to support normal growth and development and maintain a desirable body weight.
- Saturated fatty acids should provide less than 10% of total calories.
- Total fat should provide an average of no more than 30% and no less than 20% of total calories.
- Polyunsaturated fatty acids should provide up to 10% of total calories.
- Less than 300 mg of cholesterol should be consumed per day.
- Children should consume five or more daily servings of fruits and vegetables.
- Children should consume 6 to 11 daily servings of whole-grain and other grain products daily.
- Children should consume adequate amounts of dietary fiber (child's age + 5 g/day).

■ The Individualized Approach

The individualized approach to cholesterol lowering calls for the cooperative effort of all health professionals. The aim of this approach is to identify and treat children and adolescents who have high cholesterol levels and are at risk of having high cholesterol as adults and thus increased risk of CVD. Figures 7.1 and 7.2 provide flow diagrams for risk assessment and management of children and adolescents, including cut points defining acceptable, borderline, and high levels of total and LDL cholesterol. The NCEP made the following recommendations for selective screening of children and adolescents at high risk in the context of their continuing health care:

- Screen children and adolescents whose parent or grandparent had CVD less than 55 years of age.
- Screen the offspring of a parent who has been found to have a cholesterol level ≥240 mg/dL (6.2 mmol/L).
- For children and adolescents whose parental history is unobtainable, particularly for those with other risk factors, physicians may choose to measure cholesterol levels to identify those in need of individual nutritional and medical advice.
- Optional cholesterol testing may be appropriate in certain children who are judged to be at higher risk for CVD independent of family history. For example, adolescents who smoke, or consume excessive amounts of

saturated fats and cholesterol, and who are overweight may also deserve testing at the discretion of their physician. For parents who do not know their cholesterol levels, pediatricians should arrange for the parents' levels to be measured. If they are elevated, the physician should provide the appropriate counseling to the family.

These recommendations are supported by studies that have shown familial aggregation of CVD, high cholesterol levels, and other risk factors.

The NCEP guidelines did not recommend universal screening in all children because (1) overdiagnosis could result in psychological labeling; (2) there was a potential for overzealous use of medications; and (3) tracking of child-

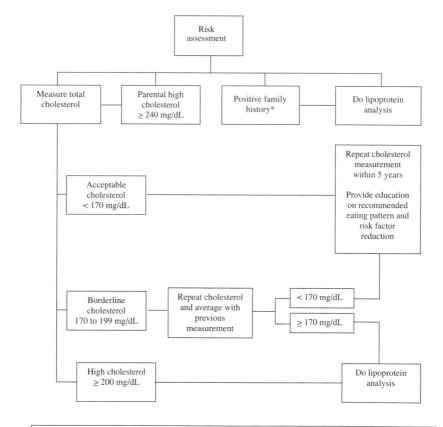

*Defined as a history of premature (< age 55 years) cardiovascular disease in a parent, the sibling of a parent, or a grandparent

FIGURE 7.1
Selective screening of children and adolescents. Algorithm for risk assessment from the National Cholesterol Education Program. Report of the Expert Panel on Blood Cholesterol in Children and Adolescents (NCEP, 1991).

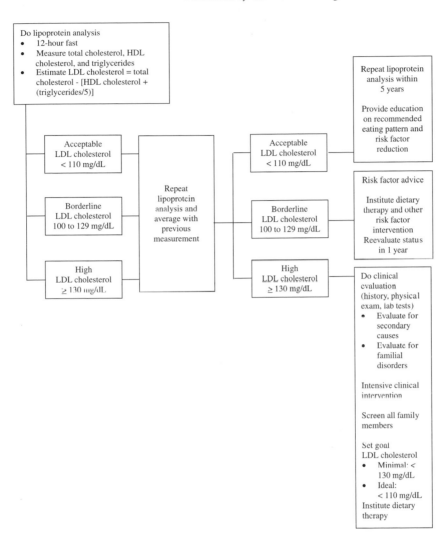

Do lipoprotein analysis
- 12-hour fast
- Measure total cholesterol, HDL cholesterol, and triglycerides
- Estimate LDL cholesterol = total cholesterol - [HDL cholesterol + (triglycerides/5)]

Acceptable LDL cholesterol < 110 mg/dL

Borderline LDL cholesterol 100 to 129 mg/dL

High LDL cholesterol ≥ 130 mg/dL

Repeat lipoprotein analysis and average with previous measurement

Acceptable LDL cholesterol < 110 mg/dL

Borderline LDL cholesterol 100 to 129 mg/dL

High LDL cholesterol ≥ 130 mg/dL

Repeat lipoprotein analysis within 5 years

Provide education on recommended eating pattern and risk factor reduction

Risk factor advice

Institute dietary therapy and other risk factor intervention Reevaluate status in 1 year

Do clinical evaluation (history, physical exam, lab tests)
- Evaluate for secondary causes
- Evaluate for familial disorders

Intensive clinical intervention

Screen all family members

Set goal LDL cholesterol
- Minimal: < 130 mg/dL
- Ideal: < 110 mg/dL
Institute dietary therapy

FIGURE 7.2

Selective screening of children and adolescents. Algorithm for classification of LDL cholesterol levels determined in Figure 7.1, and education and follow-up of children and adolescents with elevated levels. From the National Cholesterol Education Program (NCEP, 1991).

hood cholesterol percentiles into adulthood showed that of children with cholesterol levels above the 90th percentile, only 75% had elevated levels as adults. Those whose levels did not remain high may have changed their dietary habits and activities unnecessarily (Lauer and Clarke, 1990; Stuhldreher et al., 1991).

■ IDENTIFICATION AND MANAGEMENT
OF DYSLIPIDEMIA—WHAT SHOULD BE MEASURED
IN HIGH-RISK CHILDREN AND ADOLESCENTS?

The most complete approach to screening is to obtain a lipoprotein analysis which requires a 12–hour fast. This provides measures of total cholesterol, triglycerides and HDL cholesterol. LDL cholesterol can be calculated when the triglycerides are <400 mg/dL (4.5 mmol/L). Using the Friedewald formula:

$$\text{LDL cholesterol} = \left(\text{Total cholesterol} - \text{HDL cholesterol} - \frac{\text{Triglycerides}}{5} \right)$$

LDL cholesterol can also be directly measured in clinical pathology laboratories. Initial screening for most children and adolescents begins with the measurement of a fasting total cholesterol level (Fig. 7.1). If the total cholesterol level is borderline, a second measurement of total cholesterol should be obtained and averaged with the first measurement. If the average is borderline or high, a lipoprotein analysis should be obtained. Dietary therapy is the initial therapy for children and adolescents with high LDL cholesterol levels (see Chapter 8) and should be considered before pharmacologic therapy.

■ PHARMACOLOGIC THERAPY AFTER DIETARY
THERAPY TO REDUCE CHOLESTEROL LEVELS
IN CHILDREN AND ADOLESCENTS

Several algorithms for drug therapy in children have been recommended (NCEP, 1991; Ose and Tonstad, 1995; Sprecher and Daniels, 1996). We present here the recommendations of the National Cholesterol Education Program's Expert Panel on Blood Cholesterol in Children and Adolescents (NCEP, 1991). The American Heart Association has also provided guidelines for the prevention of cardiovascular disease beginning in childhood (Kavey et al., 2003), including goals for the management of cholesterol levels (Table 7.1). Prior to prescribing drug therapy, secondary causes (Table 7.2) for dyslipidemia (e.g., diabetes, hypothyroidism, obstructive liver disease, chronic renal failure) and use of drugs that increase LDL cholesterol and decrease HDL cholesterol (e.g., progestins, anabolic steroids, and corticosteroids) should be considered. If appropriate, these secondary causes should be treated.

The NCEP guidelines recommend limiting pharmacologic therapy to children ≥10 years of age whose LDL cholesterol levels have not sufficiently decreased after 6 months to 1 year on an adequate trial of diet therapy. For children and adolescents ≥10 years of age, pharmacologic therapy should be considered if the LDL cholesterol level remains ≥160 mg/dL (4.1 mmol/L) and other CVD risk fac-

TABLE 7.1
American Heart Association guidelines for cardiovascular risk
reduction: Intervention for children and adolescents with identified risk

Risk Intervention	Recommendations
Blood Cholesterol Management	
• LDL-C <160 mg/dL (<130 mg/dL is even better) is goal • For patients with diabetes, LDL-C <100 mg/dL is goal	• If LDL-C is above target level, initiate additional therapeutic lifestyle changes, particularly in diet (<7% of calories from saturated fat; <200 mg cholesterol per day), in conjunction with a trained dietitian. • Consider LDL-lowering dietary options (increase soluble fiber by using age [in years] plus 5 to 10 g up to age 15, when the total remains at 25 g/day) in conjunction with a trained dietitian. • Emphasize weight management and increased physical activity. • If LDL-C is persistently above target level, evaluate for secondary causes (thyroid-stimulating hormone, liver function tests, renal function tests, urinalysis). • Consider pharmacologic therapy for individuals with LDL >190 mg/dL with no other risk factors for CVD; or >160 mg/dL with other risk factors present (blood pressure elevation, diabetes, obesity, strong family history of premature CVD). • Bile acid–binding resins or statins are usual first-line agents. • Pharmacologic intervention for dyslipidemia should be done in collaboration with a physician experienced in treatment of disorders of cholesterol in pediatric patients.
Other Lipids and Lipoproteins	
• Fasting TG <150 mg/dL is goal HDL-C >35 mg/dL is goal	• Elevated fasting TG and reduced HDL-C are often seen in the context of overweight with insulin resistance. Therapeutic lifestyle changes should include weight management with appropriate energy intake and expenditure. Decrease intake of simple sugars. • If fasting TG are persistently elevated, evaluate for secondary causes such as diabetes, thyroid disease, renal disease, and alcohol abuse. • No pharmacologic interventions are recommended in children for isolated elevation of fasting TG unless this is very marked (treatment may be initiated at TG > 400 mg/dL to protect against postprandial TG of 1000 mg/dL or greater, which may be associated with an increased risk of pancreatitis).

CVD, cardiovascular disease; HDL-C, high-density lipoprotein cholesterol; LDL, low-density lipoprotein; TG, triglycerides.
Source: Adapted from the National Cholesterol Education Program. Report of the Expert Panel on Blood Cholesterol Levels in Children and Adolescents (NCEP, 1991), and AHA Scientific Statement: American Heart Association Guidelines for Primary Prevention of Atherosclerotic Cardiovascular Disease Beginning in Childhood (Kavey et al., 2003). Reproduced with permission. Copyright © 2003. American Heart Association.

TABLE 7.2
Causes of secondary hypercholesterolemia

Exogenous

Drugs: corticosteroids, isotretinoin (Accutane), thiazides, anticonvulsants, β blockers, anabolic steroids, certain oral contraceptives
Alcohol
Obesity

Endocrine and Metabolic

Hypothyroidism
Diabetes mellitus
Lipodystrophy
Pregnancy
Idiopathic hypercalcemia

Obstructive Liver Disease

Biliary atresia
Biliary cirrhosis

Chronic Renal Disease

Nephrotic syndrome

Storage Diseases

Glycogen storage disease
Sphingolipidoses

Others

Anorexia nervosa
Progeria
Collagen disease
Klinefelter's syndrome

Source: Adapted from the National Cholesterol Education Program, Report of the Expert Panel on Blood Cholesterol Levels in Children and Adolescents (NCEP, 1991).

tors are present (Table 7.3), or if the LDL cholesterol level remains ≥190 mg/dL (4.9 mmol/L) even if no other risk factors are present.

▪ Bile Acid Sequestrants

The NCEP recommended that bile acid sequestrants be the initial drug therapy for children and adolescents (NCEP, 1991; Sprecher and Daniels, 1996). There are several formulations of bile acid–binding resins (Table 7.4), including two powders, colestipol (Colestid) and cholestyramine (Questran). These have

TABLE 7.3
Other risk factors that contribute to earlier onset
of cardiovascular disease

• Family history of premature coronary heart disease, cerebrovascular disease, or occlusive
  peripheral vascular disease (definite onset <55 years of age in a parent, sibling of a parent, or
  grandparent)
• Cigarette smoking
• Elevated blood pressure
• Low HDL cholesterol concentration (<35 mg/dL)
• Severe obesity (≥95th percentile of weight for height)

Source: Adapted from the National Cholesterol Education Program, Report of the Expert Panel
on Blood Cholesterol Levels in Children and Adolescents, (NCEP, 1991).

proven efficacy, relative freedom from side effects, and apparent safety when used
in children and adolescents (West et al., 1980; Kwiterovich, 1986). These powders must be taken along with sufficient liquids to prevent constipation and the
powder can also be mixed with applesauce. If constipation occurs, psyllium (2
to 4 g/day) along with an appropriate amount of liquids is effective treatment
(Sprecher and Daniels, 1996). There is also a tablet formulation of Colestid, although tablets may be difficult for some children to swallow. Each tablet incorporates 1 g of active material. The Colestid powder is smaller in total volume for
the specific amount of active ingredient but is somewhat gritty. There is more
volume in cholestyramine powder and it is less gritty. The suggested starting
dosage of cholestyramine powder resin is 1 to 4 g/day for children and up to 8 g/
day for adolescents. It has been shown that 8 g of cholestyramine per day provides the largest cholesterol reduction. Doses above 8 g/day provide diminish-
ing cholesterol lowering benefit and likely increase the prevalence of side effects
(Superko et al., 1992). The cholestyramine resin may be started at 2 g/day and
increased on the basis of efficacy and tolerance (Sprecher and Daniels, 1996).
An approximate reduction of 5% in LDL cholesterol level is seen with low total
fat and saturated fat and low-cholesterol diets; the reduction in LDL cholesterol
is 15% to 19% with cholestyramine. The bile acid sequestrants are not absorbed
and do not usually cause any systemic difficulties. These agents may result in
decreased absorption of fat-soluble vitamins (vitamins A, D, E, and K) and may
decrease absorption of other medications.

In a study conducted in Norway, cholestyramine was used to treat children
6 to 11 years of age with FH and levels of LDL cholesterol >190 mg/dL (4.9 mmol/
L) or LDL cholesterol >160 mg/dL (4.1 mmol/L) who did not respond well to
diet therapy alone. The children showed normal growth patterns and there was
a significant lowering of LDL cholesterol levels in one-half of the children who
were treated (Tonstad et al., 1996). However, hydroxyvitamin D and folate levels
decreased and homocysteine levels increased in a few subjects.

TABLE 7.4
Pharmacotherapy used for hypercholesterolemia in children and adolescents

Type of Drug	Dosage Available	Adverse Reactions
Bile Acid Sequestrants		
Colestid (colestipol) provided as granules or 1 g tablets	1 packet or 1 level scoopful of Colestid granules contains 5 g colestipol hydrochloride. There is also a 1 gm tablet formulation of Colestid. The dose of the resins is not related to the body weight of a child but to the levels of LDL cholesterol after a trial of diet therapy. Children should be started on the lowest dose of resin possible and then increased one dose at a time to achieve the goal of lowering total and LDL cholesterol levels. Doses of 2–12 g/day divided for children under age 12, and 10–15 g/day divided for those ages 7 to 20 have been suggested. The drugs should be taken before, during, or after a meal when bile acids are present in the intestine.	Colestid granules and flavored Colestid granules should not be taken dry; mix with water or other fluids before ingesting. Phenylketonuria: a 7.5 g dose of flavored Colestid contains 18.2 mg of phenylalanine. Powders or tablets must be taken along with sufficient liquids to prevent constipation. The granules can also be mixed with applesauce. If constipation occurs, psyllium (2–4 g/day) along with an appropriate amount of liquids is effective. Tablets may be difficult for some children to swallow.
Cholestyramine (Questran) provided as a powder 1 package contains 4 g	The suggested starting dosage of cholestyramine powder resin is 1 to 4 g/day for children, and up to 8 g/day for adolescents. It has been shown that 8 g of cholestyramine per day provides the largest cholesterol reduction. Tablets of cholestyramine are no longer available. Doses of 375 mg capsules and 625 mg tablets Available for adults	The powder must be taken along with sufficient liquids to prevent constipation. The powder can also be mixed with applesauce. If constipation occurs, psyllium (2–4 gms/day) along with an appropriate amount of liquids is effective.
Colesevelam (Welchol) The long-term safety and effectiveness have not been established in children and adolescents.		May cause difficulty in swallowing and/or intestinal problems May interfere with absorption of fat-soluble vitamins Has not been tested in children

Inhibitors of Lipoprotein Production and Function

Nicotinic acid (niacin) immediate release Niaspan (niacin) sustained release	Crystalline nicotinic acid tablets (immediate release) are provided in 1.5 to 3 g tablets. Doses of niacin should be gradually titrated up to a maximum dose of 10 mg/kg/day divided into three doses. Niaspan tablets (sustained release) are available in 500, 750, and 1000 mg to be taken at bedtime. OTC niacin sustained-release or controlled-release tablets are available in 125, 250, and 400 mg strengths. These are sold as nutrition supplements and are not FDA-approved for treatment of hypercholesterolemia	Doses of nicotinic acid that lower cholesterol levels frequently cause flushing and may cause liver dysfunction, requiring liver function testing to observe whether the dose of niacin should be decreased or treatment stopped. ASA taken 1 hour prior to niacin can decrease flushing. Tolerance to flushing occurs over several weeks. Pruritis and gastrointestinal distress also reduce slowly with increasing doses of niacin and by avoiding administration on an empty stomach.

HMG-CoA Reductase Inhibitors

Simvastatin (Zocor) The long term safety and effectiveness have not been established in children, but have been shown in adolescents.	Available in 5, 10, 20, 40, and 80 mg tablets. Dosage is started low and increased as required to lower cholesterol. Bile acid sequestrants have been combined with pravastatin or lovastatin to enhance lowering of LDL cholesterol and triglyceride levels and to increase HDL cholesterol levels.	Patients on statins should be advised of the risk of myopathy. If muscle pains occur, measures of CK should be obtained. With increasing doses, liver dysfunction may occur. Thus measures of liver function should be obtained prior to drug use and again 6 to 12 weeks after initiation of therapy, or initiation of higher doses and periodically thereafter (e.g., every 6 months).

Inhibitor of Cholesterol Absorption

Zetia (Ezetimibe) The long-term safety and effectiveness have not been established in children and adolescents.	Zetia is provided in 10 mg tablets. The suggested dose is 1 tablet per day.	None described in children or adolescents.

ASA, acetylsalicyclic acid; CK, choline kinase; FDA, Food and Drug Administration (U.S.); HDL, high-density lipoprotein; LDL, low-density lipoprotein; OTC, over-the-counter.

Colesevelam (Welchol) was recently approved by the U.S. Food and Drug Administration (FDA) for use in lowering cholesterol levels in adults (Table 7.4). It also belongs to the bile acid resin class of drugs. In adults, Welchol has been tested as monotherapy or in combination with statins (HMG-CoA reductase inhibitors). The long-term safety and effectiveness of Welchol in children and adolescents have not yet been established.

■ Nicotinic Acid (Niacin)

When LDL cholesterol levels cannot be reduced sufficiently with bile acid sequestrants, niacin (immediate-release) (Table 7.4) has been used in children with FH. The dose necessary to lower cholesterol, however, often results in side effects such as day-time flushing and may cause liver function abnormalities (in about 10%). In adults flushing has been ameliorated by acetylsalicyclic acid (ASA) prior to niacin ingestion. In children, however, ASA use has been associated with Reye's syndrome. Therefore, nicotinic acid therapy requires perseverance and careful follow-up. Nicotinic acid has been used in adults in doses up to 3 to 6 g of product. In children the maximum is 10 mg/kg/day divided. There are listings for over-the-counter (OTC) niacin sustained-release or controlled-release tablets and capsules in 125, 250, and 400 mg strengths. These are sold as supplements and are not FDA approved for the treatment of hypercholesterolemia. The latter doses may be used to gradually increase the dose of sustained-release niacin. Niaspan (sustained-release) may be given to children if extremely high cholesterol levels warrant higher doses. Niaspan is available in three tablet strengths containing 500, 750, and 1000 mg niacin. To maximize bioavailability and reduce the risk of gastrointestinal upset, the administration of Niaspan with a low-fat meal or snack is recommended. Patients receiving nicotinic acid should have periodic measures of aminotransferases.

■ HMG-CoA Reductase Inhibitors

Some children and adolescents are unable to continue with daily doses of bile acid sequestrants because of their unwillingness to ingest the resin suspension. In these circumstances, some practitioners have recommended the use of 3-hydroxy-3-methylglutaryl-coenzyme A (HMG-CoA) reductase inhibitors. In children ≥10 years of age and older, particularly those over ≥15 years of age, who have LDL cholesterol levels ≥190 mg/dL and a family history of premature CVD, these statin agents have been used to reduce LDL cholesterol levels. In large drug trials in adult populations they have been shown to reduce LDL cholesterol levels and result in a significant decrease in not only CVD mortality but also all-cause mortality (Ducobu et al., 1992; Sinzinger et al., 1992; Lambert et al., 1996).

A number of clinical trials of statins support their safety and efficacy in children and adolescents. In the Canadian Lovastatin in Children Study, boys ≤17 years of age and younger with FH were assigned doses ranging from 10 to 40 mg/day. A reduction in LDL cholesterol of 21% to 36% was observed (Lambert et al., 1996). A number of other clinical investigations in children and adolescents have shown similar results (Stein, 1989; Ducobu et al., 1992; Coleman and Watson, 1996; Sanjad et al., 1997; Couture et al., 1998; Stefanutti et al., 1999). LDL cholesterol levels of male and female children with heterozygous FH were reduced by 23% to 33% after 12 weeks of therapy with pravastatin (5 to 20 mg/day) (Knipscheer et al., 1996). A multicenter double-blind, placebo-controlled, randomized trial of lovastatin conducted in the United States and Finland (10 to 40 mg/day) in 10- to 17-year-old males with heterozygous FH showed LDL cholesterol reductions of up to 27% without significant adverse events (Stein et al., 1999). A similar study of simvastatin (10 to 40 mg/day) in boys and girls showed LDL cholesterol reduction of 41% without adverse events (de Jongh et al., 2002). A multicenter randomized placebo-controlled trial demonstrated the safety and efficacy of atorvostatin. (10 to 20 mg/day) in children and adolescents with FH or severe hypercholesterolemia as well as LDL cholesterol reduction of 40% (McCrindle et al., 2003).

The use of these drugs has been associated with reversible elevations of hepatic amino transferases and muscle enzymes in adolescents and adults. Thus, creatine phosphokinase and aminotransferase levels should be measured periodically in patients receiving HMG-CoA reductase inhibitors (Sprecher and Daniels, 1996). In adolescent females with the potential for pregnancy, statins should be used cautiously because their teratogenic effect is unknown. Bile acid sequestrants have also been combined with statins, pravastatin or lovastatin, in doses of 2.5 to 5.0 mg/day. The statin–bile acid sequestrant combination can reduce LDL cholesterol levels by 17% (McCrindle et al., 2002).

A randomized, double-blind, placebo-controlled trial of pravastatin (20 to 40 mg/day) was conducted in more than 200 children and adolescents 8 to 18 years of age with FH (Wiegman et al., 2004). Two years of therapy induced a significant regression of carotid atherosclerosis, with no adverse effects on growth, sexual maturation, hormone levels, or liver or muscle tissue. LDL cholesterol levels were reduced by 24% in the pravastatin-treated group.

▧ Zetia (Eztimibe)

Zetia is in a class of lipid-lowering compounds that selectively inhibit the intestinal absorption of cholesterol and related phytosterols. In patients with hypercholeterolemia Zetia reduces total and LDL cholesterol, apo B, and tryglycerides and increases HDL cholesterol. By inhibiting the absorption of cholesterol by the small intestine Zetia reduces blood cholesterol, but it does not inhibit cholesterol synthesis in the liver or increase bile acid excretion. It appears to localize and act at the brush border of the small intestine, inhibiting the absorption of cholesterol, leading to a decrease in the delivery of intestinal cholesterol to the liver. This process causes a reduction of hepatic cholesterol stores and an increase of clearance from the blood. Zetia can be complementary to HMG-CoA reductase inhibitors. The long-term safety and effectiveness of Zetia in children and adolescents have not yet been established.

■ SUMMARY

- High total cholesterol, LDL cholesterol, and VLDL cholesterol levels and low HDL cholesterol levels are associated with the extent of atherosclerotic lesions in adolescents and young adults.
- High cholesterol levels aggregate in families as a result of shared environmental and genetic factors.
- Children and adolescents with elevated cholesterol levels, particularly LDL cholesterol levels, are frequently members of families in which there is a high incidence of CVD among adult relatives.
- Children and adolescents with high cholesterol levels are more likely than the general population to have high levels as adults.
- Two combined strategies have been suggested to lower cholesterol levels: (1) the population approach, serving as a major means to prevent CVD in a population later in life, recommends a diet low in total fat, saturated fat, and cholesterol for the entire population; and (2) the individualized approach, which requires the identification of children and adolescents at high risk for elevated cholesterol levels and increased risk for CVD in adult life.
- Identification of those at high risk is accomplished by measuring cholesterol levels in the children of families in which a parent or grandparent has been diagnosed with CVD at age 55 years or younger, or families in which a parent has a total cholesterol level ≥240 mg/dL. These children often (50%) have significantly elevated cholesterol levels and require dietary counseling. If diet therapy does not result in sufficient lowering of cholesterol levels after 6 to 12 months, drug therapy should be considered if LDL cholesterol level remains ≥160 mg/dL and two or more CVD risk factors (obesity, hypertension, smoking, diabetes, and physical inactivity) are present; or LDL cholesterol level remains ≥190 mg/dL even if no other risk factors are present.
- Because of potential side effects, and with consideration of the age at onset of atherosclerosis, bile acid–sequestering agents, nicotinic acid, and HMG-CoA reductase inhibitors are not recommended for routine use in children under 10 years of age.
- Children and adolescents who undergo drug therapy should be followed initially every 6 weeks to 3 months and subsequently every 3 to 6 months.

• If drug therapy is required, it should be given with careful management and follow-up because the safety and efficacy in children for some agents have yet to be established. Drug dosage should be started at low levels and gradually increased to bring about the appropriate levels of LDL cholesterol.

▧ REFERENCES

Assman, G. 1990. Genes and Dyslipoproteinemias. *Eur Heart J* 11(Suppl H):4–8.

Austin, M.A., J.E. Hokanson, and K.L. Edwards. 1998. Hypertriglyceridemia as a Cardio-vascular Risk Factor. *Am J Cardiol* 81:7B–12B.

Berenson, G.S., S.R. Srinivasan, W. Bao, W.P. Newman, III, R.E. Tracy, and W.A. Wattigney. 1998. Association between Multiple Cardiovascular Risk Factors and Arteriosclerosis in Children and Young Adults. *N Engl J Med* 338:1650–6.

Blankenhorn, D.H., S.A. Nessim, R.L. Johnson, M.E. Sanmarco, S.P. Azen, and L. Cashin-Hemphill. 1987. Beneficial Effects of Combined Colestipol-Niacin Therapy on Coronary Atherosclerosis and Coronary Venous Bypass Grafts. *JAMA* 257:3233–40.

Brensike, J.F., R.I. Levy, S.F. Kelsey, E.R. Passamani, J.M. Richardson, I.K. Loh, N.J. Stone, R.F. Aldrich, J.W. Battaglini, D.J. Moriarty, M.R. Fisher, L. Friedman, W. Friedewald, K.M. Detre; and S.E. Epstein. 1984. Effects of Therapy with Cholestyramine on Progression of Coronary Arteriosclerosis: Results of the NHLBI Type II Coronary Intervention Study. *Circulation* 69:313–24.

Breslow, J.L. 1989. Genetic Basis of Lipoprotein Disorders. *J Clin Invest* 84:373–80.

Breslow, J.L. 2000. Genetics of Lipoprotein Abnormalities Associated with Coronary Heart Disease Susceptibility. *Annu Rev Genet* 34:233–54.

Brown, G., J.J. Albers, L.D. Fisher, S.M. Schaefer, J.T. Lin, C. Kaplan, X.Q. Zhao, B.D. Bisson, V.F. Fitzpatrick, and H.T. Dodge. 1990. Regression of Coronary Artery Disease as a Result of Intensive Lipid-Lowering Therapy in Men with High Levels of Apolipoprotein B. *N Engl J Med* 323:1289–98.

Brunzell, J.D., and S.S. Deeb. 2001. Familial Lipoprotein Lipase Deficiency and Other Causes of the Chylomicronemia Syndrome. In: *The Metabolic Basis of Inherited Disease*, 8th ed. Edited by C.R. Scriver, A.L. Beaudet, W.S. Sly, D. Valle, B. Childs, K.W. Kinzler, and B. Vogelstein. New York: McGraw-Hill, pp. 2789–815.

Buchwald, H., R.L. Varco, J.P. Matts, J.M. Long, L.L. Fitch, G.S. Campbell, M.B. Pearce, A.E. Yellin, W.A. Edmiston, R.D. Smink, Jr., H.S. Sawin, Jr., C.T. Campos, B.J. Hansen, N. Tuna, J.N. Karnegis, M.E. San Marco, K. Amplatz, W.R. Castaneda-Zuniga, D.W. Hunter, J.K. Bissett, F.J. Weber, J.W. Stevenson, A.S. Leon, T.C. Chalmers, and POSCH Group. 1990. Effect of Partial Ileal Bypass Surgery on Mortality and Morbidity from Coronary Heart Disease in Patients with Hypercholesterolemia. Report of the Program on the Surgical Control of the Hyperlipidemias (POSCH). *N Engl J Med* 323: 946–55.

Canner, P.L., K.G. Berge, N.K. Wenger, J. Stamler, L. Friedman, R.J. Prineas, and W. Friedewald. 1986. Fifteen Year Mortality in Coronary Drug Project Patients: Long-Term Benefit with Niacin. *J Am Coll Cardiol* 8:1245–55.

Carlson, L.A., and G. Rosenhamer. 1988. Reduction of Mortality in the Stockholm Ischaemic Heart Disease Secondary Prevention Study by Combined Treatment with Clofibrate and Nicotinic Acid. *Act Med Scand* 223:405–18.

Civeira, F., and The International Panel on Management of Familial Hypercholesterolemia. 2004. Guidelines for the Diagnosis and Management of Heterozygous Familial Hyper-cholesterolemia. *Atherosclerosis* 173:55–68.

Coleman, J.E., and A.R. Watson. 1996. Hyperlipidemia, Diet and Simvastatin Therapy in Steroid-Resistant Nephrotic Syndrome of Childhood. *Pediatr Nephrol* 10:171–4.

Couture, P., L.D. Brun, F. Szots, M. Lelievre, D. Gaudet, J.P. Despres, J. Simard, P.J. Lupien, and C. Gagne. 1998. Association of Specific LDL Receptor Gene Mutations with Differential Plasma Lipoprotein Response to Simvastatin in Young French Canadians with Heterozygous Familial Hypercholesterolemia. *Arterioscler Thromb Vasc Biol* 18:1007–12.

Cox, D.W., D.E. Wills, F. Quan, and P.N. Ray. 1988. A Deletion of One Nucleotide Results in Functional Deficiency of Apolipoprotein CII (Apo CII). *J Med Genet* 25:649–52.

Davies, H. 1990. Atherogenesis and the Coronary Arteries in Childhood. *Int J Cardiol* 28:283–91.

Deckelbaum, R.J., E. Granot, Y. Oschry, L. Rose, and S. Eisenberg. 1984. Plasma Triglyceride Determines Structure-Composition in Low and High Density Lipoproteins. *Arteriosclerosis* 4:225–31.

de Jongh, S., L. Ose, T. Szamosi, C. Gange, M. Lambert, R. Scott, P. Perron, D. Dobbelaere, M. Saborio, M.B. Tuohy, M. Stepanavage, A. Sapre, B. Gumbiner, M. Mercuri, A.S.P. van Trotsenburg, H.D. Bakker, and J.J.P. Kastelein. 2002. Efficacy and Safety of Statin Therapy in Children with Familial Hypercholesterolemia: A Randomized, Double-Blind, Placebo-Controlled Trial with Simvastatin. *Circulation* 106:2231–7.

DISC Collaborative Research Group. 1995. The Efficacy and Safety of Lowering Dietary Intake of Total Fat, Saturated Fat, and Cholesterol in Children with Elevated LDL-Cholesterol: The Dietary Intervention Study in Children (DISC). *JAMA* 273:1429–35.

Ducobu, J., D. Brasseur, J.M. Chaudron, J.P. Deslypere, C. Harvengt, E. Muls, and M. Thomson. 1992. Simvastatin Use in Children. *Lancet* 339:1488.

Dyer, A.R., K. Liu, M. Walsh, C. Keife, D.R. Jacobs, Jr., and D.E. Bild. 1999. Ten-Year Incidence of Elevated Blood Pressure and its Predictors: The CARDIA Study (Coronary Artery Risk Development in (Young) Adults). *J Hum Hypertens* 13:13–21.

Eckel, R.H., and R.M. Krauss. 1998. American Heart Association Call to Action: Obesity as a Major Risk Factor for Coronary Heart Disease. AHA Nutrition Committee. *Circulation* 97:2099–100.

Falkner, B., K. Sherif, A.E. Sumner, and H. Kushner. 1999. Blood Pressure Increase with Impaired Glucose Tolerance in Young Adult American Blacks. *Hypertension* 34:1086–90.

Freedman, D.S., W.P Newman, III, R.E. Tracy, A.E. Voors, S.R. Srinivasen, L.S. Webber, C. Restrepo, J.P. Strong and G.S. Berenson. 1988. Black-White Differences in Aortic Fatty Streaks in Adolescence and Early Adulthood: The Bogalusa Study. *Circulation* 77:856–64.

Frick, M.H., M.O. Elo, K. Haapa, O.P. Heinonen, P. Heinsalmi, P. Helo, J.K. Huttunen, P. Kaitaniemi, P. Koskinen, V. Manninen, H. Maenpaa, M. Malkonen, M. Manttar, S. Norda, A. Pasternack, J. Pikkarainen, M. Romo, T. Sjoblom, and E. Nikkila. 1987. Helsinki Heart Study: Primary-Prevention Trial with Gemfibrozil in Middle-Aged Men with Dyslipidemia. Safety of Treatment, Changes in Risk Factors, and Incidence of Coronary Heart Disease. *N Engl J Med* 317:1237–45.

Goldstein, J.L., H. Hobbs, and M.S. Brown. 2001. Familial Hypercholesterolemia. In: *The Metabolic Basis of Inherited Disease*, 8th ed. Edited by C.R. Scriver, A.L. Beaudet, W.S. Sly, D. Valle, B. Childs, K.W. Kinzler, and B. Vogelstein. New York: McGraw-Hill, pp. 2863–911.

Gotto, Jr., A.M. 2004. Targeting High-Risk Young Patients for Statin Therapy. *JAMA* 292:377–8

Grundy, S.M. 1998. Hypertriglyceridemia, Atherogenic Dyslipidemia, and the Metabolic Syndrome. *Am J Cardiol* 81:18B–25B.

Grundy, S.M. 1999. Hypertriglyceridemia, Insulin Resistance, and the Metabolic Syndrome. *Am J Cardiol* 83:25F–29F.

Haust, M.D. 1990. The Genesis of Atherosclerosis in the Pediatric Age-Group. *Pediatr Pathol* 10:253–71.

Hennekens, C.H., M.J. Jesse, B.E. Klein, J.E. Gourly, and S. Blumenthal. 1976. Cholesterol among Children of Men with Myocardial Infarction. *Pediatrics* 58:211–7.

Kane, J.P., M.J. Malloy, T.A. Ports, N.R. Phillips, J.C. Diehl, and R.J. Havel. 1990. Regression of Coronary Atherosclerosis during Treatment of Familial Hypercholesterolemia with Combined Drug Regimens. *JAMA* 264:3007–12.

Kavey, R-E.W., S.R. Daniels R.M. Lauer, D.L. Atkins, L.L. Hayman, and K. Taubert. 2003. American Heart Association Guidelines for Primary Prevention of Atherosclerotic Cardiovascular Disease Beginning in Childhood. *Circulation* 107:1562–66.

Knipscheer, H.C., C.C. Boelen, J.J. Kastelein, D.E. van Diermen, B.E. Groenemeijer, A. van den Ende, H.R. Buller, and H.D. Bakker. 1996. Short-Term Efficacy and Safety of Pravastatin in 72 children with Familial Hypercholesterolemia. *Pediatr Res* 39:867–71.

Krauss, R.M. 1998. Atherogenicity of Triglyceride-Rich Lipoproteins. *Am J Cardiol* 81:13B–17B.

Kwiterovich, Jr., P.O. 1986. Bile Acid Sequestrant Resin Therapy in Children. In: *Pharmacologic Control of Hyperlipidemia*. Edited by R. Fears. Barcelona: Prouse Science Publishers, pp. 55–66.

Kwiterovich, Jr., P.O. 1989. Pediatric Implications of Heterozygous Familial Hypercholesterolemia. Screening and Dietary Treatment. *Arteriosclerosis* 9(Suppl I):I-111–I-20.

Kwiterovich, Jr., P.O. 1996. Disorders of Lipid and Lipoprotein Metabolism. In: *Pediatrics*, 20th ed. Edited by A.M. Rudolph, J.I.E. Hoffman, and C.D. Rudolph. Norwalk, CT: Appleton & Lange, pp. 343–51.

Kwiterovich, Jr., P.O. 2002. Clinical Relevance of the Biochemical, Metabolic, and Genetic Factors that Influence Low-Density Lipoprotein Heterogeneity. *Am J Cardiol* 90(Suppl): 30i–47i.

Kwiterovich, Jr., P.O., D.S. Fredrickson, and R.I. Levy. 1974. Familial Hypercholesterolemia (One Form of Familial Type II Hyperlipoproteinemia). A Study of its Biochemical, Genetic, and Clinical Presentation in Childhood. *J Clin Invest* 53:1237–49.

Lagstrom, H., H. Niinikoski, H. Lapinlcimu, J. Viikari, T. Ronnemaa, and O. Simell. 1998. Modifying Coronary Heart Disease Risk Factors in Children: Is it Ever too Early to Start? *JAMA* 279:1261–2.

Lambert, M., P.J. Lupin, C. Gagne, E. Levy, S. Blaichman, S. Langlois, M. Hayden, V. Rose, J.T. Clarke, B.M. Wolfe, C. Clarson, H. Parsons, D.K. Stephure, D. Potvin, and J.Lambert. 1996. Treatment of Familial Hypercholesterolemia in Children and Adolescents: Effect of Lovastatin. Canadian Lovastatin in Children Study Group. *Pediatrics* 97:619–28.

Lauer, R.M., and W.R. Clarke. 1990. Use of Cholesterol Measurements in Childhood for the Prediction of Adult Hypercholesterolemia: The Muscatine Study. *JAMA* 264:3034–8.

Lee, J., R.M. Lauer, and W.R. Clarke. 1986. Lipoproteins in the Progeny of Young Men with Coronary Artery Disease: Children with Increased Risk. *Pediatrics* 78:330–7.

Leren, T.P., K. Solberg, O.K. Rodningen, S. Tonstad, and L. Ose. 1994. Two Founder Mutations in the LDL Receptor Gene in Norwegian Familial Hypercholesterolemia Subjects. *Atherosclerosis* 111:175–82.

Lipid Research Clinics Program. 1984a. The Lipid Research Clinics Coronary Primary Prevention Trial Results. I. Reduction in Incidence of Coronary Heart Disease. *JAMA* 251:351–64.

Lipid Research Clinics Program. 1984b. The Lipid Research Clinics Coronary Primary Prevention Trial Results. II. The Relationship of Reduction in Incidence of Coronary Heart Disease to Cholesterol Lowering. *JAMA* 251:365–74.

Mahley, R.W., and S.C. Rall, Jr. 2001. Type III Hyperlipoproteinemia (Dysbetalipoproteinemia): Role of Apolipoprotein E in Normal and Abnormal Lipoprotein Metabolism. In: *The Metabolic Basis of Inherited Disease*, 8th ed. Edited by C.R. Scriver, A.L. Beaudet, W.S. Sly, D. Valle, B. Childs, K.W. Kinzler, and B. Vogelstein. New York: McGraw-Hill, pp. 2835–61.

McCrindle, B.W., E. Helden, G. Cullen-Dean, and W.T. Conner. 2002. A Randomized Cross-over Trial of Combination Pharmacologic Therapy in Children with Familial Hyperlipidemia. *Pediatr Res* 51:715–21.

McCrindle, B.W., M.B. O'Neill. G. Cullen-Dean, and E. Helden. 1997. Acceptability and Compliance with Two Forms of Cholestyramine in the Treatment of Hypercholesterolemia in Children: A Randomized Crossover Trial. *J Pediatr* 130:266–73.

McCrindle B.W., L. Ose, and A.D. Marais. 2003. Efficacy and Safety of Atorvostatin in Children and Adolescents with Familial Hypercholesterolemia or Severe Hyperlipidemia: A Muticenter, Randomized, Placebo-Controlled Trial. *J Pediatr* 143:74–80.

Moll, P.P., C.F. Sing, W.H. Weidman, H. Gordon, R.D. Ellefson, P.A. Hodgson, and B.A. Kottke. 1983. Total Cholesterol and Lipoproteins in School Children: Prediction of Coronary Heart Disease in Adult Relatives. *Circulation* 67:127–34.

[NCEP] National Cholesterol Education Program. 1991. Report of the Expert Panel on Blood Cholesterol Levels in Children and Adolescents. Bethesda, MD: U.S. Department of Health and Human Services, National Institutes of Health, National Heart, Lung and Blood Institute. NIH Publication 91–2732.

National Institutes of Health. 1998. Clinical Guidelines on the Identification, Evaluation, and Treatment of Overweight and Obesity in Adults—The Evidence Report. Bethesda, MD: National Heart, Lung, and Blood Institute. NIH Publ. No. 98–4083.

Newman, III, W.P., D.S. Freedman, A.W. Voors, P.D. Gard, S.R. Srinivasan, J.L. Cresanta, G.D. Williamson, L.S. Weber, and G.S. Berenson. 1986. Relation of Serum Lipoprotein Levels and Systolic Blood Pressure to Early Atherosclerosis: The Bogalusa Heart Study. *N Engl J Med* 314:138–44.

Ornish, D., S.E. Brown, L.W. Scherwitz, J.H. Billings, W.T. Armstrong, T.A., Ports, S.M. McLanahan, R.L. Kirkeeide, R.J. Brand and K.L. Gould. 1990. Can Lifestyle Changes Reverse Coronary Heart Disease? The Lifestyle Heart Trial. *Lancet* 336:129–33.

Ose, L. 2002. Familial Hypercholesterolemia from Children to Adults. *Cardiovasc Drug Ther* 16:289–93.

Ose, L., and S. Tonstad. 1995. The Detection and Management of Dyslipidemia in Children and Adolescents. *Acta Paediatr* 84:1213–5.

PDAY Research Group. 1990. Relationship of Atherosclerosis in Young Men to Serum Lipoprotein Cholesterol Concentration and Smoking: A Preliminary Report from the Pathological Determinants of Atherosclerosis in Youth (PDAY) Research Group. *JAMA* 264:3018–24.

Reaven, G.M. 1995. Pathophysiology of Insulin Resistance in Human Disease. *Physiol Rev* 75:473–86.

Rose, G. 1985. Sick Individuals and Sick Populations. *Int J Epidemiol* 14:32–8.

Salo, P., J. Viikari, M. Hamalainen, H. Lapinleimu, T. Routi, T. Ronnemaa, R. Seppanen, E. Jokinen, I. Valimaki, and O. Simell. 1999. Serum Cholesterol Ester Fatty Acids in 7- and 13-Month-Old Children in a Prospective Randomized Trial of a Low-Saturated Fat, Low-Cholesterol Diet: The STRIP Baby Project. Special Turku Coronary Risk Factor Intervention Project for Children. *Acta Paediatr* 88:505–12.

Sanjad, S.A., A. al-Abbad, and S. al-Shorafa. 1997. Management of Hyperlipidemia in Children with Refractory Nephrotic Syndrome: The Effect of Statin Therapy. *J Pediatr* 130: 470–4.

Schaefer, E.J. 1984. Clinical, Biochemical, and Genetic Features in Familial Disorders of High Density Lipoprotein Deficiency. *Arteriosclerosis* 4:303–22.

Schrott, H.G., W.R. Clarke, P. Abrahams, D.A. Wiebe, and R.M. Lauer. 1982. Coronary Artery Disease Mortality in Relatives of Hypertriglyceridemic School Children: The Muscatine Study. *Circulation* 65:300–5.

Sinaiko, A.R., D.R. Jacobs, Jr., J. Steinberger, A. Moran, R. Luepker, A.P. Rocchini, and R.J. Prineas 2001. Insulin Resistance Syndrome in Childhood: Associations of the

Euglycemic Insulin Clamp and Fasting Insulin with Fatness and Other Risk Factors. *J Pediatr* 139:700–7.

Sinzinger, H., P. Schmid, C.H. Pirich, I. Virgolini, B. Pesau, S. Granegger, and J. O'Grady. 1992. Treatment of Hypercholesterolemia in Children. *Lancet* 340:548–9.

Sprecher, D.L., and S.R. Daniels. 1996. Rational Approach to Pharmacologic Reduction of Cholesterol Levels in Children. *J Pediatr* 129:4–7.

Sprecher, D.L., E.J. Schaefer, K.M. Kent, R.E. Gregg, L.A. Zech, J.M. Hoeg, B. McManus, W.C. Roberts, and H.B. Brewer, Jr. 1984. Cardiovascular Features of Homozygous Familial Hypercholesterolemia: Analysis of 16 Patients. *Am J Cardiol* 54:20–30.

Stefanutti, C., G. Lucani, A. Vivenzio, and S. Di Giacomo. 1999. Diet Only and Diet Plus Simvastatin in the Treatment of Heterozygous Familial Hypercholesterolemia in Childhood. *Drug Exp Clin Res* 25:23–8.

Stein, E.A. 1989. Treatment of Familial Hypercholesterolemia with Drugs in Children. *Arteriosclerosis* 9(Suppl I):I-145–I-51.

Stein, E.A., D.R. Illingworth, P.O. Kwiterovich, Jr., C.A. Liacouras, M.A. Siimes, M.S. Jacobson, T.G. Brewster, P. Hopkins, M. Davidson, K. Graham, F. Arensman, R.H. Knopp, C. DuJovne, C.L. Williams, J.L. Isaacsohn, C.A. Jacobsen, P.M. Laskarzewski, S. Ames, and G.J. Gormley. 1999. Efficacy and Safety of Lovastatin in Adolescent Males with Heterozygous Familial Hypercholesterolemia: A Randomized Controlled Trial. *JAMA* 281:137–44.

Stuhldreher, W.L., Orchard, T.J., R.P. Donohue, L.H. Kuller, M.F. Gloninger, and A.L. Drash. 1991. Cholesterol Screening in Childhood: the 16–Year Beaver County Lipid Study Experience. *J Pediatr* 119:551–6.

Superko, H.R., P. Greenland, R.A. Manchester, N.A. Andreadis, G. Schectman, N.H. West, D. Hunninghaka, W.L. Haskell, and J.L. Probstfield. 1992. Effectiveness of Low-Dose Colestipol Therapy in Patients with Moderate Hypercholesterolemia. *Am J Cardiol* 70:135–40.

Tonstad, S., J. Knudtzon., M. Siversten, H. Refsum, and L. Ose. 1996. Efficacy and Safety of Cholestyramine in Prepubertal Children with Familial Hypercholesterolemia. *J Pediatr* 129:42–9.

U.S. Department of Health and Human Services. 1996. *Physical Activity and Health: A Report of the Surgeon General.* Atlanta, GA: U.S. Department of Health and Human Services, Centers for Disease Control and Prevention. National Center for Chronic Disease Prevention and Health Promotion.

West R.J., J.K. Lloyd, and J.V. Leonard. 1980. Long-Term Follow-Up of Children with Familial Hypercholesterolaemia Treated with Cholestyramine. *Lancet* :316:873–5.

Wiegman, A., B.A. Hutten, E. de Groot, J. Rodenburg, H.D. Bakker, H.R. Buller, E.J.G. Sijbrands, and J.J.P. Kastelein. 2004. Efficacy and Safety of Statin Therapy in Children with Familial Hypercholesterolemia. *JAMA* 292:331–7.

Wilson, P.W., R.B. D'Agostino, D. Levy, A.M. Belanger, H. Silbershatz, and W.B. Kannel. 1998. Prediction of Coronary Heart Disease Using Risk Factor Categories. *Circulation* 97:1837–47.

CHAPTER **8**

Dietary Management of Children and Adolescents with High Cholesterol

Linda Snetselaar and Ronald M. Lauer

Dietary change for managing hyperlipidemia in children and adolescents is key to the treatment of a condition that tracks into adulthood with associated morbidity and mortality end points. Studies that have focused on eating habits and parental control (Birch and Fisher, 1998) and on dietary intervention, such as the Dietary Intervention Study in Children (DISC) (1995), have taught us a great deal about behavior change. This chapter reviews information from population-oriented studies like DISC and discusses the individualized approach to changing eating habits of children. Parental control issues and strategies for altering eating behaviors in children and adolescents are also discussed.

▪ THE POPULATION APPROACH

In the population approach, the aim is to lower the average population levels of blood lipids by changing eating habits of children in a safe, acceptable, and efficacious manner. The DISC study showed that cholesterol-lowering diets administered through a population intervention approach are safe in children. The objective was to assess the efficacy, safety and acceptability of lowering dietary intake in total fat, saturated fat, and cholesterol to decrease low-density lipoprotein (LDL) cholesterol levels in children (DISC Collaborative Research Group, 1995). This six-center randomized, controlled, clinical trial included hypercholesterolemic prepubertal boys ($n = 362$) and girls ($n = 301$), 8 to 10 years of age, with LDL cholesterol levels ≥80th and <98th percentiles for age and sex, who were randomized into an intervention group ($n = 334$) and a usual-care group ($n = 329$). Dietary intervention included instruction in behavioral change to promote adherence. Figure 8.1 shows the DISC dietary prescription which included <75 mg/1000 kcal per day of cholesterol (not to exceed 150 mg/day).

The main outcome measure was LDL cholesterol level, with primary safety measures of height and serum ferritin levels at 3 years. Secondary efficacy outcomes were LDL cholesterol at 1 year and total cholesterol at 1 and 3 years. Secondary safety outcomes included red blood cell folate; serum zinc, retinal, and albumin levels; serum high-density lipoprotein (HDL) cholesterol, LDL/HDL cholesterol ratio, and total triglycerides; sexual maturation; and psychosocial health.

From baseline to year 1, the decrease in LDL cholesterol was greater in the intervention group than in the usual-care group (Fig. 8.2). After 3 years, dietary total fat (28.6% kcal), saturated fat (10.2% kcal), and cholesterol (95 mg/1000 kcal) decreased significantly in the intervention group compared to levels in the usual-care group. No significant difference ($p > 0.05$) resulted between the groups in adjusted mean height, serum ferritin, or other safety outcomes.

The DISC study demonstrated that dietary intervention is effective in achieving a modest lowering of LDL cholesterol over 3 years while maintaining adequate growth, iron stores, nutritional adequacy, and psychological well-being during the critical growth period of adolescence. The DISC study also provided support for the long-term safety, efficacy, and acceptability of lower-fat diets in high-risk pubertal children. The National Cholesterol Education Program (NCEP III) panel findings (NCEP, 1992) are in line with the DISC results. Shown in Table 8.1 are the macronutrient levels for an initial treatment strategy for children and adolescents with hyperlipidemia; the corollary food-based advice is described in Table 8.2. The dietary changes required to impact serum lipid levels in the population at large are described in Table 8.3.

Additionally, research shows that dietary modifications for cardiovascular disease (CVD) are more effective if exercise is combined with changes in eating habits (Dietz, 1998). The CARDIA Study compared the role of fiber to that of

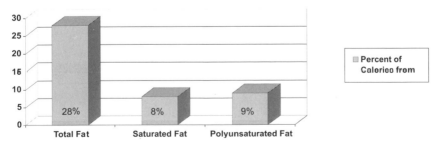

FIGURE 8.1
The Dietary Intervention Study in Children (DISC) dietary prescription.

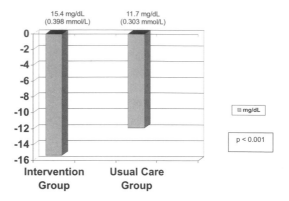

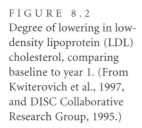

FIGURE 8.2
Degree of lowering in low-density lipoprotein (LDL) cholesterol, comparing baseline to year 1. (From Kwiterovich et al., 1997, and DISC Collaborative Research Group, 1995.)

fat and other major dietary components in the development of hyperinsulinemia, obesity, and other CVD risk factors in young healthy adults. It showed the positive effects of high-fiber diets and the importance of controlled consumption of dairy products for reduction in risk of type 2 diabetes (Pereira et al., 2002). Needless to say, the formation of healthy eating habits begins early in life.

■ THE INDIVIDUALIZED APPROACH

The individualized approach to lowering cholesterol depends on the cooperation of a team of health care professionals to identify and treat children and

TABLE 8.1
Macronutrient recommendations for therapeutic lifestyle changes

Component	Recommendation
Saturated fat	Less than 7% of total calories
Polyunsaturated fat	Up to 10% of total calories
Monounsaturated fat	Up to 20% of total calories
Total fat	25% to 35% of total calories*
Carbohydrate†	50% to 60% of total calories*
Dietary fiber	20 to 30 g /day
Protein	Approximately 15% of total calories

*ATP III allows an increase of total fat to 35% of total calories and a reduction in carbohydrates to 50% for persons with the metabolic syndrome.
†Carbohydrates should derive predominantly from foods rich in complex carbohydrates, including grain—especially whole grains—fruits, and vegetables.
Source: National Cholesterol Education Program, Adult Treatment Panel III; see www.nhlbi.nih.gov/guidelines/cholesterol/atp3_rpt.htm.

TABLE 8.2
Food-based advice for therapeutic lifestyle changes diet

Food Items to Choose More Often	Food Items to Choose Less Often
Breads and Cereals	
≥6 servings per day, adjusted to caloric needs	Many bakery products, including doughnuts, biscuits, butter croissants, Danish, pies, cookies
Breads, cereals, especially whole grain; pasta; rice; potatoes; dry beans and peas; low-fat crackers and cookies	Many grain-based snacks, including chips, cheese puffs, snack mix, regular crackers, buttered popcorn
Vegetables and Fruits	
3 to 5 servings of vegetables per day fresh, frozen, or canned, without added fat, sauce, or salt	Vegetables fried or prepared with butter, cheese, or cream sauce
2 to 4 servings of fruits per day fresh, frozen, canned, or dried	Fruits fried or served with butter or cream
Dairy Products	
2 to 3 servings per day of fat-free, ½% or 1% milk, buttermilk, yogurt, cottage cheese; fat-free and low-fat cheese	Whole or 2% milk, whole-milk yogurt, ice cream, cream, cheese
Eggs	
≤2 egg yolks per week Egg whites or egg substitute	Egg yolks, whole eggs
Meat, Fish, and Poultry	
≤5 oz per day Lean cuts: loin, leg, round Extra lean hamburger; cold cuts made with lean meat or soy protein; skinless poultry; fish	Higher-fat meat cuts: ribs, T-bone steak, regular hamburger, bacon, sausage Cold cuts: salami, bologna, hot dogs Organ meats: liver, brains, sweetbreads Poultry with skin; fried meat; fried poultry; fried fish
Fats and oils	
Amount adjusted to caloric level: unsaturated oils; soft or liquid margarines and vegetable oil spreads, salad dressings, seeds, and nuts	Butter, shortening, stick margarine, chocolate, coconut

Source: National Cholesterol Education Program, Adult Treatment Panel III; see www.nhlbi.nih.gov/guidelines/cholesterol/atp3_rpt.htm.

TABLE 8.3
Dietary CAGE questions for assessment of intake of saturated fat
and cholesterol

C	Cheese (and other sources of dairy fats—whole milk*, ice cream, cream, cream cheese, whole-fat yogurt)
A	Animal fats (hamburger, ground meat, frankfurters, bologna, salami, sausage, fried foods, fatty cuts of meat)
G	Got it away from home (high-fat meals either purchased and brought home or eaten in restaurants)
E	eat (extra) high-fat commercial products: candy, pastries, pies, doughnuts, cookies

*In infants, use of skim milk can reduce the intake of linoleic acid to less than half of that recommended. Therefore, it is currently recommended that skim milk be avoided prior to 1 year of age (American Academy of Pediatrics, 1983; Martinez et al., 1985; Ryan et al., 1987).
Source: National Cholesterol Education Program, Adult Treatment Panel III; see www.nhlbi.nih.gov/guidelines/cholesterol/atp3_rpt.htm.

adolescents at high risk of having elevated cholesterol levels and eventual CVD later as adults. Children with a family history of CVD should be screened in their regular health care setting. The application of nutrition interventions in this individualized approach depends on an understanding of infant feeding practices and food preferences from infancy to adolescence.

■ INFANT FEEDING PRACTICES AND FOOD PREFERENCES

Research has demonstrated that an infant's experience of flavor in their mother's milk or in formula affects their acceptance of foods. One study showed that infants who experienced the flavor of carrots in mother's milk spent less time feeding when given carrot-flavored cereal. This may mean that infants are less responsive to a flavor that they were exposed to in the recent past (Mennella and Beauchamp, 1999). Infants fed carrots or a variety of vegetables ate more of the carrots after the exposure period. This study also showed that daily experience with fruit initially enhanced the infants' acceptance of carrots (Gerrish and Mennalla, 2001). Another study showed that infants' preferences for flavored cereal correlated with their mothers' reported willingness to eat novel foods and flavors (Mennella and Beauchamp, 1997).

■ CHILDHOOD FOOD PREFERENCES

Birch and colleagues have identified ways in which children form food preferences (Birch and Fisher, 1998) and note that children's food preferences relate to parental involvement in their children's learning experiences about food. The determination of preference in young children may include time to experience a food. If encounters with a food are positive and repetitive, lasting preferences are formed (Birch and Marlin, 1982; Birch et al., 1982, 1987; Sullivan and Birch, 1990, 1994). Thus development of childhood preferences for healthy foods may require changes in parental behavior in food selection and preparation.

Well-meaning parents may force eating habits on small children to increase their consumption of lower-fat foods. Such child-feeding techniques that encourage children to eat specific foods can result in a negative preference for those foods (Birch and Marlin, 1982; Birch et al., 1982, 1984; Newman and Taylor 1992). For example, often when low-fat diets are recommended, parents will encourage children to eat more fruits and vegetables. Researchers have noted, however, that when parents force their children to eat vegetables the children have a lower preference for vegetables (Hertzler, 1983).

Often parents will withhold foods they feel are high in saturated fat or sugar with the good intention of forming healthy eating habits (Eppright et al., 1972; Stanek et al., 1990). Researchers have documented that limiting a food used as a reward increased the child's preference for that food (Birch et al., 1980). They also found that when the mother restricted a food, it was more likely to be eaten in an "unrestricted" setting, such as a friend's home (Birch and Marlin, 1982; Birch et al., 1982).

Achieving a lower fat intake may be a challenge to parents trying to alter their children's intake. Because children eat foods they like and avoid foods they dislike, food preferences are especially important in determining what is eaten (Birch, 1979a, 1979b; Domel et al., 1993, 1996; Fisher and Birch, 1995). Fisher and Birch (1995) served the same diet consisting of ≈33% of calories from fat to a group of children. The actual fat intake, however, ranged from 25% to 42% of energy, showing the importance of food preference on actual eating habits.

Studies of toddlers have shown that repeated opportunities to consume new foods result in increased preference and intake of that food (Birch and Marlin, 1982; Birch et al., 1982, 1990; Sullivan and Birch, 1990, 1994). Often 5 to 10 exposures are required. These findings underscore the importance of early experience with foods and food acceptance; children like and eat what is familiar.

Child feeding practices that encourage restricting foods may decrease a child's use of appetite as a signal to eat or to stop eating, thus affecting the amount of total calories eaten (Birch et al., 1991, 1993). When children are rewarded for eating, their responsiveness to the energy content of the foods, dictated by appetite, decreases (Birch et al., 1987).

An alternate way to control child feeding practices requires a division of responsibility. The parent is responsible for supplying the child with a healthful selection of foods and a positive, upbeat eating atmosphere. The child is responsible for deciding when and how much to eat (Satter, 1986, 1996).

■ ASSESSING CHILDREN'S EATING HABITS

With this knowledge of early childhood eating preferences and how they are formed, we move to childhood with its existing habits and preferences. Knowing what a child currently eats can be a guide to where change in eating behavior might occur.

A variety of methods exist to assess children's eating habits. Van Horn and colleagues (1993) have described their experience of assessing fat intake in children in the DISC study. Prior to the dietary intake assessment in DISC, most studies reported that children younger than 10 years of age had difficulty identifying foods, remembering what they ate, and estimating portion sizes (Meredith et al., 1951; Eppright et al., 1952; Emmons and Hayes, 1973; Frank et al., 1977; Persson and Carlgren, 1984; Baranowski et al., 1986). Researchers have now applied the same techniques used in adults to collect children's dietary data, including a parent's version of intake (Eck et al., 1989; Treiber et al., 1990). One study found that for school-age children, a combination of the parent's observations and the child's recall offered the most complete and accurate data (Eck et al., 1989). Standardized training results in comparable information for both children's self-report and the parent's recall of their child's intake (Van Horn et al., 1990). This training becomes more important when children consume many meals away from home, as they grow older.

■ CHANGING DIETARY HABITS OF ADOLESCENTS

The DISC study began by focusing on group-based dietary intervention. In the initial stages of the study, this type of education-based intervention worked well. As the study progressed, dietary adherence began to decrease. To solve this problem more focused interventions with motivational interviewing strategies based on the transtheoretical model of change were initiated (Prochaska and DiClemente, 1982). This model includes tailored approaches. First, detailed individual feedback looking at compliance over time is assessed by the adolescent. Second, the adolescent is asked to evaluate his or her adherence to diet by selecting a degree of adherence between 1 and 12 on a ruler. With this information the nutrition counselor assigns a category: 1, ready to change; 2, not ready to change; or 3, unsure of readiness to change.

This method of achieving behavior change is especially appropriate for adolescents, as they are typically in an exploratory or initiation phase with health-compromising behaviors (Jaffe et al., 1988). During this time in their lives, adolescents progress through stages of behavior initiation, acquiring habits that parallel key concepts in the stages of change model (Werch and DiClemente, 1994). Researchers have shown that motivational interviewing is beneficial in early stages of change (Rollnick and Morgan, 1991; Grimley et al., 1995), thus it may be equally beneficial for adolescents who are considering experimenting with or changing a behavior.

As adolescents struggle to acquire an identity separate from their family and other adults, they commonly resist and resent persons in positions of authority and turn their attention to peers for approval and reinforcement (Christopher et al., 1993). Because motivational interviewing has at its core the patient-centered helping style, it provides opportunities to increase adolescents' sense of control over their lives, thus circumventing the usual resistance to adult figures (Tober, 1991).

Motivational interviewing can be tailored to the individual needs and attitudes of adolescents, including having little patience for things in which they have no interest. This model allows the behavioral intervention to focus on unique needs, circumstances, and readiness to change. Use of motivational interviewing in the DISC study showed that it could be beneficial, as eating behaviors to reduce intake of total fat and specifically saturated fat were successfully modified (Berg-Smith et al., 1999).

Initially, the assessment involves determining a person's level of readiness to change level (ready, unsure, not ready). Using a ruler or just a scale concept the interviewer asks, "On a scale of 1 to 12, how ready are you to make new changes to eat less fat?" (1 = not ready to change; 12 = very ready to change).

During an interview adolescents may move from one readiness-to-change category to another. This means that the caregiver must be ready to move back and forth between category-specific strategies. Clues that an adolescent has changed the readiness to change category might be confusion, detachment, or resistance during discussions. Such clues are the caregiver's prompt to determine if readiness to change has lessened; tailoring the discussion to a different stage of change as necessary.

It is crucial to remember that every counseling session does not have to end with adolescent agreement. A decision to think about change is a successful conclusion to a motivational interviewing session.

■ Counseling Sessions for Individuals
Not Ready to Change

The not-ready-to-change intervention involves three goals: (1) facilitating the adolescent's ability to consider change; (2) reducing the adolescent's resistance to the change; and (3) identifying steps to change that are tailored to the individual adolescent's needs. Several communication skills that will help in achieving these goals include open-ended questions, reflective listening, affirming, summarizing, and eliciting self-motivational statements, all discussed below.

An open-ended question requires more than a "yes" or "no" answer. It is answered by explaining or discussing a particular topic. Examples of open-ended questions are the following:

• Tell me how your dietary change experiences are going."
• "What do you like about the changes you have made so far in your diet? What problems are connected with making these changes?"

Listening in a reflective way involves identifying feelings that surface during a description of problems that result from changing eating habits. This type of listening is more than just paraphrasing words an adolescent has spoken. Reflective listening includes a guess at what the adolescent feels, restated as a statement, not a question. Through this skill, what the adolescent feels is communicated and then paraphrased as a statement. Use of this skill enables the nutrition counselor to more fully understand true adolescent feelings. For example:

Adolescent: "I really want to do well with my diet but my friends seem to entice me to eat out and their selection of places is not a good fit for my new eating pattern."
Caregiver: "You feel frustrated because you really want to change your eating habits but at the same time you want to be spontaneous with friends."

Adolescents often feel at odds with authority figures and see adults as less than supportive. Through the skill of affirmation, the counselor tells the adolescent that he or she understands and is with the adolescent in difficult times when diet change is not easy. Another important concept is normalization: the caregiver tells the adolescent that he or she is perfectly within reason and that it is very normal to have such reactions and feelings. For example:

• "I know that it is difficult for you to talk with me about this problem you are having with dietary change, but thank you for making this effort."
• "You have had an incredible schedule with sports, academics and being the lead in your school play. I feel that you have done extremely well given your circumstances."
• "Many of the teens I talk with express the same problems. I can understand why you are having difficulty."

Summarizing key concepts discussed during the session ensures that the counselor understands issues that are often complex. A summarizing statement will help an adolescent only if it is simple and straightforward. In the case of teens, the summary may often involve descriptions of negative feelings.

The four communication skills described above are important to the final strategy, eliciting self-motivational statements. The goals of these statements are threefold:

1. To acknowledge that a problem exists, for example:
   "I know that your friends are always eating out after school, what specifically makes this a problem for you?"

"Tell me from your point of view as a teen, in what ways following your diet has been a problem."

2. To acknowledge that there is concern about the problem, for example:

"When you give in to your teenage friends and eat high fat foods, how do you feel?"

"Describe your concerns when you just can't eat what you would like to eat after a basketball game."

"What are your concerns if you don't make a change in the foods you are eating?"

3. To affirm that in the future, positive steps can be taken to correct the problem, for example:

"If you could eat in a way that is healthy all the time, what would need to be different for you?"

"What do you see as advantages to making dietary changes that reduce saturated fat?"

"If you decided to make a change in late night snacking while you study, what would need to happen?"

"You have done many things in sports that require devotion and dedication. What makes you think that if you decided to make a change you could do it?"

"What encourages you to change if you want to?"

"If you decided to change, what strategies would help you maintain that change?"

It is important to be tentative when approaching a teen about problem eating behaviors: "Would you be willing to continue our discussion and talk about the possibility of change?" To allow time for a thoughtful discussion about eating habits, the counselor should ask open-ended questions or command statements, such as the following:

- "Tell me why you picked _____ on the ruler."
- "What would need to happen for you to move from a 3 to a 12 on the ruler? What might I do to help you get there?"

Teens are very responsive to helping, attentive adults. To demonstrate this helping attitude the counselor should summarize statements about (1) past progress, (2) difficulties, (3) reasons for change, and (4) what would help in moving forward. This summarization will allow the teen to rethink the rationale for change.

Counselors often strive for goal setting behaviors in adolescents. In this stage of change, forcing goal setting behaviors will only cause feelings of defeat for both the teen and counselor. To address this frustration, the counselor might say something like the following:

"I can understand why this is a difficult time for you to make changes in your eating habits. Just being able to state the problems you are having is a very positive step forward. Things do change in our lives. When you are ready to discuss changes I am always available. Based on decisions you have made in the past, I know you will come back to me when the time is right."

A crucial topic to cover prior to ending the session is the confidence and hope you have in the teen's ability to make changes. A follow-up contact should be established.

As counselors, dealing with teens can be frustrating. Counselors should avoid the urge to push, coax, persuade, confront, or direct the adolescent. Moving from one stage of change to another for a teen may not occur in the office setting. One should *not* expect a teen to commit to major changes during a visit. In fact, in this stage it may mean that the teen is merely trying to please the counselor. In summary, the counselor should strive for an open, caring environment that allows the teen to feel in control of making changes related to eating habits.

■ Counseling Sessions for Individuals
Unsure about Change

The goal in this stage is to build readiness to change, so that major steps can be taken to alter dietary adherence. In this stage, teens are ambivalent about making a change in their eating habits. To explore this ambivalence, the counselor should ask the teen to list the pros and cons of making changes in eating habits. For example:

• "Tell me some of the things you like about old higher-saturated fat eating habits."
• "What are some of the good things about changing your eating habits?"

The caregiver's goal is to help the teen consider change. This will occur by guiding the teen to a discussion about what life might be like after a change. By anticipating the advantages and disadvantages of modifying eating habits, the teen has the chance to see both sides of the issue of dietary change. To generate a discussion with the teen, the caregiver might begin with the following:

"I can see why you're not totally sure of making new or additional changes in the way you eat. Imagine that you decided to make a change. What could that be like and what specifically would you want to do?"

Finally, the nutrition counselor should summarize the positive and negative aspects of making a change and include statements that describe potential plans for change.

It is important to negotiate change with the teen. Initially, the counselor should set broad goals, with specific goals to follow, with questions such as "How would you like things to be different?" and "What do you want to change?"

The teen might be asked to list strategies for dietary change. If one does not work, others might. Then the teen is asked to formulate a plan and write it down. To conclude the session, the counselor can ask, "What do you plan to do between now and the next visit?"

The final statement should give the teen courage to make decisions: "I will not force you into achieving your goals. You have said that you are unsure. Take your time and know that I am always available to help you."

Counseling Sessions for Individuals Ready to Change

Meeting the goal of this stage requires collaboration with the teen to set a plan for action. The nutrition counselor should facilitate this plan by providing tools to use in meeting goals.

Questioning about change involves helping the teen confirm and rationalize the decision to make a change. Using the ruler again, the counselor can ask, "Why did you choose a 3 instead of a 1 or a 12? Give me some ideas for why you think you are ready to change."

The counselor should focus on helping the teen identify a first step in making a change: "What specifically could you do at school to make a change in your eating habits? Is this a truly workable plan? How will things be different for you if you make these changes?"

Goal setting becomes very important in this stage. Often teens will want to push ahead too fast. Realistic and achievable short-term goals are important. So, the counselor might suggest, "Let's do things gradually. What is a short-term goal that you know is positioned for success?"

Following the setting of a short-term achievable goal, the specifics of how to be successful should be mapped out and barriers to success identified. Doing this early will allow the teen to formulate ideas to overcome barriers or avoid them. It is important to identify supportive family and friends to call on when eating healthful foods becomes a problem. It is also important to help the teen identify when a plan is successful. The teen should be asked to write down the plan for future discussions.

Finally, the session is closed by the counselor giving encouraging comments and praising the teen for identifying the specifics of the plan, with emphasis on the fact that the teen is the expert on his or her own behavior: "You have come so far. It's clear that you are an expert on what is good for you. Keep in mind that change is gradual. If this plan doesn't work, there are others to try."

As with all of the stages, the counselor should avoid giving advice. It is critical that the teen be allowed to express ideas for goals that will achieve the greatest success. The counselor should encourage the teen to feel in control of changing eating behaviors. "I could give you a variety of goals, but what do you think will work best for you?"

In summary, changing eating habits for teens who have elevated lipids can be a highly successful endeavor. Keys to positive change include allowing the teen to make decisions about how to alter eating habits, proceeding gradually with change, and emphasizing that goal setting should depend on a teen's specific category of readiness to change. Specific goals should be set only when the teen is ready to change.

■ SUMMARY

* Dealing with dietary change in pediatric age groups requires an understanding of current eating habits.
* Preferences for which food to select are formed when the infant moves from bottle to solid food.
* As the child becomes older, changing behavior may require special motivational skills that set the stage for positive eating behaviors targeting prevention of the eventual problems associated with hyperlipidemia.

Sample meals that are reduced in fat are available from the National Heart, Lung and Blood Institute (2000). In these sample meals for families, whole grains, fruits, and vegetables are emphasized.

■ REFERENCES

American Academy of Pediatrics, Committee on Nutrition. 1983. *Pediatrics* 72:253–5.

Baranowski, T., R. Dwarkin, J.C. Henske, D.R. Clearman, J.K. Dunn, P.R. Nader, and P.C. Hooks.·1986. The Accuracy of Children's Self Reports of Diet: Family Health Project. *J Am Diet Assoc* 86:1381–5.

Berg-Smith, S.M., V.J. Stevens, K.M. Brown, L. Van Horn, N. Gernhofer, E. Peters, R. Greenberg, L. Snetselaar, L. Ahrens, and K. Smith, for the Dietary Intervention Study in Children (DISC) Research Group. 1999. A Brief Motivational Intervention to Improve Dietary Adherence in Adolescents. *Health Educ Res* 14:399–410.

Birch, L.L. 1979a. Dimensions of Preschool Children's Food Preferences. *J Nutr Educ* 11:77–80.

Birch, L.L. 1979b. Preschool Children's Food Preferences and Consumptions Patterns. *J Nutr Educ* 11:189–92.

Birch, L.L., D. Birch, D. Marlin, and L. Kramer. 1982. Effects of Instrumental Eating on Children's Food Preferences. *Appetite* 3:125–34.

Birch, L.L., and J.O. Fisher. 1998. Development of Eating Behaviors among Children and Adolescents. *Pediatrics* 101:539–49.

Birch, L.L., S.L. Johnson, G. Andersen, J.C. Peters, and M.C. Schulte. 1991. The Variability of Young Children's Energy Intake. *N Engl J Med* 324:232–5.

Birch, L.L., S.L. Johnson, M.B. Jones, and J.C. Peters. 1993. Effects of a Non-Energy Fat Substitute on Children's Energy and Macronutritient Intake. *Am J Clin Nutr* 58:326–33.

Birch, L.L., and D.W. Marlin. 1982. I Don't Like It; I Never Tried It: Effects of Exposure to Food on Two-Year-Old Children's Food Preferences. *Appetite* 4:353–60.

Birch, L.L., D.W. Marlin, and J. Rotter. 1984. Eating as the "Means" Activity in a Contingency: Effects on Young Children's Food Preference. *Child Dev* 55:432–9.

Birch, L.L., L. McPhee, B.C. Shoba, E. Pirok, and L. Steinberg. 1990. What Kind of Exposure Reduces Children's Food Neophobia? *Appetite* 26:546–51.

Birch, L.L., L. McPhee, B.C. Shoba, L. Steinberg, and R. Krehbrel. 1987. Clean Up Your Plate: Effects of Child Feeding Practices on the Conditioning of Meal Size. *Learn Motiv* 18:301–17.

Birch, L.L., S. Zimmerman, and H. Hind. 1980. The Influences of Social-Affective Context on Preschool Children's Food Preferences. *Child Dev* 51:856–61.

Christopher, J., D. Nangle, and D. Hansen. 1993. Social Skills Interventions with Adolescents. *Behav Mod* 17:314–38.

Dietz, Jr., W.H. 1998. Health Consequences of Obesity in Youth: Childhood Predictors of Adult Disease. *Pediatrics* 101:549–54.

DISC Collaborative Research Group. 1995. Efficacy and Safety of Lowering Dietary Intake of Total Fat, Saturated Fat, and Cholesterol in Children with Elevated LDL-Cholesterol: The Dietary Intervention Study in Children (DISC). *JAMA* 273:1429–35.

Domel, S.B., T. Baronowski, H. Davis, S.B. Leonard, P. Riley, and J. Baronowski. 1993. Measuring Fruit and Vegetable Preferences among 4th and 5th Grade Students. *Prev Med* 22:866–79.

Domel, S.B., W.O. Thomson, H.C. Davis, T. Baronowski, S.B. Leonard, and J. Baronowski. 1996. Psychosocial Predictors of Fruit and Vegetable Consumption among Elementary School Children. *Health Educ Res* 11:299–308.

Eck, L.H., R.C. Klesges, and C.L. Hanson. 1989. Recall of a Child's Intake from One Meal: Are Parents Accurate? *J Am Diet Assoc* 89:784–9.

Emmons, L., and M. Hayes. 1973. Accuracy of 24-hr Recalls of Young Children. *J Am Diet Assoc* 62:409–15.

Eppright, E.S., H.M. Fox, B.A. Fyer, G.H. Lamkin, V.M. Vivian, and E.S. Fuller. 1972. Nutrition of Infants and Preschool Children in the North Central Region of the United States of America. *World Rev Nutr Diet* 14:269–332.

Eppright, E.S., M.B. Patton, A.L. Marlatt, and M.L. Hathaways. 1952. Dietary Study Methods, V: Some Problems in Collecting Dietary Information about Groups of Children. *J Am Diet Assoc* 28:43–8.

Fisher, J.A., and L.L. Birch. 1995. Three to 5 Year-Old Children's Fat Preferences and Fat Consumption are Related to Parental Adiposity. *J Am Diet Assoc* 95:759–64.

Frank, G., G.S. Berenson, P.E. Schilling, and M.C. Moore. 1977. Adapting the 24-hr Recall for Epidemiologic Studies of School Children. *J Am Diet Assoc* 71:26–31.

Gerrish, C.J., and J.A. Mannella. 2001. Flavor Variety Enhances Food Acceptance in Formula-Fed Infants. *Am J Clin Nutr* 73:1080–5.

Grimley, D., V. Prochaska, W. Velicer, and G. Prochaska. 1995. Contraception and Condom Use Adoption and Maintenance: A Stage Paradigm Approach. *Health Educ Quart* 22:20–35.

Hertzler, A.A. 1983. Children's Food Patterns—A Review. II. Family and Group Behavior. *J Am Diet Assoc* 83:555–60.

Jaffe, A., S. Radius, and M. Gall. 1988. Health Counseling for Adolescents: What They Want, What They Get and Who Gives It. *Pediatrics* 82:481–5.

Kwiterovich., Jr., P.O., B.A. Barton, R.P. McMahon, E. Obarzanek, S. Hunsberger, D. Simons-Morton, S.Y. Kimm, L.A. Friedman, N. Lasser, A. Robson, R. Lauer, V. Stevens, L. Van Horn, S. Gidding, L. Snetselaar, V.W. Hartmuller, M. Greenlick, and F. Franklin, Jr. 1997. Effects of Diet and Sexual Maturation on Low-Density Lipoprotein Cholesterol during Puberty: The Dietary Intervention Study in Children (DISC). *Circulation* 96:2526–33.

Martinez, G.A., A.S. Ryan, and D.J. Malec. 1985. Nutrient Intakes of American Infants and Children Fed Cow's Milk or Infant Formula. *Am J Dis Child* 139:1010–8.

Mennella, J.A., and G.K. Beauchamp. 1997. Mothers' Milk Enhances the Acceptance of Cereal during Weaning. *Pediatr Res* 41:188–92.

Mennella, J.A., and G.K. Beauchamp. 1999. Experience with a Flavor in Mother's Milk Modifies the Infant Acceptance of Flavored Cereal. *Dev Psychobiol* 35:197–203.

Meredith, A., A. Matthews, M. Zickefoose, E. Weagley, M. Wayave, and E.G. Brown. 1951. How Well Do School Children Recall What they Have Eaten?" *J Am Diet Assoc* 27:749–51.

[NCEP] National Cholesterol Education Program. 1992. Highlights of the Report of the Expert Panel on Blood Cholesterol Levels in Children and Adolescents. *Pediatrics* 89:495–501.

National Heart, Lung, and Blood Institute. 2000. The Practical Guide. Identification, Evaluation, and Treatment of Overweight and Obesity in Adults. NIH Publication 00–4084. Available at: http://emall.nhlbihin.net.

Newman, J., and A. Taylor. 1992. Effect of a Means: End Contingency on Young Children's Food Preferences. *J Exp Child Psychol* 64:200–16.

Pereira, M.A., D.R. Jacobs, L. Van Horn, M.L. Slattery, A.I. Kartashov, and D.S. Ludwig. 2002. Dairy Consumption, Obesity, and the Insulin Resistance Syndrome in Young Adults: The CARDIA Study. *JAMA* 287:2081–9.

Persson, L.A., and G. Carlgren. 1984. Measuring Children's Diets: Evaluation of Dietary Assessment Techniques in Infancy and Childhood. *Int J Epidemiol* 13:506–17.

Prochaska, J., and C. DiClemente. 1982. Transtheoretical Therapy: Toward a More Integrative Model of Change. *Psychother Theory Res Prac* 19:276–88.

Rollnick, S., and M. Morgan. 1991. Motivational Interviewing: Increasing Readiness to Change. In *Psychotherapy and Substance Abuse: A Practitioner's Handbook*. Edited by A.M. Washton. New York: Guilford Press, pp. 179–91.

Ryan, A.S., G.A. Martinez, and F.W. Kreiger. 1987. Feeding Low-Fat Milk during Infancy. *Am J Phys Anthropol* 73:539–48.

Satter, E.M. 1986. The Feeding Relationship. *J Am Diet Assoc* 86:352–6.

Satter, E.M. 1996. Internal Regulation and the Evaluation of Normal Growth as a Basis for Prevention of Obesity in Children. *J Am Diet Assoc* 96:860–4.

Stanek, K., D. Abbott, and S. Cramer. 1990. Diet Quality and the Eating Environment of Preschool Children. *J Am Diet Assoc* 90:1582–6.

Sullivan, S., and L. Birch. 1990. Pass the Sugar; Pass the Salt: Experience Dictates Preference. *Dev Psychol* 26:546–51.

Sullivan, S.A., and L.L. Birch. 1994. Infant Dietary Experience and Acceptance of Solid Food. *Pediatrics* 93:271–7.

Tober, G. 1991. Motivational Interviewing with Young People. In: *Motivational Interviewing*. Edited by W.R. Miller and S. Rollnick. New York: Guilford Press, pp. 248–59.

Treiber, F., S. Leonard, G. Frank, L. Musante, H. Davis, W. Strong, and M. Levy. 1990. Dietary Assessment Instruments for Preschool Children: Reliability of Parental Responses to the 24-Hour Recall and Food Frequency Questionnaire. *J Am Diet Assoc* 90:814–20.

Van Horn, L., N. Gernhofer, A. Moag-Stahlberg, R. Farris, G. Hartmuller, V. Lasser, P. Stumbo, S. Craddick, and C. Ballew. 1990. Dietary Assessment in Children using Electronic Methods: Telephones and Tape Recorders. *J Am Diet Assoc* 90:412–6.

Van Horn, L.V., P. Stumbo, A. Moag-Stahlberg, E. Obarzanek, V. Hartmuller, R.P. Farris, S.Y.S. Kimm, L. Frederick, L. Snetselaar, and K. Liu. 1993. The Dietary Intervention Study in Children (DISC): Dietary Assessment Methods for 8–10 Year-Olds. *J Am Diet Assoc* 93:1396–403.

Werch, C.H., and C.C. DiClemente. 1994. A Multi-component Stage Model for Matching Drug Prevention Strategies and Messages to Youth Stage of Use. *Health Educ Res* 9:37–46.

Blood Pressure in Childhood and Adolescence

CHAPTER 9

The Epidemiology of Childhood Blood Pressure

Trudy L. Burns and Stephen R. Daniels

In adults, high blood pressure has been associated with cerebrovascular disease, myocardial infarction, renal disease, and other cardiovascular end points (MacMahon et al., 1990). In the Framingham Study, blood pressure was positively associated with the annual incidence of coronary heart disease, ischemic cerebrovascular disease, congestive heart failure, and intermittent claudication when subjects were followed over an 18-year period (Kannel, 1975). A 10 mmHg increase in systolic blood pressure (SBP) was associated with a 20% increase in age-adjusted risk of cardiovascular events in the age group 35 to 64 years and a 13% increase in the age group 65 to 94 years (Kannel, 1998). Similar increases in risk were associated with a 10 mmHg increase in diastolic blood pressure (DBP). In the Seven Countries Study, there was a significant association ($r = 0.69$) between SBP and the 10-year age-standardized rates of coronary death (Keys, 1980). Hypertension is second only to diabetes mellitus as a cause of end-stage renal disease (National High Blood Pressure Education Program, 1996). As many as 1 billion individuals worldwide are estimated to have high blood pressure, which is associated with the highest attributable risk of death throughout the world (World Health Organization, 2002).

The mechanism by which blood pressure elevation contributes to the process of development of cardiovascular disease is not completely known. One possibility is the fact that elevated blood pressure causes greater shear stress on the endothelium, which results in injury and dysfunction. This effect may be increased when endothelial cell membranes are stiffened due to increased blood levels of low-density lipoprotein cholesterol. In this setting, high pressure and turbulent blood flow may result in injury to endothelial cells and ultimately a denuded endothelium. This may be the substrate for the development of atherosclerotic plaques.

The etiology of human hypertension is heterogeneous. It can be classified as primary (also called essential) or secondary. Secondary hypertension occurs as part of a defined process such as renal artery stenosis. The pathophysiology of primary hypertension is also heterogeneous and may be due to increased plasma renin activity or sodium dependency (salt sensitivity), among other factors. It is estimated that essential hypertension makes up 92% to 95% of cases of hypertension in adults. Chronic renal disease is the most common cause of secondary hypertension in adults (Rudnick et al., 1977; Danielson and Dammstrom, 1981; Sinclair et al., 1987).

The prevalence of elevated blood pressure in children and adolescents is relatively low compared with that in adults. In the mid-1960s investigators began to characterize the blood pressure distribution in children and adolescents and to consider whether high blood pressure begins in childhood. Suggestive evidence for its origin early in life resulted from observations that (1) peer rank order of blood pressure is maintained during childhood (Beaglehole et al., 1977; Clarke et al., 1978; Levine et al., 1978; Hiat et al., 1982; Prineas et al., 1984; Shear et al., 1986; Lauer and Clarke, 1989; Mahoney et al., 1991; Nelson et al., 1992; Lauer et al., 1993), so children and adolescents with high blood pressure are likely to become adults with high blood pressure, i.e., there is tracking of blood pressure; and (2) there is familial aggregation of blood pressure (Biron and Mongeau, 1978; Ward et al., 1979; Annest et al., 1979; Morton et al., 1980; Moll et al., 1983; Zinner et al., 1985; Munger et al., 1988), so children of parents with high blood pressure are likely to have high blood pressure.

On the basis of blood pressure standards established using a national database of blood pressure measurements for subjects between 1 and 17 years of age from several different racial groups, it is now clear that primary hypertension is detectable in children and adolescents and that its prevalence is increasing, due in large part to the increasing prevalence of overweight and obesity in this age group (Falkner et al., 1996, 2004; Sorof and Daniels, 2002; Muntner et al., 2004).

This chapter will define high blood pressure in children, adolescents, and adults, and describe the trend toward increased blood pressure levels in children and adolescents. It will also characterize the degree of tracking of blood pressure during childhood and into young adulthood. Finally, the importance of considering a family history of hypertension when evaluating young patients with elevated blood pressure is emphasized.

▩ DEFINITION OF HIGH BLOOD PRESSURE IN ADULTS

In adults the prevalence of hypertension (high blood pressure) has been said to range from 20% to 40%. In part, this range can be attributed to the use of different cut points to define blood pressure elevation. It is also due to secular trends in the population levels of blood pressure (Burt et al., 1995a). These trends are encouraging in that the most recent survey data show a decrease in the prevalence of hypertension. Nevertheless, there may be as many as 60 million adults with SBP ≥140 mmHg or DBP ≥90 mmHg (cut points for stage 1 hypertension) in the United States and Canada (Davidson, 1991). The most recent blood pressure guidelines proposed by the Joint National Committee on Prevention, Evaluation, and Treatment of High Blood Pressure for adults aged 18 and older are displayed in Table 9.1 (Chobanian et al., 2003). Classification of blood pressure by use of these cut points should be based on the average of at least two seated blood pressure readings from each of two or more visits. The pre-hypertensive category was added to the most recent classification to identify adults who are at high risk for developing hypertension.

Treatment of blood pressure elevation in adults has been demonstrated to decrease the risk of cardiovascular disease end points. The Veterans Administration Cooperative Study (1967) was the first to show that treatment of individuals with DBP between 115 and 129 mmHg was associated with a significant reduction in cardiovascular risk. More recently, the Treatment of Mild Hypertension Study (TOMHS) showed a 33% reduction in cardiovascular events after four years in subjects who received antihypertensive drug therapy in addition to lifestyle modification, compared to those who received lifestyle modification and placebo (Neaton et al., 1993).

Despite mounting evidence of the benefit of treatment of hypertension, this has not always resulted in widespread clinical practice. For example, on the basis of data from the first portion of the Third National Health and Nutrition

TABLE 9.1

Classification of blood pressure (mmHg) for adults aged 18 and older from the Joint National Committee on Prevention, Evaluation, and Treatment of High Blood Pressure

SBP	DBP	Classification
<120	and <80	Normal
120–139	or 80–89	Prehypertension
140–159	or 90–99	Stage 1 hypertension
≥160	or ≥100	Stage 2 hypertension

*Based on the average of at least two seated blood pressure measurements from two or more visits.
Source: Chobanian et al. (2003).
Reproduced with permission from the Seventh Report of the Joint National Committee on Prevention, Detection, Evaluation, and Treatment of High Blood Pressure. Copyright © 2003. American Heart Association.

Examination Survey (1988–1991, NHANES III) it was estimated that 31% of 43 million hypertensive adults in the United States (SBP ≥140 mmHg or DBP ≥90 mmHg) were completely unaware of the problem (Burt et al., 1995b). Only 69% of individuals who were aware that they had hypertension (53% of the total) were receiving medication. However, the problem extends even further because only 45% of those on treatment (24% of the population with hypertension) had blood pressure controlled below 140/90 mmHg. There were differences by ethnic group, with only 14% of Hispanic-Americans with hypertension achieving control of blood pressure compared to 24% of white Americans and 25% of African-Americans. This represents a major public health challenge for the United States. Further evidence of this problem is the fact that despite the improvement of antihypertensive agents and their availability, the rates of hospitalization for congestive heart failure are increasing in the United States. The treatment of hypertension has been cited as a major reason for the decline in mortality rates from coronary heart disease and stroke in the United States. Unfortunately, in recent years the decline has slowed or even begun to reverse, particularly for African-Americans (Falkner et al., 1996).

■ DEFINITION OF ELEVATED BLOOD PRESSURE IN CHILDREN AND ADOLESCENTS

Routine physical examination of children over 3 years of age should include measurement of blood pressure with appropriate measuring methodologies (Morgenstern, 2002; Falkner et al., 2004; also see Chapter 10). In children, blood pressure is classified according to reference standards. The Report of the Task Force on Blood Pressure Control in Children, published in 1977, provided the first national reference standards for blood pressure measurements in children and adolescents (National Heart, Lung, and Blood Institute [NHLBI], 1977). Ten years later, the second task force used a total of 72,429 blood pressure measurements from participants (birth to 20 years of age) in nine large epidemiologic studies to produce revised age- and sex-specific blood pressure percentiles for infants, preteen children, and adolescents (NHLBI, 1987). Blood pressure in children is considerably lower than in adults, but it increases steadily throughout childhood and adolescence. At birth, the SBP of a full-term infant is approximately 70 mmHg and by 1 month of age it is approximately 85 mmHg (Zinner et al., 1985). The establishment of normative data for children and adolescents is a challenge because of the tendency for blood pressure to vary with so many different factors including age, height, weight, cuff bladder size, type of equipment, patient position at the time of measurement, and even season (Rocchini et al., 1988; Gutin et al., 1990; Rosner et al., 1993). In the clinic setting, height and weight should be used to assess the medical significance of blood pressure measurements because height especially is positively associated with blood pressure in these age groups (Lauer et al., 1985). If a child is tall and proportionally heavy for their age, a blood pressure level that is elevated for their age is to be expected and this is normal. For children who are tall and lean, elevated pressures for age are also normal. High blood pressure is commonly observed in children with excessive weight for height, but overweight is considered to be an abnormal cause of higher than normal blood pressure and it is unlikely that such children have another cause for their high blood pressure. Blood pressure levels in children also relate directly to the degree of sexual maturation as assessed by Tanner Indices (Lauer et al., 1984). Thus, children who are relatively short for their age but have accelerated sexual maturation may be expected to have a higher blood pressure than that of their height-matched peers.

Because of the importance of height in the determination of blood pressure level, the blood pressure tables were revised again by the third task force (Falkner et al., 1996), which used more than 81,000 blood pressure measurements for participants 1 to 17 years of age to produce percentiles that were age-, sex-, and height-specific. With this update, percentiles were determined for fifth-phase (fifth Korotkoff phase) DBP regardless of the age of the participant (Falkner et al., 1996), unlike the previous reference percentiles, which were based on fourth-phase DBP for children between 3 and 12 years of age. The new percentiles allowed for a more precise classification of blood pressure that accounted for the effect of height and differential rates of growth in children and adolescents by relating blood pressure to age as well as height. For the most recent update of the blood pressure reference standards (Falkner et al., 2004) the authors used 83,091 measurements for 63,227 participants from eight large epidemiologic studies, as well as NHANES III and NHANES 1999–2000. The blood pressure percentiles are based on calculation of height percentiles from the 2000 Centers for Disease Control and Prevention (CDC) growth charts (www.cdc.gov/growthcharts/).

The most recent blood pressure percentiles for children and adolescents, while specific for age, sex, and height, do not account for weight or body mass index (BMI). There is a strong association between blood pressure and BMI, and both blood pressure and BMI, when elevated, increase cardiovascular risk. Therefore, the establishment of blood pressure percentiles based on weight or BMI would incorrectly control for the pathologic influence of overweight on blood pressure. The percentiles are not race or ethnicity group–specific either, because the magnitude of the race and ethnicity group differences in this age range is not clinically relevant (Falkner et al., 2004).

The most recent percentile tables and blood pressure classification criteria for children and adolescents are reproduced in Tables 10.1 and 10.2 in Chapter 10. Blood pressure in males is slightly higher than that in females during the first decade of life. The difference between males and females begins to widen around the onset of puberty, and blood pressure is significantly higher in males by the end of the teenage years. Within a given age and sex group, blood pressure percentiles increase as height percentiles increase, and blood pressure percentiles increase steadily during childhood and adolescence. Use of these percentiles helps to prevent misclassification so that very tall non-overweight children are not automatically considered to be hypertensive and very short children with high normal blood pressure are differentiated from those with frank hypertension. If a child or adolescent has a SBP and/or DBP ≥95th percentile for their age (or ≥120/≥80 mmHg regardless of their age) on at least three occasions, especially if they are not tall or overweight, it is likely that the elevated blood pressure is the result of a pathologic process. These individuals need further evaluation for secondary causes and for lifestyle or medical interventions (see Chapters 10 and 11). Just as with body size (see Chapter 12), health care providers should plot blood pressure measurements for their young patients against age-, sex-, and height-specific blood pressure percentiles so that trends can be monitored and clinical care decisions can be made.

■ PREVALENCE OF ELEVATED BLOOD PRESSURE IN CHILDREN AND ADOLESCENTS

Because blood pressure elevation is defined by the 95th percentile (see Table 10.1 in Chapter 10), one might expect that the prevalence of elevated blood pressure in children and adolescents is 5%. However, because patients are required to have persistent elevation of blood pressure (on three separate, consecutive examinations), the prevalence is actually lower, probably in the range of 1% to 3%. In a study of junior high school children in Minneapolis, Minnesota, most school children who had blood pressure in the upper percentiles of the distribution at an initial screening did not have persistently elevated blood pressure. After two measurements at an initial screening, significant DBP elevation was found in 3.5% and significant SBP or DBP elevation was found in 4.2% of the participants. After a re-screening visit, the prevalence of blood pressure above the 95th percentile on both measurements was 0.3% for SBP, 0.8% for DBP, and 1.1% for SBP or DBP elevation (Sinaiko et al., 1989). Sorof et al. (2004) measured the blood pressures of 5102 children (13.5 ± 1.7 years of age; white, Hispanic, African-American and Asian) in eight Houston public schools. Those with blood pressure >95th percentile had their blood pressures remeasured 1 to 2 weeks later and again 1 to 2 weeks later if the second measurement was >95th percentile. Three different measurements were obtained at each screening. The prevalence after the first, second, and third screenings was 19.4%, 9.5%, and 4.5%, respectively. In an earlier study, Rames et al. (1978) found that less than 1% of children in the Muscatine Study had blood pressure persistently above 140/90 mmHg (the adult criterion for stage 1 hypertension, see Table 9.1).

Hypertension in children may be due to an identifiable pathologic process. An underlying cause can be found for some hypertensive children up to 10 years of age. The relative prevalence of different forms of hypertension in pediatric patients has been controversial. Prevalence estimates from several studies are summarized in Table 9.2. As can be seen, the estimated prevalence of primary and secondary forms of hypertension varies widely, likely because of selection

TABLE 9.2
Prevalence of causes of persistent hypertension in children in six studies

Cause	Rance et al. (1974) Toronto		Gill et al. (1975) London		New (1979) New York		Rocchini (1984) Michigan		Rames et al. (1978) Iowa		Londe (1978) St. Louis	
	N	(%)	N	(%)	N	(%)	N	(%)	N	(%)	N	(%)
Secondary												
Renal disease	66	(73)	78	(78)	62	(61)	20	(31)	2	(40)	7	(5)
Coarctation	—	—	15	(15)	13	(13)	5	(8)	2	(40)	—	—
Endocrine	8	(9)	—	—	6	(6)	4	(6)	—	—	—	—
Miscellaneous	2	(2)	5	(5)	7	(7)	4	(6)	1	(20)	—	—
Total secondary	76	(83)	98	(98)	88	(87)	33	(51)	5	(12)	7	(5)
Primary												
Obese			1	(50)	6	(46)	20	(62)	23	(64)	69	(55)
Total primary	15	(17)	2	(2)	13	(13)	32	(49)	36	(88)	125	(95)
Total	91		100		101		65		41		132	

or referral bias. The studies from Toronto, London, and New York were studies of children with substantial blood pressure elevation who were evaluated in the hospital. The study from Michigan was conducted in a preventive cardiology referral clinic. The study from Iowa was a population-based study, and the study from St. Louis was conducted in a primary pediatric practice. Thus, it is more likely that the latter two studies present a more generalizable view of the prevalence of different forms of hypertension. It is noteworthy that the prevalence of primary hypertension presented in those studies is very similar ($\approx$95%) to that found in adult populations.

Recent investigations have suggested that primary hypertension in children has become increasingly common in association with obesity and other risk factors, including insulin resistance, dyslipidemia, a positive family history of hypertension, a sedentary lifestyle, and an ethnic predisposition to hypertensive disease. Numerous studies have reported higher blood pressures and greater hypertension prevalence in obese than in lean children in U.S. (Freedman et al., 1999; Morrison et al., 1999a; Rosner et al., 2000; Sorof et al., 2002; Sorof et al., 2004) and other populations (Guillaume et al., 1996; Paradis et al., 2004). This recent increase in the prevalence of primary hypertension reflects a shift from what used to be a higher prevalence due to secondary causes in this age group. The early clinical course of hypertension in obese adolescents appears to be characterized by a preponderance (94%) of systolic hypertension (Sorof et al., 2002).

The most comprehensive study of the association between overweight and blood pressure to date was conducted by Rosner et al. (2000), using pooled data from eight large epidemiologic studies including more than 47,000 U.S. children 5 to 17 years of age. The major purpose of the analysis was to describe the blood pressure differences between black and white children in relation to body size. There were few substantive racial differences in SBP or DBP. However, regardless of race, sex, or age, the odds of elevated blood pressure were significantly higher for children in the upper decile relative to the lower decile of BMI, with the odds ratios for systolic hypertension (>95th percentile) ranging from 2.5 (95% CI 2.0–3.1) to 3.7 (95% CI 3.1–4.3). Because there are no consistent blood pressure differences between black and white children, the substantially higher prevalence of hypertension in black adults than in white adults must result from changes in the later teenage or early adult years.

The Quebec Child and Adolescent Health and Social Survey (QCAHS) was a school-based, multistage, stratified, cluster sample survey of Quebec children and adolescents 9, 13, and 16 years of age conducted during the first 5 months of 1999 (Paradis et al., 2003). Paradis et al. (2004) used the age-, sex-, and height-specific 90th and 95th percentile reference values from the National High Blood Pressure Education Program (NHLBI, 1996) to classify the 3589 participants as having high normal (between the 90th and 94th percentile) or elevated ($\geq$95th percentile) blood pressure. The proportion of 9-, 13-, and 16-year-old males with high normal or elevated SBP was 12%, 22%, and 30%, respectively; the corresponding percentages for females were 14%, 19%, and 17%. Less than 1% of the males or females had high normal or elevated DBP. The mean BMI for participants with elevated SBP was 4 to 6 kg/m^2 higher than that in participants with SBP less than the 25th percentile in all age and gender groups.

Sorof et al. (2004) screened a multiethnic group of 5102 students 10 to 19 years of age from the Houston public schools for hypertension and overweight. The ethnic distribution was 44% white, 25% Hispanic, 22% African-American, and 7% Asian. Students with an average SBP or DBP (based on three seated blood pressure measurements at the initial screen) >95th percentile (as defined in Falkner et al., 1996) were asked to return 1 to 2 weeks later for repeat blood pressure measurements, and again 1 to 2 weeks later if their SBP or DBP was still >95th percentile at the second screen. The prevalence of elevated blood pressure was 19.4%, 9.5%, and 4.5%, respectively, after the initial, second, and third screens. Hispanics (25%) had the highest prevalence of elevated blood pressure at the initial screen; Asians (16%) had the lowest. Based on the third screen, there was no significant ethnic difference with 5.6% of Hispanics, 4.6% of African-Americans, 4.1% of whites, and 3.7% of Asians having persistently elevated blood pressure. The prevalence in males after the third screen (5.7%) was significantly higher ($p < 0.001$) than the prevalence in females (3.4%). The strongest determinant of hypertension was BMI, with a four- to fivefold increase in the prevalence of hypertension after the initial and third screens for students with BMI ≥95th percentile (initial 38%, third 11%) compared to those with BMI ≤5th (initial 9%, third 2%) age- and sex-specific percentile.

The prevalence of high blood pressure and the association with overweight was investigated in 2416 Milanese boys and girls 6 to 11 years of age by Genovesi et al. (2005). Based on the 95th percentiles of the U.S. normative standards, the overall prevalence of high blood pressure was 4.2% (5.4% of 1210 females and 3.1% of 1206 males; $p < 0.005$). The percentage of those with high blood pressure was significantly greater among overweight than in normal-weight children ($p < 0.0001$).

Interestingly, there is a significant inverse association between birth weight and the risk of hypertension in adulthood (Barker et al., 1993; Law and Barker, 1994). Systolic blood pressure shows a negative association with birth weight beginning in the first decade of life. This association becomes stronger with increasing age (Law et al., 1993).

Recently, Law et al. (2002) measured the blood pressures of 346 British men and women 22 years of age whose body size had been measured at birth and for the first 10 years of life. They found that lower birth weight and greater weight gain between 1 and 5 years of age, but not weight gain during the first year of life, were associated with higher SBP at age 22. The effects of birth weight and weight gain between 1 and 5 years of age on young adult SBP were independent, so young adults who had the lowest birth weights and the greatest weight gain had the highest blood pressures. The strength of the association between birth weight and young adult SBP was not altered with further adjustment for young adult BMI. On the other hand, the association between weight gain between

1 and 5 years of age and young adult SBP was considerably attenuated with BMI adjustment, largely because those who gained the most weight between 1 and 5 years of age were more likely to have higher BMI at age 22, which is also associated with higher SBP.

▦ TRENDS IN BLOOD PRESSURE LEVELS OF CHILDREN AND ADOLESCENTS

As mentioned in the previous section, primary hypertension in children is becoming increasingly more common, especially in association with an increase in BMI. Luepker et al. (1999) surveyed public school children, 10 to 14 years of age, in Minneapolis, Minnesota in 1986 and again in 1996. They found that SBP was significantly higher in 1996 than in 1986 in all ethnicity and sex groups. However, DBP was lower in the more recent survey. The increase in SBP was associated with an increase in BMI between the two surveys. These results are similar to those found by Morrison et al. (1999b) in the Princeton School District in Cincinnati, Ohio. In that study, average SBP and DBP were higher in 1989–90 than in 1973–75. However, the prevalence of elevated SBP was not significantly different between the two surveys, while the prevalence of elevated DBP decreased from 2.7% to 0.6% from 1973–75 to 1989–90 ($p < 0.01$). Morrison et al. also observed a trend for increasing body mass index between the surveys.

Muntner et al. (2004) characterized blood pressure levels among participants 8 to 17 years of age from NHANES 1999–2000 ($n = 2086$) and from NHANES III (1988–94, $n = 3496$). All of the participants had three valid systolic and diastolic measurements along with height and weight measurements. They also evaluated the relationship between BMI trends and blood pressure levels. The trend in blood pressure was assessed separately for children 8 through 12 years of age and for adolescents 13 through 17 years of age. Mean age-, race-, and sex-adjusted SBP was 1.4 mmHg (95% CI 0.6–2.2; $p < 0.001$) higher and mean adjusted DBP was 3.3 mmHg (95% CI 2.1–4.5; $p < 0.001$) higher in 1999–2000 than in 1988–1994. After additional adjustment for BMI, mean SBP was 1.0 mmHg higher (95% CI 0.2–1.8; $p < 0.01$) and mean DBP was 2.9 mmHg higher (95% CI 1.7–4.1; $p < 0.001$). In NHANES III, 28.2% of the participants were at or above the 85th age- and sex-specific BMI percentile based on the 2000 CDC Growth Charts; in 1999–2000, it was 31.8% of the participants.

▦ TRACKING OF BLOOD PRESSURE LEVELS FROM CHILDHOOD AND ADOLESCENCE INTO ADULTHOOD

The persistence of rank order of blood pressure has been referred to as *tracking*. There is a continuous rise in blood pressure from infancy through adolescence, and at any given age there is a wide distribution of blood pressure measurements. If blood pressure levels were to maintain rank order from early childhood into adult life, then those with initially high pressures would likely be destined to be adults with hypertension. Thus there would be a very good chance that childhood pressure in the upper part of the distribution would be associated with increased cardiovascular morbidity and mortality in adult life. This association makes the recent increase in the prevalence of elevated blood pressure in children and adolescents particularly worrisome.

Many longitudinal studies during childhood and from childhood into young adulthood have shown that there is a degree of peer rank order consistency of blood pressure level, i.e., that children tend to maintain a given blood pressure percentile as they grow older. The blood pressure correlation coefficients from some of these studies are summarized in Table 9.3. Although all of the studies indicate that there is indeed tracking of blood pressure, there is considerable lability of blood pressure rank over time. For an individual child, the prediction of future blood pressure from early measurements of blood pressure is certainly not as precise as is the prediction of future height and weight from early measurements (Clarke et al., 1978).

Data from the Muscatine Study show that 45% of young adults (20 to 30 years of age) with high SBP (>90th percentile) had at least one childhood SBP measurement that was >90th percentile ($p < 0.001$) (Lauer and Clarke, 1989). The comparable figure for DBP was 40% ($p < 0.001$). Among the young adult participants for whom three or more SBP measurements were obtained during childhood and adolescence, 6% of those with no high childhood SBP measurements had high SBP as young adults, 17% of those with only one high measurement during childhood and adolescence had high SBP as young adults, and 24% of those with two or more high blood pressure measurements during childhood and adolescence had high SBP as young adults ($p < 0.001$). The Bogalusa Heart Study also showed that 40% of children and adolescents 5 to 14 years of age at baseline with SBP above the age-, race-, and sex-specific 80th percentile were also above the 80th percentile 15 years later as young adults (Bao et al., 1995). Another 23% had young adult SBP between the 60th and 80th percentile. Cook et al. (2000) demonstrated that tracking correlations between blood pressure measurements obtained over a 4-year period (each year, three measurements at each of four visits spaced 1 week apart) in a cohort of children who were 8 to 15 years of age at baseline and again when the cohort members were 18 to 26 years of age, are improved when the multiple childhood measurements were averaged vs. the measurements for only one of the years. Using only 1 year of childhood measurements, the tracking coefficients were 0.49 in boys and 0.59 in girls for SBP and 0.39 and 0.48, respectively, for DBP. In contrast, the corresponding tracking coefficients were 0.55, 0.66, 0.47, and 0.57 when all of the childhood measurements were averaged.

These observations and others like them support the hypothesis that hypertension begins during childhood. However, it is not possible to precisely identify

TABLE 9.3

Association between initial and follow-up blood pressure measurements during childhood and into young adulthood

Reference	Age at Initial Examination	Length of Follow-up	Correlation Coefficient	
			Systolic	Diastolic
During Childhood				
de Swiet et al. (1976)	4 to 6 days	4 to 6 weeks	0.20***	—
Clarke et al. (1978)	5 to 16 years	2 years	0.41***	0.27***
		4 years	0.35***	0.21***
		6 years	0.30***	0.18***
Kuller et al. (1980)	High school students			
	Boys	17 years	0.44***	0.19**
	Girls	17 years	0.39***	0.19**
Hiat et al. (1982)	6 to 11 years	3 to 4 years	0.25 to 0.65**	0.09 to 0.60**
Childhood to Young Adulthood				
Lauer and Clarke (1989)†	7 to 18 years			
	Boys	3 to 18 years	0.27 to 0.37*	0.13 to 0.26*
	Girls	3 to 18 years	0.21 to 0.39*	0.17 to 0.31*
Bao et al. (1995)	5 to 14 years	15 years	0.36 to 0.50***	0.19* to 0.42***

$*p < 0.05; **p < 0.01; ***p < 0.001.$
†Two very extreme correlation coefficients for age 7 to 8 diastolic blood pressure in boys and girls were not included in the summary range.

those children who will have primary hypertension as adults. From a prevention perspective, therefore, it is important to consider elevated blood pressure during childhood and adolescence as a risk factor even before many of the clinical manifestations of hypertension become more apparent during adulthood.

▪ HIGH BLOOD PRESSURE AS A RISK FACTOR FOR CARDIOVASCULAR DISEASE IN CHILDREN AND ADOLESCENTS

Hypertension in adolescents is associated with fatty streaks and fibrous plaques in the aorta and in coronary arteries at autopsy (Enos et al., 1953; McNamara et al., 1971; Berenson et al., 1998; McGill et al., 2001; also see Chapter 1), with central nervous system end-organ damage (Lande et al., 2003) and with increased echocardiographic left ventricular mass and diastolic dysfunction (Daniels et al., 1998).

Elevated blood pressure has been shown to be associated with the early stages of the development of cardiovascular disease in children and adolescents. In the

Bogalusa Heart Study, investigators performed autopsies on 204 young people age 2 to 39 years who died from a variety of causes, primarily trauma (Newman et al., 1986; Berenson et al., 1998). Of those subjects, 93 had participated in epidemiologic studies at a younger age and had data available on cardiovascular risk factors in childhood. The investigators found that BMI, SBP, DBP, and serum lipid and lipoprotein concentrations were strongly associated with the extent of fatty streaks and fibrous plaques in the aorta and coronary arteries. The presence of multiple risk factors was associated with an even greater increase in the extent of development of atherosclerosis. Subjects with 0, 1, 2, and 3 or 4 risk factors had an average 1.3%, 2.5%, 7.9%, and 11.0% of the coronary surface covered with fatty streaks, respectively. For fibrous plaques the corresponding numbers were 0.6%, 0.1%, 2.4%, and 7.2% (Berenson et al., 1998). Data from The Muscatine Study and The Bogalusa Heart Study have also proven useful in understanding the early stages of the development of atherosclerosis (see Chapters 4 and 5).

Blood pressure elevation has been associated with increased echocardiographically determined left ventricular mass in adults. Left ventricular hypertrophy appears to be an independent risk factor for the development of cardiovascular disease (Levy et al., 1990). Left ventricular hypertrophy has been found to be prevalent in children and adolescents with essential hypertension. Daniels et al. (1998) studied 130 young individuals with persistent blood pressure elevation above the 90th percentile. They found that 55% of patients with hypertension had left ventricular mass index (LVM in g/height in $m^{2.7}$; de Simone et al., 1995) above the 90th percentile, 14% had left ventricular mass index above the 99th percentile, and 8% had left ventricular mass index above a cut point of 51 $g/m^{2.7}$ that has been associated with a fourfold increase in risk of adverse cardiovascular end points in adults with hypertension (de Simone et al., 1995).

Blood pressure elevation in children and adolescents presents an increased risk of adverse effects on the heart and vascular system. These effects may be magnified when blood pressure elevation is combined with other risk factors, such as obesity, diabetes mellitus, dyslipidemia, and cigarette smoking.

■ FAMILIAL AGGREGATION OF BLOOD PRESSURE AND FAMILIAL HISTORY OF HYPERTENSION

Population studies show that blood pressure is a unimodally distributed quantitative trait that aggregates in families. Blood pressure variation likely results from the interaction of genetic and environmental factors, but the challenge remains of determining how environmental factors interact with molecular genetic factors within an individual or within a population to produce the distribution of blood pressures that is observed. At this point, the genetic mutations that have been identified are primarily associated with rare forms of hypertension. One of the major research questions is whether there are genes that are responsible for relatively large effects on blood pressure variability among individuals or whether the genetic component results from the combined effects of many genes, each with an individually smaller effect on blood pressure variation.

Numerous investigations conducted in many different countries have demonstrated that blood pressure aggregates in families (Ward et al., 1979; Morton et al., 1980; Moll et al., 1983). The fraction of SBP variability that was attributed to genetic variability in these studies was between 0.24 and 0.34, while the fraction attributable to variation in common environment was between 0.11 and 0.20. Estimates of the genetic and environmental contributions to DBP were similar. However, inferences regarding the role of genetic factors in familial aggregation are problematic, because the effects of shared genetic factors are confounded by the effects of shared environmental factors. A familial influence on blood pressure levels can be identified as early as the newborn period (Zinner et al., 1985). Adoption studies have demonstrated much stronger correlations between biologic siblings than between adoptive siblings, and between parents and their biologic children then between parents and their adoptive children (Annest et al., 1979; Biron and Mongeau, 1979). These observations provide an even stronger indication that the familial aggregation of blood pressure is determined at least to some extent by shared genetic factors.

While only limited progress has been made in the identification of the specific genetic factors that may confer susceptibility to the common forms of hypertension, it is clear that children from families with hypertension tend to have higher blood pressures than children from normotensive families (Munger et al., 1988), and that the adult relatives of children with persistent elevated blood pressure and relative weight are at higher risk of cardiovascular disease mortality than adult relatives of randomly selected children (Burns et al., 1992). In the absence of identified genetic factors, a family history should be used as a surrogate measure. For children and adolescents, a family history should include the first-degree relatives of the parents, i.e., the grandparents, aunts, and uncles of the children. The recent increase in "obesity hypertension" makes the consideration of family history extremely important as a component of the clinical care in this age group (Sorof and Daniels, 2002).

■ SUMMARY

- Blood pressure elevation in children and adolescents is not innocuous.
- Measurement of blood pressure is recommended yearly after 3 years of age.
- The diagnosis of hypertension in children now uses the fifth Korotkoff sound to define DBP and depends on height.
- Blood pressure is considerably lower in children than in adults and increases steadily throughout the first two decades of life.
- There are no significant blood pressure differences between ethnic groups until late adolescence.

- Greater weight, greater height, and a family history of hypertension are associated with higher blood pressure levels in children and adolescents.
- The roots of essential hypertension extend back into childhood.
- Familial aggregation of blood pressure has been demonstrated from early infancy, and children with higher blood pressure levels are more likely to come from families with a history of hypertension.
- Although it is generally agreed that early essential hypertension poses little immediate risk to most children, evidence from studies in children and adolescents has shown cardiac ventricular and hemodynamic changes consistent with an adverse effect of mild hypertension before the third decade of life.
- Since blood pressure is not transmitted in a simple genetic fashion, direct genetic intervention is impossible. However, environmental influences can be considered in counseling. The high correlation of blood pressure among relatives and the knowledge that tracking of blood pressure occurs should be useful in counseling parents and children with high blood pressure. This knowledge should influence parents to alter the family lifestyle related to salt and caloric intake.
- If cardiovascular disease morbidity and mortality are to be prevented, then children with elevated blood pressure must be identified and appropriately treated.

◼ REFERENCES

Annest, J.L., C.F. Sing, P. Biron, and J.G. Mongeau. 1979. Familial Aggregation of Blood Pressure and Weight in Adoptive Families. II. Estimation of the Relative Contributions of Genetic and Common Environmental Factors to Blood Pressure Correlations between Family Members. *Am J Epidemiol* 110:492–503.

Bao, W., S.A. Threefoot, S.R. Srinivasan, and G.S. Berenson. 1995. Essential Hypertension Predicted by Tracking of Blood Pressure During Childhood: The Bogalusa Heart Study. *Am J Hypertens* 8:657–65.

Barker, D.J.P., C.N. Hales, C.H.D. Fall, C. Osmond, K. Phipps, and P.M.S. Clark. 1993. Type 2 (Non-Insulin-Dependent) Diabetes Mellitus, Hypertension and Hyperlipidemia (Syndrome X): Relation to Reduced Fetal Growth. *Diabetologia* 36:62–7.

Beaglehole, R., C.E. Salmond, and E.F. Eyles. 1977. A Longitudinal Study of Blood Pressure in Polynesian Children. *Am J Epidemiol* 105:87–9.

Berenson, G.S., S.R. Srinivasan, W. Bao, W.P. Newman, 3rd, R.E. Tracy, and W.A. Wattigney. 1998. Association between Multiple Cardiovascular Risk Factors and Atherosclerosis in Children and Young Adults. The Bogalusa Heart Study. *N Engl J Med* 338:1650–6.

Biron, P., and J.G. Mongeau. 1978. Familial Aggregation of Blood Pressure and its Components. *Pediatr Clin North Am* 25:29–33.

Burns, T. L., P. P. Moll, and R. M. Lauer. 1992. Increased Familial Cardiovascular Mortality in Obese Schoolchildren: The Muscatine Ponderosity Family Study. *Pediatrics* 89:262–8.

Burt, V.L., J.A. Cutler, M. Higgins, M.J. Horan, D. Labarthe, P. Whelton, C. Brown, and E.J. Roccella. 1995a. Trends in the Prevalence, Awareness, Treatment, and Control of Hypertension in the Adult US Population: Data from the Health Examination Surveys, 1960–1991. *Hypertension* 26:60–9.

Burt, V.L., P. Wheaton, E.J. Roccella, C. Brown, J.A. Cutler, M. Higgins, M.J. Horan and D. LaBarthe. 1995b. Prevalence of Hypertension in the US Adult Population. Results from the Third National Health and Nutrition Examination Survey, 1988–1991. *Hypertension* 25:305–13.

Chobanian, A.V., G.L. Bakris, H.R. Black, W.C. Cushman, L.A. Green, A.L. Izzo, D.W. Jones, B.J. Materson, S. Oparil, J.T. Wright, Jr., and E.J. Rocella. 2003. Seventh Report of the Joint National Committee on Prevention, Detection, Evaluation, and Treatment of High Blood Pressure. *Hypertension* 42:1206–52.

Clarke, W.R., H. Schrott, P.E. Leaverton, W.E. Connor, and R.M. Lauer. 1978. Tracking of Blood Lipids and Blood Pressure in Children: The Muscatine Study. *Circulation* 58:626–34.

Cook, N.R., M.W. Gillman, B.A. Rosner, J.O. Taylor, and C.H. Hennekens. 2000. Combining Annual Blood Pressure Measurements in Childhood to Improve Prediction of Young Adult Blood Pressure. *Stat Med* 19:2625–40.

Daniels, S.R., J.M.H. Loggie, P. Khoury, and T.R. Kimball. 1998. Left Ventricular Geometry and Severe Left Ventricular Hypertrophy in Children and Adolescents with Essential Hypertension. *Circulation* 97:1907–11.

Danielson, M., and B. Dammstrom. 1981. The Prevalence of Secondary and Curable Hypertension. *Acta Med Scand* 209:451–5.

Davidson, D.M. 1991. Hypertension. In: *Preventive Cardiology*. Baltimore, MD: Williams and Wilkins, pp. 58–82.

de Simone, G., R.G. Devereux, S.R. Daniels, M.J. Koren, R.A. Meyer, and J.H. Laragh. 1995. Effect of Growth on Variability of Left Ventricular Mass: Assessment of Allometric Signals in Adults and Children and their Capacity to Predict Cardiovascular Risk. *J Am Coll Cardiol* 25:1056–62.

de Swiet, M., P. Fayres, and E.A. Shinebourne. 1976. Blood Pressure Survey in a Population of Newborn Infants. *BMJ* 2:9–11.

Enos, W.F., R.H. Holmes, and J. Beyer. 1953. Coronary Disease among United States Soldiers Killed in Action in Korea. Preliminary Report. *JAMA* 152:1090–3.

Falkner, B., S.R. Daniels, J.T. Flynn, S. Gidding, L.A. Green, J. Inglefinger, R.M. Lauer, B.Z. Morgenstern, R.J. Portman, R.J. Prineas, A.P. Rocchini, B. Rosner, A.R. Sinaiko, N. Stettler, E. Urbina, E.J. Roccella. 2004. The Fourth Report on the Diagnosis, Evaluation and Treatment of High Blood Pressure in Children and Adolescents. *Pediatrics* 114(2 Suppl):555–76.

Falkner, B., S.R. Daniels, M.J. Horan, J.M.H. Loggie, R.J. Prineas, B. Rosner, A.R. Sinaiko, E.J. Roccella, and D.E. Anderson. 1996. Update on the 1987 Task Force Report on High Blood Pressure in Children and Adolescents: A Working Group Report from the National High Blood Pressure Education Program. *Pediatrics* 98:649–58.

Freedman, D.S., W.H. Dietz, S.R. Srinivasan, and G.S. Berenson. 1999. The Relation of Overweight to Cardiovascular Risk Factors among Children and Adolescents: The Bogalusa Heart Study. *Pediatrics* 103:1175–82.

Genovesi, S.A., M.C. Giussani, F.A. Pieruzzi, F.A. Vigorita, C.A. Arcovio, S.B. Cavuto, and A.A. Stella. 2005. Results of Blood Pressure Screening in a Population of School-Aged Children in the Province of Milan: Role of Overweight. *J Hypertens* 23:493–7.

Gill, D.G., B.M. de Costa, J.S. Cameron, M.C. Joseph, C.S. Ogg, and C. Chantler. 1976. Analysis of 100 Children with Severe and Persistent Hypertension. *Arch Dis Child* 51:951–6.

Guillaume, M., L. Lapidus, F. Beckers, A. Lambert, and P. Bjorntorp. 1996. Cardiovascular Risk Factors in Children from the Belgian Province of Luxembourg. The Belgian Luxembourg Child Study. *Am J Epidemiol* 144:867–80.

Gutin, B., C. Basch, S. Shea, I. Contento, M. DeLozier, J. Rips, M. Irigoyen, and P. Zybert. 1990. Blood Pressure, Fitness and Fatness in 5- and 6-Year-Old Children. *JAMA* 264:1123–7.

Hiat, H.I., S. Lemeshow, and K.D. Rosenman. 1982. A Longitudinal Study of Blood Pressure in a National Survey of Children. *Am J Public Health* 72:1285–7.

Kannel, W.B. 1975. Role of Blood Pressure in Cardiovascular Disease. The Framingham Study. *Angiology* 26:1–14.

Kannel, W.B. 1998. Hypertension: Epidemiological Appraisal. In: *Preventive Cardiology: A Guide For Clinical Practice.* Edited by K. Robinson. Armonk, NY: Futura Publishing, pp. 1–14.

Keys, A. 1980. *Seven Countries. A Multivariable Analysis of Death and Coronary Heart Disease.* Cambridge, MA: Harvard University Press.

Kuller, L.H., M. Crook, M.J. Almes, K. Detre, G. Reese, and G. Rutan. 1980. Dormont High School (Pittsburgh, Pennsylvania) Blood Pressure Study. *Hypertension* 2(Suppl I):109–16.

Lande, M.B., J.M. Kaczorowski, P. Aunger, G.J. Schwartz, and M. Weitzman. 2003. Elevated Blood Pressure and Decreased Cognitive Function among School-Age Children and Adolescents in the United States. *J Pediatr* 143:720–4.

Lauer, R.M., A.R. Anderson, R. Beaglehole, and T.L. Burns. 1984. Factors Related to Tracking of Blood Pressure in Children. *Hypertension* 6:307–14.

Lauer, R.M., T.L. Burns, and W.R. Clarke. 1985. Assessing Children's Blood Pressure. Considerations of Age and Body Size: The Muscatine Study. *Pediatrics* 75:1081–90.

Lauer, R. M., and W. R. Clarke. 1989. Childhood Risk Factors for High Adult Blood Pressure: The Muscatine Study. *Pediatrics* 84:633–41.

Lauer, R.M., W.R. Clarke, L.T. Mahoney, and J. Witt. 1993. Childhood Predictors for High Adult Blood Pressure. The Muscatine Study. *Pediatr Clin North Am* 40:23–40.

Law, C.M., and D.J. Barker. 1994. Fetal Influences on Blood Pressure. *J Hypertens* 12:1329–32.

Law, C.M., M. de Swiet, C. Osmond, P.M. Fayers, D.J. Barker, A.M. Cruddas, and C.H. Fall. 1993. Initiation of Hypertension in Utero and its Amplification Throughout Life. *BMJ* 306:24–7.

Law, C.M., A.W. Shiell, C.A. Newsome, H.E. Syddall, E.A. Shinebourne, P.M. Fayers, C.N. Martyn, and M. de Swiet. 2002. Fetal, Infant, and Childhood Growth and Adult Blood Pressure. A Longitudinal Study from Birth to 22 Years of Age. *Circulation* 105:1088–92.

Levine, R.S., C.H. Hennekens, B. Klien, and M.J. Jesse. 1978. Tracking Correlations of Blood Pressure Levels in Infancy. *Pediatrics* 61:121–5.

Levy, D., R.J. Garrison, D.D. Savage, W.B. Kannel, and W.P. Castelli. 1990. Prognostic Implications of Echocardiographically Determined Left Ventricular Mass in The Framingham Heart Study. *N Engl J Med* 322:1561–6.

Londe, S. 1978. Causes of Hypertension in the Young. *Pediatr Clin North Am* 25:55–65.

Luepker, R.V., D.R. Jacobs, R.J. Prineas, and A.R. Sinaiko. 1999. Secular Trends of Blood Pressure and Body Size in a Multi-Ethnic Adolescent Population: 1986 to 1996. *J Pediatr* 134:665–6.

MacMahon, S., R. Peto, J. Cutler, R. Collins, P. Sorlie, J. Neaton, R. Abbott, J. Godwin, A. Dyer, and J. Stamler. 1990. Blood Pressure, Stroke and Coronary Heart Disease. I. Prolonged Differences in Blood Pressure—Prospective Observational Studies Corrected for the Regression Dilution Bias. *Lancet* 335:765–74.

Mahoney, L.T., W.R. Clarke, T.L. Burns, and R.M. Lauer. 1991. Childhood Predictors of High Blood Pressure. *Am J Hypertens* 4:608S–610S.

McGill, Jr., H.C., C.A. McMahan, A.W. Zieske, G.T. Malcom, R.E. Tracy, and J.P. Strong. 2001. Effects of Nonlipid Risk Factors on Atherosclerosis in Youth with a Favorable Lipoprotein Profile. *Circulation* 103:1546–50.

McNamara, J.J., M.A. Molot, J.F. Stremple, and R.T. Cutting. 1971. Coronary Artery Disease in Combat Casualties in Vietnam. *JAMA* 216:1185–7.

Moll, P.P., E. Harburg, T.L. Burns, M.A. Schork, and F. Ozgoren. 1983. Heredity, Stress and Blood Pressure, a Family Set Approach: The Detroit Project Revisited. *J Chron Dis* 36:317–28.

Morgenstern, B. 2002. Blood Pressure, Hypertension and Ambulatory Blood Pressure Monitoring in Children and Adolescents. *Am J Hypertens* 15:64S–66S.

Morrison, J.A., B.A. Barton, F.M. Biro, S.R. Daniels, and D.L. Sprecher. 1999a. Overweight, Fat Patterning, and Cardiovascular Disease Risk Factors in Black and White Boys. *J Pediatr* 135:451–7.

Morrison, J.A., F.W. James, D.L. Sprecher, P.R. Khoury, and S.R. Daniels. 1999b. Sex and Race Differences in Cardiovascular Disease Risk Factor Changes in Schoolchildren, 1975–1990: The Princeton School Study. *Am J Public Health* 89:1708–14.

Morton, N.E., C.L. Gulbrandsen, D.C. Rao, G.G. Rhoads, and A. Kagan. 1980. Determinants of Blood Pressure in Japanese-American Families. *Hum Genet* 53:261–6.

Munger, R. G., R. J. Prineas and O. Gomez-Marin. 1988. Persistent Elevation of Blood Pressure among Children with a Family History of Hypertension: The Minneapolis Children's Blood Pressure Study. *J Hypertens* 6:647–53.

Muntner, P., J. He, J.A. Cutler, R.P. Wildman, and P.K. Whelton. 2004. Trends in Blood Pressure among Children and Adolescents. *JAMA* 291:2107–13.

National Heart, Lung, and Blood Institute. 1977. Report of the Task Force on Blood Pressure Control in Children. *Pediatrics* 59(Suppl):797–820.

National Heart, Lung, and Blood Institute. 1987. Report of the Second Task Force on Blood Pressure Control in Children. *Pediatrics* 79:1–25.

National High Blood Pressure Education Program Working Group. 1996. 1995 Update of the Working Group Reports on Chronic Renal Failure and Renovascular Hypertension. *Arch Intern Med* 156:1938–47.

Neaton, J.D., R.H. Grimm, Jr., R.J. Prineas, J. Stamler, G.A. Grandits, P.J. Elmer, J.A. Cutler, J.M. Flack, J.A. Schoenberger, and R. McDonald. 1993. Treatment of Mild Hypertension Study. Final Results. *JAMA* 270:713–24.

Nelson, M.J., D.R. Ragland, and S.L. Syme. 1992. Longitudinal Prediction of Adult Blood Pressure from Juvenile Blood Pressure Levels. *Am J Epidemiol* 136:633–45.

New, M.I. 1979. Report of the Hypertension Task Force: Part A, Pediatrics. Washington, DC: U.S. Department of Health, Education and Welfare Public Health Service. NIH Publication No. 79–1628.

Newman, 3rd, W.P., D.S. Freedman, A.W. Voors, P.D. Gard, S.R. Srinivasan, J.L. Cresanta, G.D. Williamson, L.S. Webber, and G.S. Berenson. 1986. Relation of Serum Lipoprotein Levels and Systolic Blood Pressure to Early Atherosclerosis: The Bogalusa Heart Study. *N Engl J Med* 314:138–44.

Paradis, G., M. Lambert, J. O'Loughlin, C. Lavallee, J. Aubin, P. Berthiaume, M. Ledoux, E. Delvin, E. Levy, and J.A. Hanley. 2003. The Quebec Child and Adolescent Health and Social Survey: Design and Methods of a Cardiovascular Disease Risk Factor Survey for Youth. *Can J Cardiol* 19:523–31.

Paradis, G., M. Lambert, J. O'Laughlin, C. Lavallee, J. Aubin, E. Delvin, E. Levy, and J.A. Hanley. 2004. Blood Pressure and Adiposity in Children and Adolescents. *Circulation* 110:1832–8.

Prineas, R.J., R.F. Gillum, and O. Gomez-Marin. 1984. The Determinants of Blood Pressure in Children: The Minneapolis Children's Blood Pressure Study. NHLBI Workshop in Juvenile Hypertension. Edited by J.M.H. Loggie, M.J. Horan, A.B. Gruskin, J.B. Dumbard, and R.F. Havlick. New York: Biomedical Information Service, pp. 21–35.

Rames, L.K., W.R. Clark, W.E. Connor, M.A. Reiter, and R.M. Lauer. 1978. Normal Blood Pressure and the Evaluation of Sustained Blood Pressure Elevation in Childhood: The Muscatine Study. *Pediatrics* 61:245–51.

Rance, C.P., G.S. Arbus, J.W. Balfe, and S.W. Kooh. 1974. Persistent Systemic Hypertension in Infants and Children. *Pediatr Clin North Am* 21:801–24.

Rocchini, A. 1984. Childhood Hypertension: Etiology, Diagnosis, and Treatment. *Pediatr Clin North Am* 31:1259–73.

Rocchini, A.P., V. Katch, J. Anderson, J. Hinderliter, D. Becque, M. Martin, and C. Marks. 1988. Blood Pressure in Obese Adolescents: Effect of Weight Loss. *Pediatrics* 82:16–23.

Rosner, B., R. Prineas, S.R. Daniels, and J. Loggie. 2000. Blood Pressure Differences between Blacks and Whites in Relation to Body Size among US Children and Adolescents. *Am J Epidemiol* 151:1007–19.

Rosner, B., R.J. Prineas, J.M. Loggie, and S.R. Daniels. 1993. Blood Pressure Nomograms for Children and Adolescents, by Height, Sex, and Age, in the United States. *J Pediatr* 123:871–86.

Rudnick, K.V., D.L. Sackett, S. Hirst, and C. Holmes. 1977. Hypertension in Family Practice. *CMAJ* 3:492–7.

Shear, C. L., G. L. Burke, D. S. Freedman, and G. S. Berenson. 1986. Value of Childhood Blood Pressure Measurements and Family History in Predicting Future Blood Pressure Status: Results from 8 Years of Follow-up in The Bogalusa Heart Study. *Pediatrics* 77:862–9.

Sinaiko, A.R., O. Gomez-Marin, and R.J. Prineas. 1989. Prevalence of 'Significant' Hypertension in Junior High School-Aged Children: The Children and Adolescent Blood Pressure Program. *J Pediatr* 114:664–9.

Sinclair, A.M., C.G. Isles, I. Brown, H. Cameron, G.D. Murray, and J.W. Robertson. 1987. Secondary Hypertension in a Blood Pressure Clinic. *Arch Intern Med* 147:1289–93.

Sorof, J., and S. R. Daniels. 2002. Obesity Hypertension in Children. A Problem of Epidemic Proportions. *Hypertension* 40:441 7.

Sorof, J., D. Lai, J. Turner, T. Poffenbarger, and R.J. Portman. 2004. Overweight, Ethnicity, and the Prevalence of Hypertension in School-Aged Children. *Pediatrics* 113:475–82.

Sorof, J.M., T. Poffenbarger, K. Franco, L. Bernard, and R.J. Portman. 2002. Isolated Systolic Hypertension, Obesity, and Hyperkinetic States in Children. *J Pediatr* 140:660–6.

Veterans Administration Cooperative Study Group on Antihypertensive Agents. 1967. Effects of Treatment on Morbidity in Hypertension. Results in Patients with Diastolic Blood Pressures Averaging 115 through 129 mmHg. *JAMA* 202:116–22.

Ward, R.H., R.G. Chin, and I.A.M. Prior. 1979. Genetic Epidemiology of Blood Pressure in a Migrating Isolate: Prospectus. In: *Genetic Analysis of Common Diseases: Applications to Predictive Factors in Coronary Disease*. Edited by C.F. Sing, and M. Skolnick. New York: Alan R. Liss, pp. 675–709.

World Health Organization. 2002. Reducing Risks, Promoting Healthy Life. In: *World Health Report*. 2002. Geneva: World Health Organization.

Zinner, S.H., B.A. Rosner, W. Oh, and E.H. Kass. 1985. Significance of Blood Pressure in Infancy: Familial Aggregation and Predictive Effect on Later Blood Pressure. *Hypertension* 7.411–6.

CHAPTER 10

Identification and Management of Children and Adolescents with High Blood Pressure

Stephen R. Daniels

Research has clearly shown that blood pressure elevation is associated with increased cardiovascular disease (CVD) morbidity and mortality in adults. This finding has led to a clinical mandate to identify adults with hypertension and treat them appropriately (Joint National Committee, 1997). More recently, it has become clear that the origins of acquired cardiovascular disease may occur in childhood and adolescence (see Chapter 1). As knowledge in this area has increased, an approach to identification and management of pediatric patients with high blood pressure has been developed.

For children and adolescents, the degree to which doctors routinely and appropriately measure blood pressure and are able to treat hypertension is not completely known. Kluger et al. (1991) found that both family physicians (21%) and pediatricians (14%) mislabeled blood pressures at the age specific 90th percentile as normal. This occurred more commonly when the patient was young and the cut point was lower. In this survey, blood pressure was the cardiovascular risk factor that was most often assessed by primary care physicians; however, cigarette smoking was the risk factor that received the most patient counseling. In a more recent national survey of 1036 eligible physicians selected from a national probability sample, Kimm et al. (1998) found that almost all physicians with pediatric patients performed routine blood pressure measurements. Nearly all pediatricians initiated blood pressure measurements in patients younger than age 5, while other practitioners tended to initiate blood pressure measurement at older ages. Dietary management of blood pressure elevation was the first-line therapy in all physician categories. Low-sodium diet (45.3%) and weight reduction were the two most frequently prescribed nonpharmacologic therapies. Only a minority (25.5%) of physicians indicated that they treated blood pressure elevation in children with medication. It is likely that many children and adolescents go without routine measurement of blood pressure. It also appears that blood pressure measurements in young patients may not be interpreted correctly and that young patients who need therapy may not get it.

■ MEASUREMENT OF BLOOD PRESSURE

To recognize hypertension, it is important to measure blood pressure correctly. While in theory this seems simple, in practice it proves to be quite difficult. Many health care professionals have not been appropriately trained to measure blood pressure and others have developed bad habits in measurement that may lead to inaccurate measurements.

The Second National Heart, Lung, and Blood Institute (NHLBI) Task Force on Blood Pressure Control in Children (1987), the update by the National High Blood Pressure Education Program (NHBPEP) (Falkner et al., 1996), and the Fourth Report of the NHBPEP (Falkner et al., 2004) all recommend auscultation as the method by which blood pressure should be measured in pediatric patients. Auscultatory measurement has been the gold standard for measurement and is the method used in the large epidemiologic studies on which the current standards are based. Because there is a subjective component to measurement of blood pressure by auscultation the examiner must be trained to perform measurements in a standardized fashion and must have adequate hearing to be able to discern the Korotkoff phases. To perform measurements of blood pressure it is necessary to have a mercury column sphygmomanometer or an aneroid device calibrated to a mercury column. Some concern about the presence of mercury in the hospital setting has led to replacement of mercury column sphygmomanometers with electronic devices. In a position statement the American Heart Association has recommended the general use of mercury manometers or aneroid devices as the instruments of choice until other instruments are better validated (Jones et al., 2001). If mercury instruments cannot be reintroduced for regular use, in settings where aneroid or electronic devices are used exclusively physicians should insist on the use of mercury instruments for routine calibration of the equipment used.

Most electronic blood pressure–measuring devices have not been adequately validated over a wide range of ages, blood pressures, and clinical conditions (Carney et al., 1999; Yarrows and Brook, 2000). In studies of pediatric patients, systematic differences have been found between blood pressure measurement with electronic devices and auscultation (Park et al., 2001). Electronic devices have been touted as a way of reducing human error in blood pressure measurement, such as hearing impairment, digit preference, and too-rapid deflation of the blood pressure cuff. Electronic devices leave ample room for human error in choice of cuff size, placement of the cuff, and other aspects of measurement. At present, electronic devices are best reserved for blood pressure monitoring in situations where frequent measurements are made and clinical interest is focused on trends in change of blood pressure over time. It is likely that electronic devices will improve over time; however, currently auscultation with a mercury column sphygmomanometer remains the method of choice.

A critical aspect of blood pressure measurement is the choice of an appropriate size cuff. This is particularly true for children and adolescents, who have a spectrum of arm shapes and sizes. The necessary equipment includes a total of six blood pressure cuffs—three pediatric cuffs of different sizes, a standard adult cuff, an oversized cuff, and a thigh cuff for measurement of blood pressure in the leg and for use in the arm for patients who are very overweight.

The approach to determining the optimum cuff size recommended by the National High Blood Pressure Education Program (Falkner et al., 2004) is to use a cuff with a bladder width that is approximately 40% of the upper arm circumference midway between the shoulder and the elbow. In practice this will be a cuff that will encircle 80% to 100% of the arm and will cover approximately 66% of the distance between the shoulder and the elbow. Manufacturers of blood pressure cuffs usually include lines on the cuff indicating the range of arm sizes for which that cuff bladder will be correct.

Use of a cuff that is too small will result in a blood pressure measurement that is falsely elevated because the pressure inside the cuff is intended to equal the pressure exerted on the artery. When the cuff is too small, the pressure in the cuff may be high, but the pressure on the artery is considerably lower. A cuff that is too big may result in a falsely low blood pressure measurement. Even more important, a cuff that is too large may impinge on the axilla or may cover the antecubital fossa, leading to further difficulty with blood pressure measurement.

Generally, blood pressure should be measured in the right arm after a resting period of 3 to 5 minutes. Blood pressure measured with the patient in a sitting position with the arm resting on a solid surface at heart level has become the standard. However, it may also be useful to measure blood pressure with the patient supine or standing. Measurement of blood pressure in the leg may be helpful in evaluating the presence of vascular anomalies, such as coarctation of the aorta. Blood pressure should be recorded at least twice on each occasion with the average used to estimate the level of blood pressure.

When auscultation is used, it is appropriate for the first cuff inflation to be used to determine the point at which the pulse is obliterated. For the second inflation, the blood pressure cuff should be inflated to a point 20 mmHg above the pressure at which the pulse is obliterated. The cuff should then be deflated at the slow rate of 2 to 3 mmHg/second. A period of 1 minute should occur between cuff inflations. When automated blood pressure measuring devices are used, the first measurement should usually be discarded, as it is often invalid. The first inflation with an automated device is similar to the inflation used to find the pressure at which the pulse is obliterated.

The *Korotkoff phases* refer to the sounds heard by auscultation when the blood pressure is measured. The first Korotkoff phase is the onset of snapping tones heard with each heart beat as the cuff is deflated. The fourth Korotkoff phase occurs when there is a muffling of sounds, and the fifth Korotkoff phase occurs when the sounds disappear completely.

Systolic blood pressure is determined by the onset of the Korotkoff sounds. The recommendation of the National High Blood Pressure Education Program is that diastolic blood pressure for children and adolescents be determined by the onset of the fifth Korotkoff phase, or the disappearance of sound. This brings the recommendation in line with the long-standing recommendation for adults. In the past, the recommendation has been to use the onset of the fourth Korotkoff phase, or the muffle of sounds. The fourth phase is somewhat more difficult to determine as it involves a qualitative assessment of sounds. This can lead to lower reliability when observers are not extensively trained and standardized. Nevertheless, there is controversy regarding which measure of diastolic blood pressure is better from an epidemiologic perspective. Biro et al. (1996) showed that classification of children as having normal or elevated blood pressure may differ substantially according to whether the onset of the fourth or fifth Korotkoff phase is used. This difference in criteria may affect as many as 60% of children with potential blood pressure elevation. Elkasabany et al. (1998) found that correlation of adult systolic and diastolic blood pressure was higher with the childhood fourth Korotkoff phase than with the fifth Korotkoff phase diastolic blood pressure in the Bogalusa Heart Study. This means that childhood fourth Korotkoff phase diastolic blood pressure may be a better predictor of adult blood pressure elevation.

■ AMBULATORY BLOOD PRESSURE MONITORING

Ambulatory blood pressure monitoring has been used widely for the evaluation of adults with hypertension, but it has not been used as often in children and adolescents. In adults, ambulatory blood pressure monitoring has been used as a means to evaluate white coat hypertension (Verdecchia, 1999). Ambulatory blood pressure measurements have also been found to be a useful predictor of target organ effects (Fagard et al., 1995). In children, ambulatory blood pressure measurements have also been found to correlate with hypertensive target organ changes (Belsha et al., 1998). Ambulatory monitoring has seen only limited research use in pediatric populations, in part because it has been unclear which measures of blood pressure over 24 hours are the best ones to use and because there have been limited normative data. Research in this area has begun to change that scenario.

Soergel et al. (1997) published the results of a large study of healthy children in Europe that begin to define normal 24-hour blood pressure data. In the United States, Harshfield et al. (1991) investigated ambulatory blood pressure patterns in children and adolescents. Their data suggest that there may be ethnic differences in ambulatory blood pressure patterns, with a blunted nocturnal decline in blood pressure observed in African-American youths (Harshfield et al., 1994).

It remains unknown which 24-hour blood pressure variables are most likely to be useful in the clinic setting for children and adolescents. Examination of mean 24-hour blood pressure values may be misleading because of the differences in blood pressure from the awake (higher) to the sleep (lower) states. The degree to which blood pressure declines at night may be important to evaluate and has been shown to be related to target organ abnormalities (Young et al., 1998). More sophisticated analytic techniques such as blood pressure load, the hyperbaric index, and measures of blood pressure variability, in addition to blood pressure level, may be quite important and may be different for children than for adults.

At present, the clinical use of 24-hour ambulatory monitoring in children and adolescents is often limited to the evaluation of white coat hypertension. Lurbe et al. (2004) have developed an algorithm for the use of 24-hour monitoring to identify white coat hypertension and evaluate the severity of blood pressure elevations. Further research is necessary to extend its utility into the diagnosis and treatment of hypertension in children and adolescents.

◼ ASSESSMENT OF BLOOD PRESSURE

There are no outcome-based standards for the assessment of blood pressure in children and adolescents. The traditional and current approach is to compare a patient's measurements with percentile ranks generated from epidemiologic studies of large numbers of healthy children. Clinical use of this approach relies on the concept that blood pressure tracks over time; an individual who is in an upper percentile for blood pressure at one point in time is likely to remain in the upper percentiles over time. There are a number of studies that support the concept of tracking for blood pressure (Clarke et al., 1978, Lauer et al., 1984, Lauer and Clarke, 1989). This approach also relies on the fact that higher blood pressure in children and adolescents is related to the early stages of development of target organ abnormalities, demonstrated in studies of abnormal left ventricular mass and geometry (Daniels et al., 1998).

Because body size is the strongest correlate of blood pressure in children and adolescents, blood pressure is classified on the basis of sex, age, and height. This approach provides standards that allow for differences in the rate of growth among children. Under the previous standards, tall children were prone to be overdiagnosed with blood pressure elevation, whereas shorter children could be underdiagnosed. The current approach avoids the potential for misclassification by height and does not allow for the influence of overweight, which is thought to result in a pathologic increase in blood pressure in children.

The classification of blood pressure including the definition of hypertension is presented in Table 10.1. When using this approach to classification, practitioners should remember that blood pressure varies widely throughout the day because of diurnal variation, physical activity, stress, and other factors. Any one blood pressure measurement should be interpreted with caution; blood pressure must be elevated on several occasions before a diagnosis of hypertension is made. The definition of stage 1 hypertension requires that the systolic or diastolic blood pressure be persistently above the 95th percentile. Stage 2 hypertension requires that blood pressure be above the 99th percentile, by 5 mmHg or more. Stage 2 hypertension is severe and may require more immediate clinical evaluation and treatment.

To interpret a blood pressure measurement, the first step is to determine whether it was measured correctly. The second step is to measure the child's height and record the height percentile from the Centers for Disease Control and Prevention (CDC) growth charts for the child. The third step is to use tables of blood pressure standards (Table 10.2A for boys, Table 10.2B for girls). To use these tables, the appropriate table should be chosen according to the patient's sex and whether the blood pressure of interest is the systolic or diastolic blood pressure. Next, the height percentile can be located across the top and the age can be located on the left edge of the table. Using these two variables, the appropriate box in the table can be located that provides the 90th and 95th percentiles for children of that sex, age, and height. The measured blood pressure should then be compared to the values in the table to determine if the measured blood pressure is above the 90th or 95th percentile.

TABLE 10.1
Classification of blood pressure in children and adolescents

*Blood Pressure Level Based on Percentile**	*Classification*
<90th percentile	Normal blood pressure
90th to 95th percentile or if blood pressure exceeds 120/80 mmHg even if it is below the 90th percentile†	Pre-hypertension
>95th percentile Persistent on at least 3 separate occasions	Stage 1 hypertension
>99th percentile plus 5 mmHg	Stage 2 hypertension

*From the Fourth Report on the Diagnosis, Evaluation and Treatment of High Blood Pressure in Children and Adolescents (Falkner et al., 2004).
†This occurs typically at age 12 years for systolic blood pressure and at age 16 years for diastolic blood pressure.

TABLE 10.2A
Blood pressure levels for boys by age and height percentile

Age (Years)	BP Percentile*	Systolic BP (mmHg) Percentile of Height							Diastolic BP (mmHg) Percentile of Height						
		5th	10th	25th	50th	75th	90th	95th	5th	10th	25th	50th	75th	90th	95th
1	90th	94	95	97	99	100	102	103	49	50	51	52	53	53	54
	95th	98	99	101	103	104	106	106	54	54	55	56	57	58	58
	99th	105	106	108	110	112	113	114	61	62	63	64	65	66	66
3	90th	100	101	103	105	107	108	109	59	59	60	61	62	63	63
	95th	104	105	107	109	110	112	113	63	63	64	65	66	67	67
	99th	111	112	114	116	118	119	120	71	71	72	73	74	75	75
5	90th	104	105	106	108	110	111	112	65	66	67	68	69	69	70
	95th	108	109	110	112	114	115	116	69	70	71	72	73	74	74
	99th	115	116	118	120	121	123	123	77	78	79	80	81	81	82
7	90th	106	107	109	111	113	114	115	70	70	71	72	73	74	74
	95th	110	111	113	115	117	118	119	74	74	75	76	77	78	78
	99th	117	118	120	122	124	125	126	82	82	83	84	85	86	86
9	90th	109	110	112	114	115	117	118	72	73	74	75	76	76	77
	95th	113	114	116	118	119	121	121	76	77	78	79	80	81	81
	99th	120	121	123	125	127	128	129	84	85	86	87	88	88	89
11	90th	113	114	115	117	119	120	121	74	74	75	76	77	78	78
	95th	117	118	119	121	123	124	125	78	78	79	80	81	82	82
	99th	124	125	127	129	130	132	132	86	86	87	88	89	90	90

13	90th	117	118	120	122	124	125	126	75	75	76	77	78	79	79
	95th	121	122	124	126	128	129	130	79	79	80	81	82	83	83
	99th	128	130	131	133	135	136	137	87	87	88	89	90	91	91
15	90th	122	124	125	127	129	130	131	76	77	78	79	80	80	81
	95th	126	127	129	131	133	134	135	81	81	82	83	84	85	85
	99th	134	135	136	138	140	142	142	88	89	90	91	92	93	93
17	90th	127	128	130	132	134	135	136	80	80	81	82	83	84	84
	95th	131	132	134	136	138	139	140	84	85	86	87	88	88	89
	99th	139	140	141	143	145	146	147	92	93	93	94	95	96	97

BP, blood pressure.

*The 90th percentile is 1.28 SD, 95th percentile is 1.645 SD, and 99th percentile is 2.326 SD over the mean.

Source: Fourth Report on the Diagnosis, Evaluation and Treatment of High Blood Pressure in Children and Adolescents (Falkner et al., 2004).

TABLE 10.2B
Blood pressure levels for girls by age and height percentile

Age (Years)	BP Percentile*	Systolic BP (mmHg) Percentile of Height							Diastolic BP (mmHg) Percentile of Height						
		5th	10th	25th	50th	75th	90th	95th	5th	10th	25th	50th	75th	90th	95th
1	90th	97	97	98	100	101	102	103	52	53	53	54	55	55	56
	95th	100	101	102	104	105	106	107	56	57	57	58	59	59	60
	99th	108	108	109	111	112	113	114	64	64	65	65	66	67	67
3	90th	100	100	102	103	104	106	106	61	62	62	63	64	64	65
	95th	104	104	105	107	108	109	110	65	66	66	67	68	68	69
	99th	111	111	113	114	115	116	117	73	73	74	74	75	76	76
5	90th	103	103	105	106	107	109	109	66	67	67	68	69	69	70
	95th	107	107	108	110	111	112	113	70	71	71	72	73	73	74
	99th	114	114	116	117	118	120	120	78	78	79	79	80	81	81
7	90th	106	107	108	109	111	112	113	69	70	70	71	72	72	73
	95th	110	111	112	113	115	116	116	73	74	74	75	76	76	77
	99th	117	118	119	120	122	123	124	81	81	82	82	83	84	84
9	90th	110	110	112	113	114	116	116	72	72	72	73	74	75	75
	95th	114	114	115	117	118	119	120	76	76	76	77	78	79	79
	99th	121	121	123	124	125	127	127	83	83	84	84	85	86	87
11	90th	114	114	116	117	118	119	120	74	74	74	75	76	77	77
	95th	118	118	119	121	122	123	124	78	78	78	79	80	81	81
	99th	125	125	126	128	129	130	131	85	85	86	87	87	88	89

Age	BP percentile														
13	90th	117	118	119	121	122	123	124	76	76	76	77	78	79	79
	95th	121	122	123	124	126	127	128	80	80	80	81	82	83	83
	99th	128	129	130	132	133	134	135	87	87	88	89	89	90	91
15	90th	120	121	122	123	125	126	127	78	78	78	79	80	81	81
	95th	124	125	126	127	129	130	131	82	82	82	83	84	85	85
	99th	131	132	133	134	136	137	138	89	89	90	91	91	92	93
17	90th	122	122	123	125	126	127	128	78	79	79	80	81	81	82
	95th	125	126	127	129	130	131	132	82	83	83	84	85	85	86
	99th	133	133	134	136	137	138	139	90	90	91	91	92	93	93

BP, blood pressure

*The 90th percentile is 1.28 SD, 95th percentile is 1.645 SD, and 99th percentile is 2.326 SD over the mean.

Source: Fourth Report on the Diagnosis, Evaluation and Treatment of High Blood Pressure in Children and Adolescents (Falkner et al., 2004).

■ CAUSES OF BLOOD PRESSURE ELEVATION

Hypertension can be caused by a number of disease processes, including renal, cardiovascular, neurogenic, oncologic, endocrinologic, and iatrogenic. The most common form of hypertension in adults and adolescents is a form for which no cause can currently be identified. This is usually referred to as *primary* or *essential* hypertension. The term *essential hypertension* derives from a time in the first half of the twentieth century when blood pressure elevation was thought to be a normal part of the aging process. In fact, it was believed that higher blood pressure was essential to maintain blood flow through arteries hardened by age. It is now understood that this is a pathologic process, which should be prevented or treated.

Primary hypertension probably has a genetic etiology because it tends to cluster in families. However, specific genes that cause primary hypertension have not been identified. Primary hypertension may result from the combined effects of a number of genes and environmental influences, such as diet and lack of physical activity. In children and adolescents, it is common for primary blood pressure elevation to be associated with obesity, although the mechanism by which obesity results in elevation remains to be completely elucidated. One possibility is that the insulin resistance that is often associated with obesity may also have an impact on blood pressure by altering either sodium and water homeostasis or the neurohormonal control of vascular tone (Rocchini et al., 1988, 1989). Thus, primary hypertension in some patients may be part of the metabolic or insulin resistance syndrome (Reaven, 1988).

The variety of potential secondary causes of blood pressure elevation are listed in Table 10.3. Some forms of secondary hypertension are more likely to result in acute blood pressure elevation, while others are more likely to be associated with chronic blood pressure elevation. Many of the secondary forms of hypertension result in much higher blood pressure than is usually found in primary hypertension. Some may result in a hypertensive emergency requiring rapid treatment of the blood pressure elevation.

■ CLINICAL EVALUATION OF CHILDREN WITH BLOOD PRESSURE ELEVATION

The evaluation of a pediatric patient with blood pressure elevation involves the assessment of whether the blood pressure elevation is persistent, evaluation of the level of severity of blood pressure elevation, determination of the likelihood of secondary hypertension, and assessment of the presence of target organ effects. Much can be accomplished with a detailed history, including the family history and a comprehensive physical examination. Some laboratory testing may be helpful, depending on the results of the history and physical examination. The ultimate goal of evaluation of the patient is to determine the most appropriate approach to management.

TABLE 10.3

Causes of blood pressure elevation in children and adolescents

Cause

Renal

Acute glomerulonephritis (a)
Acute renal failure (a)
Hemolytic uremic syndrome (a)
Congenital defects (c)
Chronic pyelonephritis (c)
Hydronephrosis (c)
Hypoplastic kidney (c)
Collagen vascular disease (c)

Endocrine

Hyperthyroidism (systolic) (c)
Primary aldosteronism (c)
Diabetes mellitus (c)

Vascular

Renovascular trauma (a)
Coarctation of the aorta (c)
Renal artery stenosis (c)
Takayasu arteritis (c)
Arteriovenous fistula (c)
Neurofibromatosis (c)
Tuberous sclerosis (c)

Neurogenic

Increased intracranial pressure (a)
Guillain-Barre syndrome (a)
Dysautonomia (c)

Metabolic

Hypercalcemia (a)
Hypernatremia (a)

Drugs

Cocaine (a)
Phencyclidine (PCP) (a)
Amphetamines (a)
Nonsteroidal anti-inflammatory drugs (c)
Oral contraceptives (c)
Anabolic steroids (c)
Corticosteroids (c)

Miscellaneous

Burns (a)
Leg traction (a)
Heavy metal poisons (c)

Oncologic

Pheochromocytoma (c, episodic)
Neuroblastoma (c, episodic)

a, acute blood pressure elevation; c, chronic blood pressure elevation.

Table 10.4 presents important aspects of the patient's present complaint, past medical history, review of systems, and family history. It is important to address each of these issues in detail. Important aspects of the physical examination are outlined in Table 10.5. As can be seen, the history and physical examination may provide important clues to the presence of secondary forms of hypertension. In general, the younger the patient, the higher the blood pressure, and the less family history of hypertension, the higher the index of suspicion for a possible secondary form of hypertension.

The physical examination may also provide clues to the presence of target-organ abnormalities. This can be aided by selected laboratory tests. Table 10.6 provides a list of possible manifestations of target organ abnormalities.

The standard approach to laboratory evaluation in the patient with persistent blood pressure elevation is the urinalysis, blood urea nitrogen (BUN), creatinine, electrolytes, and complete blood count. In addition, a plasma fasting lipid profile is useful because risk factors for cardiovascular disease may cluster in both individuals and in families.

■ TREATMENT OF CHILDREN WITH HYPERTENSION

The general approach to evaluation and treatment of blood pressure elevation is outlined in Figure 10.1. Once the diagnosis of primary hypertension is established and if the patient does not have severe blood pressure elevation, non-pharmacologic treatment is usually the first line of therapy (see Chapter 11). Pharmacologic therapy is initiated when children have severe hypertension or chronic hypertension that does not respond to nonpharmacologic therapy, particularly if there is evidence of target-organ abnormality or a strong family history of cardiovascular disease. For secondary forms of hypertension, the management of blood pressure elevation is similar, but treatment should also be directed at the underlying cause of blood pressure elevation.

For therapy to be successful, it is important for families to recognize that blood pressure elevation is usually asymptomatic, that effective therapy can control blood pressure but does not cure the disorder, and that a combination of lifestyle changes and medication may be needed. Good compliance with the prescribed regimen and consistent clinical follow-up are necessary for successful treatment.

■ NONPHARMACOLOGIC TREATMENT

Because many pediatric patients with primary hypertension are overweight, the first approach to management of hypertension should be weight management. The principles of weight management are discussed in Chapters 13 and 14. In-

TABLE 10.4
Important historical information

Information	Relevance
Present Illness	
Headaches, dizziness, epistaxis, visual problems	Nonspecific symptomatology, usually not etiologically helpful. Often not related to blood pressure elevation
Past Medical History	
Neonatal history	Use of umbilical artery catheter suggests need to evaluate renal vasculature and kidneys
Review of Systems	
Snoring, abnormal breathing pattern during sleep	Obstructive sleep apnea
Abdominal pain, dysuria, frequency, nocturia, enuresis	May suggest underlying renal disease
Joint pain and swelling, facial or peripheral edema	Suggests connective tissue disease and/or other forms of nephritis
Weight loss, failure to gain weight with good appetite, sweating, flushing, fevers, palpitations	In combination, symptoms suggest pheochromocytoma
Muscle cramps, weakness, constipation	May suggest hypokalemia and hyperaldosteronism
Age of onset of menarche, sexual development, regularity of menstrual periods	May be helpful in suggesting endocrinopathy, polycystic ovary syndrome
Ingestion of prescription and over-the-counter drugs, contraceptives, illicit drugs	Drug-induced hypertension
Family History	
Family history of early complications of hypertension and/or atherosclerosis factors	Suggests likely course of hypertension and/or presence of other coronary artery disease
Family history of hypertension, preeclampsia, toxemia, renal disease, tumors	Important in essential hypertension, inherited renal disease, and some endocrine diseases

Source: Adapted from the Report of the Second Task Force on Blood Pressure Control in Children, (NHLBI, 1987).

vestigators have shown that weight loss is accompanied by decreased blood pressure in adults (MacMahon et al., 1985) and in adolescents (Rocchini et al., 1989). In adults, blood pressure appears to fall at a rate of 1 mmHg/kg of body weight loss and is associated with reduction of both systolic and diastolic blood pressure. The effect of weight loss appears to be independent of changes in dietary

TABLE 10.5
Important physical examination findings

Physical Findings	Relevance
General	
Pale mucous membranes, facial or pretibial edema	Renal disease
Pallor, evanescent flushing, increased sweating at rest	Pheochromocytoma vs. hyperdynamic essential hypertension
Café–au-lait spots, neurofibromas	Neurofibromatosis
Moon face, hirsutism, buffalo hump, truncal obesity, striae	Cushing's syndrome
Webbing of the neck, low hairline, wide-spaced nipples, wide carrying angle	Turner's syndrome (coarctation of the aorta)
Elfin facies, poor growth, retardation	William's syndrome (coarctation of the aorta, renal artery stenosis)
Thyroid enlargement	Hyper- or hypothyroidism
Cardiovascular	
Absent or delayed femoral pulses, low leg pressure relative to arm blood pressure	Coarctation of the aorta
Heart size, rate, rhythm, murmurs, respiratory difficulty, hepatomegaly	(1) Murmur-coarctation; (2) tachycardia and/ or arrhythmia–pheochromocytoma; (3) large heart or heart failure; prolonged or severe hypertension
Bruits over great vessels	Arteritis or arteriopathy
Abdomen	
Epigastric bruit	Renovascular diseases isolated or associated with William's syndrome, neurofibromatosis, or arteritis
Unilateral or bilateral masses	Wilm's tumor, neuroblastoma, pheochromocytoma, polycystic kidneys, other tumors
Neurologic	
Hypertensive funduscopic changes	Chronic hypertension
Bell's palsy	Chronic hypertension
Neurologic deficits (e.g., hemiparesis)	Chronic or severe acute hypertension with stroke

Source: Adapted from the Report of the Second Task Force on Blood Pressure Control in Children (NHLBI, 1987).

TABLE 10.6
Manifestation of target-organ abnormalities

Organ System	Manifestation and Evaluation
Cardiac	Left ventricular hypertrophy by echocardiography
	Left ventricular dysfunction by echocardiography
Renal	Renal insufficiency
	Microalbuminuria
	Proteinuria
	Elevated serum creatinine
Vascular	Retinopathy
	Arteriolar narrowing, tortuosity, hemorrhages, or exudates
Neurologic	Seizures (can be seen with accelerated hypertension)

intake of sodium and in physical activity. However, there may be a threshold of weight loss that must be achieved before blood pressure reduction is seen. Some investigators have also found a "floor effect," or a degree of weight loss beyond which no further reduction in blood pressure occurs (Cohen and Flamenbaum, 1985).

Another important nonpharmacologic approach is the reduction of dietary sodium (see Chapter 11). Moderate dietary sodium restriction appears to carry little risk and may benefit some patients with blood pressure elevation. Those patients who benefit from sodium restriction are said to be salt-sensitive. In adults, almost 50% of patients who restrict their intake of sodium to 2 g (5 to 6 g of salt) will have a reduction of blood pressure of approximately 5 mmHg (Cutler et al., 1991). Epidemiologic evidence from Japan suggests that reduction of salt intake across the whole population can lead to a reduction in the prevalence of hypertension and cardiovascular outcomes (Perry, 1990).

Other dietary approaches to blood pressure reduction, including increasing calcium and potassium intake, have been investigated but currently are not clinically recommended. One dietary factor that is often overlooked in adolescents is the intake of alcohol. It is clear that high intake of alcohol is associated with blood pressure elevation in adults (Maheswaran et al., 1991), so adolescent patients should be questioned about alcohol intake and counseled to avoid alcoholic beverages.

Another important aspect of the nonpharmacologic treatment of hypertension is physical activity. An increase in physical activity is beneficial from the standpoint of weight management, and chronic physical activity may have an independent blood pressure–lowering effect (Nelson et al., 1986). This effect seems to be present for both aerobic and resistance (weight training) forms of exercise. Because systolic blood pressure rises sharply during acute exercise some concerns have been raised about recommendations for athletes with elevated

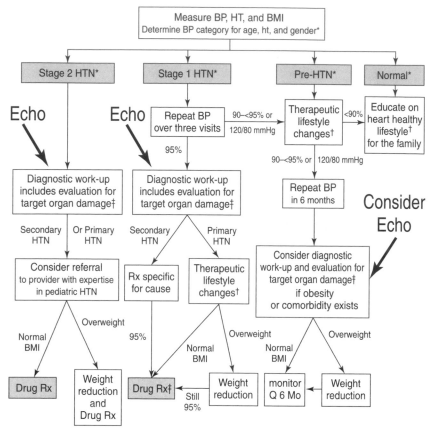

F I G U R E   1 0 . 1
Management algorithm for evaluating hypertension in children and adolescents. BMI, body mass index; BP, blood pressure; HT, height; HTN, hypertension. *New National Institutes of Health definition; †Diet including sodium restriction and exercise. ‡Especially if younger, have very high blood pressure, or have little or no family history, or if diabetic or have other risk factors.
Source: From the Fourth Report on the Diagnosis, Evaluation and Treatment of High Blood Pressure in Children and Adolescents (Faulkner et al., 2004).

blood pressure. Athletes with blood pressure elevation that is not severe should be allowed to participate in competitive athletics (American Academy of Pediatrics, 1997). In some cases it may be useful to perform a graded exercise test and follow the blood pressure response to exercise. If the blood pressure rises above normal ranges for exercises, athletic participation of the patient may not be advised. However, the blood pressure response to the standard exercise test is not necessarily equivalent to that seen during practice or competition (Palantini et al., 1990). Children and adolescents with severe hypertension should be restricted from competition until their blood pressure is controlled. In this situation, the goal should be to institute appropriate therapy and monitor blood pressure in the clinic. When blood pressure has been controlled, it is acceptable for the patient to return to athletics.

■ PHARMACOLOGIC MANAGEMENT OF HYPERTENSION

The decision to use medication to treat blood pressure elevation in children and adolescents should not be taken lightly. Those patients with primary hypertension may ultimately need long-term treatment. Compliance may be difficult because patients feel no adverse effects from their blood pressure elevation. Nevertheless, patients with persistent blood pressure elevation that has not been ameliorated by nonpharmacologic treatment, and especially those with evidence of target organ abnormalities such as left ventricular hypertrophy, should be considered candidates for drug treatment. Such treatment should be individualized according to the patient's age, level of blood pressure, past medical history and family history.

The goal of antihypertensive pharmacologic therapy is to reduce blood pressure below the 95th percentile. If chronic renal disease or diabetes mellitus is present, it is appropriate to be more aggressive and aim to lower blood pressure below the 90th percentile. The Fourth Report on the Diagnosis, Evaluation and Treatment of High Blood Pressure in Children and Adolescents (Falkner et al., 2004) provides guidelines for the use of antihypertensive medications; a number of classes of antihypertensive agents are available for use in pediatrics (Table 10.7). The usual approach is to initially use a diuretic, β-adrenergic blocking agent, calcium channel antagonist, or an angiotensin-converting enzyme (ACE) inhibitor. The lowest appropriate dose is usually the starting point, with titration of dosage upward to achieve control of blood pressure as necessary.

There is considerable clinical experience with using β-adrenergic blocking agents and diuretics for treatment of hypertension in children, and increasing information is available on the use of calcium channel blockers and ACE inhibitors. No long-term clinical trials have been conducted to establish the benefit of pharmacologic treatment of primary hypertension with any class of antihypertensive agents in pediatric patients (Kay, 2001). An increasing number of short-term clinical trials have evaluated the safety of these agents and their ability to lower blood pressure. ACE inhibitors have become primary agents for antihypertensive therapy because of their blood pressure-lowering effect and their beneficial effects on cardiac function and structure and renal function. They may be especially useful in patients with diabetes mellitus. In selecting any agent, physicians should take into consideration any contraindications and possible side effects (Table 10.8).

In some clinical situations, it may be appropriate to pharmacologically treat children with less severe levels of hypertension. For example, children with

TABLE 10.7

Antihypertensive drug therapy for chronic hypertension in children

| Drug* | Dose (mg/kg/day) | | Dosing Interval (hours) |
	Initial	Maximum	
Adrenergic-Blocking Agents			
α/β blocker			
Labetalol	1–3 mg/kg/day	10 mg/kg/day Up to 2.4 g/day	q 12
α blocker			
Prazosin	0.05–0.1 mg/kg/day	0.5–1 mg/kg/day	q 8
β-adrenergic blockers			
Atenolol	0.5 mg/kg/day	2 mg/kg/day Up to 100 mg/day	q 12–24
Propranolol	1 mg/kg/day	4 mg/kg/day	q 6–12
Alpha agonist	*Children ≥12 years*		
Clonidine	0.2 mg/day	2.4 mg/day	q 12
Angiotensin Converting Enzyme Inhibitors			
Captopril	0.3–0.5 mg/kg/dose (>12 months old)	6 mg/kg/day	q 8
Lisinopril	0.07 mg/kg/day Up to 5 mg/day	0.6 mg/kg/day up to 40 mg/day	q 24
Calcium Antagonists	*Children 6–17 years*		
Amlodipine	2.5 mg/dose	10 mg/day	q 24
Nifedipine (extended release)	0.25–0.5 mg/kg/day	3 mg/kg/day up to 120 mg/day	q 12–24
Diuretics			
Furosemide	0.5–2.0 mg/kg/dose	6 mg/kg/day	q 6–24
Hydrochlorothiazide	1 mg/kg/day	3 mg/kg/day Up to 50 mg/day	q 12
Spironolactone	1 mg/kg/day	3 mg/kg/day Up to 100 mg/day	q 12–24
Triamterine	1–2 mg/kg/day	3 mg/kg/day Up to 300 mg/day	q 12
Vasodilators			
Hydralazine	0.75 mg/kg/day	7.5 mg/kg/day Up to 200 mg/day	q 6

*Other drugs are available in some classes, but data on dosage in children have not been published.
Source: Fourth Report on the Diagnosis, Evaluation and Treatment of High Blood Pressure in Children and Adolescents (Faulkner et al., 2004).

TABLE 10.8
Choice of antihypertensive therapy

Class of Agent	Contraindications	Clinically Apparent Side Effects	Less Apparent Side Effects
ACE inhibitors	Pregnancy Bilateral renovascular disease	Chronic cough Rash Disturbance of taste	Hyperkalemia Proteinuria Leukopenia
β blockers	Asthma Heart Block Type 1 diabetes mellitus	Bronchospasm Fatigue Lack of awareness of hypoglycemia	Glucose intolerance Increased triglycerides Decreased HDL-C
Calcium-channel blockers	Heart failure	Flushing Pretibial edema Constipation Gingival hyperplasia	AV conduction abnormality
Diuretics	Preexisting hypovolemia Type 1 diabetes mellitus	Weakness, palpitations	Hypokalemia Glucose intolerance Hypercholesterolemia Hyperuricemia

ACE, angiotensin-converting enzyme; AV, atrioventricular; HDL-C, high-density lipprotein cholesterol.

diabetes mellitus and chronic renal disease are at increased risk of progression of renal abnormalities. These patients should have their blood pressure lowered below the 95th percentile to preserve renal function.

▪ HYPERTENSIVE EMERGENCIES

Children and adolescents with severe blood pressure elevation are at risk for short-term complications of hypertension, such as encephalopathy and cardiac failure. Such patients need immediate attention and referral to a physician experienced in the management of severe hypertension. Parenteral medications are often the agents used in this setting; however, in pediatric patients, oral nifedipine may also be used effectively (Sinaiko and Daniels, 2001). The most commonly used agents for treatment of hypertension emergencies are presented in Table 10.9. For accelerated hypertension in children with target organ abnormalities, particularly congestive heart failure, blood pressure should be lowered aggressively to the 95th percentile. However, too rapid reduction of blood pressure to too low a level may lead to a reduction in myocardial perfusion and other organ system problems. Such treatment should only occur in closely monitored settings so that appropriate titration of the blood pressure level can be achieved.

TABLE 10.9
Drug therapy for hypertensive emergencies in children

Drug	Dose
Sodium nitroprusside (vasodilator)	0.3 mg/kg/minute IV initially; may be increased stepwise to 8 mg/kg/minute maximum
Labetalol (α and β blocker)	0.2–1 mg/kg/dose up to 40 mg/dose IV; may be increased incrementally to 1 mg/kg/dose until response received; 0.25–3 mg/kg/hour maintenance, IV infusion
Esmolol (β blocker)	100–500 µg/kg/minute; IV infusion
Hydralazine (vasodilator)	0.2–0.6 mg/kg/dose IV prn; may be repeated two times if no response
Nifedipine (short acting) (calcium channel blocker)	0.1–0.2 mg/kg oral prn, may be repeated if no response
Minoxidil (vasoldilator)	0.1–0.2 mg/kg/dose oral

Source: Fourth Report on the Diagnosis, Evaluation and Treatment of High Blood Pressure in Children and Adolescents (Faulkner et al., 2004).

▨ SUMMARY

- In adults, much cardiovascular disease morbidity and mortality can be attributed to underrecognition and undertreatment of hypertension.
- Blood pressure elevation may begin in childhood and adolescence and may be associated with the early stages of development of cardiovascular disease.
- It is imperative that children with blood pressure elevation be recognized and treated appropriately.
- Management of children with hypertension can present challenges, but effective treatment can be achieved by both nonpharmacologic and pharmacologic means.

▨ REFERENCES

American Academy of Pediatrics Committee on Sports Medicine and Fitness. 1997. Athletic Participation by Children and Adolescents Who Have Systemic Hypertension. *Pediatrics* 99:637–8.

Belsha, C.W., T.G. Wells, K.L. McNiece, P.M.Seib, J.K. Plummer, and P.L. Berry. 1998. Influence of Diurnal Blood Pressure Variations on Target Organ Abnormalities in Adolescents with Mild Essential Hypertension. *Am J Hypertens* 11:410–7.

Biro, F.M., S.R. Daniels, B.A. Barton, G.H. Payne, and J.A. Morrison. 1996. Differential Classification of Blood Pressure by Fourth and Fifth Korotkoff Phases in School-Aged Girls. The National Heart, Lung and Blood Institute Growth and Health Study. *Am J Hypertens* 9:242–7.

Carney, S.L., A.H. Gillie, S.L. Green, O. Patterson, M.S. Taylor, and A.J. Smith. 1999. Hospital Blood Pressure Measurement: Staff and Device Assessment. *J Qual Clin Pract* 19:95–8.

Clarke, W.R., H.G. Schrott, P.E. Leaverton, W.E. Connor, and R.M. Lauer. 1978. Tracking of Blood Lipids and Blood Pressures in School Age Children: The Muscatine Study. *Circulation* 58:626–34.

Cohen, W., and W. Flamenbaum. 1985. Obesity and Hypertension. Demonstration of a 'Floor Effect'. *Am J Med* 80:177–81.

Cutler, J.A., D. Follmann, P. Elliott, and I. Suh. 1991. An Overview of Randomized Trials of Sodium Reduction and Blood Pressure. *Hypertension* 17:127–33.

Daniels, S.R., J.M.H. Loggie, P. Khoury, and T.R. Kimball. 1998. Left Ventricular Geometry and Severe Left Ventricular Hypertrophy in Children and Adolescents with Essential Hypertension. *Circulation* 97:1907–11.

Elkasabany, A.M., E.M. Urbina, S.R. Daniels, and G.S. Berenson. 1998. Prediction of Adult Hypertension by K4 and K5 Diastolic Blood Pressure in Children: The Bogalusa Heart Study. *J Pediatr* 132:687–92.

Fagard, R., J.A. Staessen, and L. Thijs. 1995. The Relationships between Left Ventricular Mass and Daytime and Night-Time Blood Pressures: A Meta-Analysis of Comparative Studies. *J Hypertens* 13:823–9.

Falkner, B., S.R. Daniels, J.T. Flynn, S. Gidding, L.A. Green, J. Inglefinger, R.M. Lauer, B.Z. Morgenstern, R.J. Portman, R.J. Prineas, A.P. Rocchini, B. Rosner, A.R. Sinaiko, N. Stettler, E. Urbina, E.J. Roccella. 2004. The Fourth Report on the Diagnosis, Evaluation and Treatment of High Blood Pressure in Children and Adolescents. *Pediatrics* 114(2 Suppl):555–76.

Falkner, B., S.R. Daniels, M.J. Horan, J.M.H. Loggie, R.J. Prineas, B. Rosner, A.R. Sinaiko, E.J. Roccella, and D.E. Anderson. 1996. Update on the Task Force Report (1987) on High

Blood Pressure in Children and Adolescents: A Working Group Report from the National High Blood Pressure Education Program. *Pediatrics* 98:649–58.

Harshfield, G.A., B.S. Alpert, D.A. Pulliam, G.W. Somes, and D.K. Wilson. 1994. Ambulatory Blood Pressure Recordings in Children and Adolescents. *Pediatrics* 94:180–4.

Harshfield, G.A., D.A. Pulliam, B.S. Alpert, B. Stapleton, E.S. Willey, and G.W. Somes. 1991. Ambulatory Blood Pressure Patterns in Children and Adolescents: Influence of Renin-Sodium Profiles. *Pediatrics* 87:94–100.

Joint National Committee. 1997. The Sixth Report of the Joint National Committee on Prevention, Detection, Evaluation, and Treatment of High Blood Pressure. *Arch Intern Med* 157:2413–46.

Jones, D.W., E.D. Frohlich, C.M. Grim, C.E. Grim, and K.A. Taubert. 2001. Mercury Sphygmomanometers Should Not Be Abandoned: An Advisory Statement from The Council for High Blood Pressure Research, American Heart Association. *Hypertension* 37:185–6.

Kay, J.D., A.R. Sinaiko, and S.R. Daniels. 2001. Pediatric Hypertension. *Am Heart J* 142:422–32.

Kimm, S.Y., G.H. Payne, M.P. Stylianou, M.A. Waclawiw, and C. Lichtenstein. 1998. National Trends in the Management of Cardiovascular Disease Risk Factors in Children: Second NHLBI Survey of Primary Care Physicians. *Pediatrics* 102:e61

Kluger, C.Z., J.A. Morrison, and S.R. Daniels. 1991. Preventive Practices for Adult Cardiovascular Disease. *J Fam Pract* 33:65–72.

Lauer, R.M., and W.R. Clarke. 1989. Childhood Risk Factors for High Adult Blood Pressure: The Muscatine Study. *Pediatrics* 84:633–41.

Lauer, R.M., W.R. Clarke, and R. Beaglehole. 1984. Level, Trend and Variability of Blood Pressure during Childhood: The Muscatine Study. *Circulation* 69:242–9.

Lurbe, E., J. Sorof, and S.R. Daniels. 2004. Clinical and Research Aspects of Ambulatory Blood Pressure Monitoring in Children. *J Pediatr* 144:7–16.

MacMahon, S.W., F.J. MacDonald, L. Bernstein, G. Andrews, and R.B. Blacket. 1985. Comparison of Weight Reduction with Metoprolol in Treatment of Hypertension in Young Overweight Patients. *Lancet* 325:1233–6.

Maheswaran, R., J.J. Gill, P. Davies, and D.G. Beevers. 1991. High Blood Pressure due to Alcohol. A Rapidly Reversible Effect. *Hypertension* 17:787–92.

National Heart, Lung, and Blood Institute. 1987. Report of the Second Task Force on Blood Pressure Control in Children. *Pediatrics* 79:1–25.

Nelson, L., G.L. Jennings, M.D. Esler, and P.I. Korner. 1986. Effect of Changing Levels of Physical Activity on Blood Pressure and Haemodynamics in Essential Hypertension. *Lancet* 328:473–6.

Palantini, P., L. Mos, P. Mormino, L. Munari, M. Del Torre, F. Valle, E. Scaldalai and A.C. Pessina. 1990. Intra-Arterial Blood Pressure Monitoring in the Evaluation of the Hypertensive Athlete. *Eur Heart J* 11:348–54.

Park, M.K., S.W. Menard, and C. Yuan. 2001. Comparison of Auscultatory and Oscillometric Blood Pressures. *Arch Pediatr Adolesc Med* 155:50–3.

Perry, I.J. 1990. What has Caused the Widespread Decline in Stroke Mortality?" *J Irish Coll Physicians Surg* 19:257–9.

Reaven, G.M.. 1988. Banting Lecture: Role of Insulin Resistance in Human Disease. *Diabetes* 37:1595–1607.

Rocchini, A.P., V. Katch, J. Anderson, J. Hinderliter, D. Becque, M. Martin and C. Marks. 1988. Blood Pressure in Obese Adolescents: Effect of Weight Loss. *Pediatrics* 82:16–23.

Rocchini, A.P., J. Key, D. Bondie, R. Chico, C. Moorehead, V. Katch, and M. Martin. 1989. The Effect of Weight Loss on the Sensitivity of Blood Pressure to Sodium in Obese Adolescents. *N Engl J Med* 321:580–5.

Sinaiko, A.R., and S.R. Daniels. 2001. The Use of Short-Acting Nifedipine in Children with Hypertension: Another Example of the Need for Comprehensive Drug Testing in Children. *J Pediatr* 139:7–9.

Soergel, M., M. Kirschtein, C. Busch, T. Danne, J. Gellermann, R. Holl, F. Krull, H. Reichert, G.S. Reusz and W. Rascher. 1997. Oscillometric Twenty-Four-Hour Ambulatory Blood Pressure Values in Healthy Children and Adolescents: A Multicenter Trial Including 1141 Subjects. *J Pediatr* 130:178–84.

Verdecchia, P. 1999. White-Coat Hypertension in Adults and Children. *Blood Pressure Monitor* 4:175–9.

Yarrows, S.A., and R.D. Brook. 2000. Measurement Variation among Twelve Electronic Home Blood Pressure Monitors. *Am J Hypertens* 13:276–82.

Young, L.A., T.R. Kimball, S.R. Daniels, D.A. Standiford, P.R. Khoury, S.M. Eichelberger, and L.M. Dolan. 1998. Nocturnal Blood Pressure in Young Patients with Insulin-Dependent Diabetes Mellitus: Correlation with Cardiac Function. *J Pediatr* 133:46–50.

CHAPTER 11

Dietary Management of Children and Adolescents with High Blood Pressure

Linda Van Horn and Eileen Vincent

Hypertension (systolic blood pressure [SBP] >140 mmHg or diastolic blood pressure [DBP] >90 mmHg) is a major risk factor for cardiovascular disease and is estimated to affect over 60 million adults at a cost of 14 billion dollars annually (Gillman and Ellison, 1993; Fernandes and McCrindle, 2000). Pre-hypertension (SBP of 120–139 mmHg or DBP of 80–89 mmHg) is estimated to affect another 45 million individuals and is strongly associated with development of hypertension with increasing age (Chobanian et al., 2003). Although hypertension in childhood is typically secondary to some other pathological condition, growing evidence from landmark studies including the Muscatine, Bogalusa, and Cardiovascular Risk in Young Finns studies confirms that blood pressure in youth tracks into adulthood (Webber et al., 1983; Lauer et al., 1984; Lauer and Clarke, 1989; Raitakari et al., 1994; Muntner et al., 2004). This phenomenon may be even more pronounced in certain ethnic groups (Rosner et al., 2000). For example, the Pathobiological Determinants of Atherosclerosis in Youth (PDAY) research group reported that, based on autopsy studies, more extensive raised lesions were found in blacks than in whites with hypertension (McGill et al., 2000; also see Chapter 1). Concerns about these associations are further magnified by evidence of increased levels of blood pressure in children and adolescents, ages 8 to 17 years, from the National Health and Nutrition Examination Survey (NHANES) conducted in 1988–94 and 1999–2000 (Muntner et al., 2004).

The first report of the Task Force on Blood Pressure Control in Children (National Heart, Lung and Blood Institute [NHLBI], 1977), following published results of the Muscatine study (Lauer et al., 1975), provided guidelines for detection and treatment of hypertension in children and established normal blood pressure levels. As further blood pressure data have accumulated, these guidelines have been updated several times (NHLBI, 1987; Rosner et al., 1993; Falkner et al., 1996, 2004). The dietary recommendations for prevention and treatment of high blood pressure in children, by contrast, are generally adapted from research in adults. Simons-Morton and colleagues (Simons-Morton et al., 1997; Simons-Morton and Obarzanek, 1997) reviewed existing research on diet and blood pressure in children and reported that given the paucity of data on this subject, no conclusive dietary recommendations could be made. Unlike the elegant series of studies, Dietary Approaches to Stopping Hypertension (DASH), in adults (Sacks et al., 1995, 2001; Appel et al., 1997), there have been no comparable controlled feeding studies in children. Pediatricians and other health care providers have depended largely on clinical judgment to determine how best to adapt the adult-based findings to their pediatric patients. This chapter summarizes and updates research on diet and blood pressure in children. Because of the relatively limited data on this subject, extrapolations are made from adult-based studies for dietary strategies appropriate for children.

■ CORRELATES OF BLOOD PRESSURE

A variety of factors have been linked to elevated blood pressure levels, including diet and anthropometric and behavioral variables (Kuczmarski et al., 1994). Body mass index (BMI) levels influence blood pressure but the impact may also vary by race, by sex, and by degree of fatness (Folsom et al., 1991). In children, as in adults, as body mass increases, blood pressure increases (Sorof et al., 2002), with the strongest associations being at the highest levels of BMI (Solomon and Manson, 1997; Must et al., 1999). Among children with BMI above the 97th percentile, elevated blood pressure and insulin were reported to be twice as common as among children with BMI between the 95th to 97th percentile (Freedman et al., 1999). Weight loss is associated with reductions in blood pressure (Clarke et al., 1986; Rocchini et al., 1988). Fortunately, long term maintenance of weight loss in children has also been documented (Epstein et al., 1990), making childhood an especially appropriate time to address problems in both weight and blood pressure.

Studies of Seventh Day Adventist (SDA) and non-SDA lacto ovo vegetarian adults have reported significantly lower blood pressure levels in these groups than in omnivorous adults (Rouse and Beilin, 1984). When comparing SDA and non-SDA adolescents, a significant direct association was found only between body weight and blood pressure, with weaker associations between exercise, diet, religiosity, type A behavior, and anger (Kuczmarski et al., 1994). The authors speculated that possible protective effects of the vegetarian diet may not emerge until adulthood. Similarly, despite established differences between blacks and whites in the prevalence of hypertension in adults, few ethnic differences in either SBP or DBP appear in childhood (Rosner et al., 2000).

In a study of the metabolic syndrome in childhood, Arslanian and Suprasongsin (1996) reported that among prepubertal children, DBP was negatively associated with insulin sensitivity and positively associated with insulin levels, independent of adiposity. The authors proposed that the roots of the metabolic syndrome begin in childhood with diet influencing insulin levels (see Chapter 15). Direct associations between weight and insulin resistance and between insulin resistance and blood pressure in children have been documented in the Minneapolis Children's Blood Pressure Study and the Bogalusa Heart Study (Taittonen et al., 1996; Sinaiko et al., 1997,1999). The rate of weight gain during childhood was found to be a more powerful predictor of adult cardiovascular risk than absolute weight at any point in time (Sinaiko et al., 1999).

Elevated SBP combined with hyperinsulinemia, elevated triglycerides, low high-density lipoprotein (HDL) cholesterol, and elevated body fat measurements was an identified risk factor for metabolic syndrome among children and adolescents in the European Youth Heart Study (Andersen et al., 2003). This study also demonstrated that a fitness level 1.2 SD below and BMI 1.6 SD above the targeted pediatric population mean were highly significant across sex, age groups, and five defined risk factors for metabolic syndrome. These findings support the importance of establishing healthy lifestyle habits early in life as a proactive approach toward prevention of chronic diseases such as hypertension in adulthood.

■ FETAL ORIGINS

Fetal origins of adult hypertension and the influence of maternal diet and rate of maternal weight gain have now been repeatedly documented (Barker et al., 1989; Law et al., 1993; Adair et al., 2001; Loos et al., 2001). Recent studies suggest that maternal diet quality even more than quantity affects a child's blood pressure in later life (Roseboom et al., 1999). Protein and carbohydrate balance during late pregnancy was found to be associated with blood pressure levels in offspring 40 years later, independent of current body weight (Campbell et al., 1996). Other studies are inconclusive (Stanner et al., 1997; Leary et al., 2005).

In a large cohort from the Cebu (Philippines) Longitudinal Health and Nutrition Survey, maternal nutrition also appeared to have a sex-specific influence on blood pressure during adolescence (Adair et al., 2001). The mother's protein intake (expressed as percent of protein calories) during pregnancy was inversely correlated with SBP among male offspring at 16 years of age. But maternal dietary fat intake was significantly associated with lower SBP and DBP levels in the teenage girls studied. Additionally, lower maternal body fat levels negatively impacted blood pressure levels in these male and female Filipino adolescents. These findings suggest that the mother's available energy stores as well as diet composition during pregnancy may have lifelong effects on a child's blood pressure.

A follow-up study of children 13 to 16 years of age who were born pre-term and randomly assigned to either banked breast milk or formula reported significantly lower (mean 81.9 vs. 86.1 mmHg; 95% CI -6.6 to -1.6, $p = 0.001$) mean arterial pressure in those who received breast milk (Singhal et al., 2001). Thus diet appeared to influence blood pressure, perhaps starting in utero. Additional studies are needed to confirm these findings. More recently, results from the Avon Longitudinal Study of Parents and Children (ALSPAC) showed no evidence of an association between material diet in late pregnancy and offspring blood pressure at age 7½ years (Leary et al., 2005).

■ RECOMMENDED TREATMENT OF HYPERTENSION IN CHILDREN AND ADOLESCENTS

Nonpharmacologic therapy is the preferred approach to treatment of high blood pressure in children (Falkner et al., 1996; Gidding et al., 2005). Among children with frank hypertension (see Table 10.1 in Chapter 10) and high normal blood pressure (90th to 95th percentile), dietary intervention is advocated prior to or as a complement to drug therapy (Berenson et al., 1998). Because body size and especially overweight influence high blood pressure, weight loss is the single most important strategy for improving both SBP and DBP levels (Rocchini et al., 1988; Falkner et al., 1996; Lobstein et al., 2004; Reinehr et al., 2004). Likewise, prevention of excessive weight gain during normal growth and development is strongly advocated. Blood pressure is also directly related to physical fitness (Fraser et al., 1983; Hansen et al., 1991). Studies on weight control in children that have successfully demonstrated effective approaches to weight loss consistently incorporate a combined diet plus physical activity regimen that can be sustained over the lifetime (Vandongen et al., 1995).

■ PRIMARY PREVENTION

Prevention of high blood pressure in children is strongly advocated (Falkner et al., 1996; Simons-Morton et al., 1997; Gidding et al., 2005). Previous discussion and public health recommendations have generally focused on population-based vs. high-risk intervention approaches (Prineas et al., 1985). Population-based approaches are favored, especially when the suspected cause is environmental. The whole society benefits by shifting to an eating pattern that is more consistently associated with lower blood pressure levels (Prineas et al., 1985; National High Blood Pressure Education Program Working Group on High Blood Pressure in Children and Adolescents, 2004). A leftward shift in the distribution, i.e., a reduction, of blood pressure across the whole population could result in reduced incidence of hypertension overall (Chobanian et al., 2003). Opponents of this population-based approach resent the concept of changing everyone's diet to benefit presumably a relative few. Resolution of this debate may lie in broadening the overriding assumptions. Key questions are not only who is susceptible and who is not, but also whether there are potential benefits beyond blood pressure control that are conferred by adopting a prevention-type diet. Given the growing epidemic of obesity in this country, a population-wide improvement in calorie balance, including increased physical activity, could be the single most beneficial strategy toward reducing overall risk of hypertension and other chronic diseases. A diet lower in sodium, fat, and sugar and higher in fiber, fruits, and vegetables would benefit the vast majority of the American public including children. Successful implementation of such an environmental approach requires major cooperation among school systems, parents, and the medical community (Perry et al., 1988; Simons-Morton et al., 1991; Luepker et al., 1996; Nader et al., 1996; Webber et al., 1996; Burke et al., 1998; also see Chapter 18).

DIET AND BLOOD PRESSURE STUDIES

Despite growing research interest in diet and blood pressure, there are far fewer studies documenting the impact of dietary changes on children than there are on adults. Simons-Morton and Obarzanek (1997) reviewed more than 40 studies examining relationships between dietary nutrients and blood pressure in children and adolescents. A summary of these results, expanded to include new research reported since their review, is presented below.

Sodium

Sodium, the subject of 25 observational and 12 intervention studies, has been the most extensively studied nutrient related to blood pressure in children (Simons-Morton and Obarzanek, 1997). Methodologic limitations were cited in most of these studies, prohibiting conclusive findings, but the authors provided consistent evidence that higher sodium intake is related to higher blood pressure in children and adolescents.

Of all the observational studies on sodium, nine studies had multiple measures of sodium intake including urinary and dietary measures, considered the gold standard for determining objective outcomes (Cooper et al., 1980; Faust, 1982; Liebman et al., 1986; Geleijnse et al., 1990; Jones et al., 1990; Gillman et al., 1992). In black and white obese and non-obese children and adolescents, a positive relationship was consistently reported between sodium and both DBP and SBP. A study in 956 ten-year-old Israeli school children reported increased blood pressure levels associated with higher sodium and nitrate levels that were measured in their drinking water (Pomeranz et al., 2000). Both systolic and mean arterial blood pressures were raised.

Likewise, of all the documented pediatric dietary intervention studies, the majority have focused on sodium. Simons-Morton and Obarzanek (1997) identified 12 intervention studies (Gillum et al., 1981; Trevisan et al., 1981; Cooper et al., 1984; Calabrese and Tuthill, 1985; Howe et al., 1985, 1991; Tuthill and Calabrese, 1985; Tochikubo et al., 1986; Miller et al., 1988; Sinaiko et al., 1993), with 2 (Tochikubo et al., 1986; Miller et al., 1988) reporting reduced blood pressure levels following reduced sodium intake. One study (Rocchini et al., 1989) reported differences on the basis of body size, with significantly lower mean blood pressure in obese but not non-obese boys following a low-sodium diet. Conversely, in a crossover study of children in a Seventh Day Adventist boarding school, Cooper et al. (1984) reported greater reductions in SBP among children with BMI less than 23 following lower sodium intake. In another two-school crossover study, Ellison et al. (1989) reported lower blood pressure with lower sodium intake, based on regression analyses adjusted for sex and baseline blood pressure. Similarly, in a follow-up study 15 years after a randomized trial of lower vs. normal sodium intake in newborn Dutch infants, adjusted SBP was 3.6 mmHg lower and DBP was 2.2 mmHg lower in the lower-sodium group than in the control group (Geleijnse et al., 1997). Overall, in a summary of available data from studies with the most rigorous methodologic conditions, Simons-Morton and Obarzanek (1997) concluded that higher sodium intake was related to higher blood pressure in children and adolescents.

Subsequent to this review, the Child and Adolescent Trial on Cardiovascular Health (CATCH) was conducted in 96 schools across the United States (Luepker et al., 1996). The CATCH study was designed to assess the impact of school foodservice modifications, such as reductions in fat and salt, as part of an environmental, school-based approach to improve diet and physical activity levels in children (Luepker et al., 1996). While the CATCH intervention successfully achieved dietary and other environmental changes, blood pressure, body size, and cholesterol measures were not significantly different between control and intervention groups after 2 years. Self-reported lifestyle changes persisted after 3 years among 3714 (73%) of the initial cohort of 5106 students that participated in a follow-up study (Nader et al., 1999). Despite this 3-year sustained adherence, no significant differences were noted among physiologic outcomes, including blood pressure, in these young, healthy cohorts. Whether such lifestyle changes made in youth and sustained throughout young adulthood will ultimately affect risk for cardiovascular disease in later adulthood has yet to be studied and documented.

As described by Falkner and Michel (1997), the typical intake of sodium in the United States far exceeds the nutrient requirement. According to secular trends, intake of sodium among children, adolescents, and adults has increased. Although blood pressure sensitivity to sodium is apparent in certain subgroups, it may be linked to other risk factors such as race, family history, and obesity. Just as these risk factors may cluster, dietary sodium may be only one of several other nutrients or dietary factors that collectively influence blood pressure if not initially then over time (Simon et al., 1994; Falkner and Michel, 1997). Data from the DASH-Sodium Trial, in which three sodium levels were tested among hypertensive and normotensive adults, indicated improvements in blood pressure in both groups and across different ethnic and weight subgroups (Appel et al., 1997; Vollmer et al., 2001) when sodium was reduced. As a primary prevention strategy, reducing sodium intake among children appears prudent. Sodium intake of 1.5 g/day was recommended for adults by the Institute of Medicine (2004) and the DASH results further document that nutrient needs can easily be met at this level of sodium intake following a Western-type diet (Lin et al., 2003).

Potassium

Reviews of the adult literature have concluded that potassium has an inverse effect on blood pressure (Cappuccio and MacGregor, 1991). Results from randomized trials using potassium supplements have been inconsistent (Grimm et al., 1990; Whelton et al., 1995), but evidence from the DASH trial reaffirmed the benefit of potassium-rich foods in adults (Appel et al., 1997, Karanja et al., 1999; Sacks et al., 2001). In a review of 12 observational studies on potassium and blood pressure conducted between 1980 and 1996 (Simons-Morton and Obarzanek, 1997), no clear associations could be identified, because of measurement differences and other inadequate methodology. Some of the more reliable studies used urinary measures of potassium excretion as an objective measure (Cooper et al., 1980; Watson et al., 1980; Armstrong, 1982; Staessen et al., 1983; Connor et al., 1984; Zhu et al., 1987; Knuiman et al., 1988; Gilejinse et al., 1990; Wu et al., 1991) but others did not (Liebman et al., 1986; Jenner et al., 1988; Gillman et al., 1992; Simon et al., 1994). Simons-Morton and Obarzanek (1997) concluded that among the existing observational studies in children, about one-half reported an inverse association between potassium and blood pressure; in one case the reverse was true. Only two relatively small intervention studies tested the effects of dietary potassium supplements of 35 to 80 mmol/dL (Miller et al., 1987; Sinaiko et al., 1993). No significant effects of potassium supplementation on blood pressure were reported. Whether a diet increased in potassium-rich foods can favorably affect children's blood pressure just as the DASH diet did in adults has yet to be studied.

▦ Calcium

Of the eight studies on calcium that were identified by Simons-Morton and Obarzanek (1997), only three were considered properly controlled because they reported urinary calcium, the objective measure of calcium intake (Staessen et al., 1983; Zhu et al., 1987; Knuiman et al., 1988). None of these three studies found a significant association between calcium and blood pressure in this age group.

Only one randomized controlled trial involving a 600 mg calcium-supplemented beverage has been published (Gillman et al., 1995). The authors reported a small, nonsignificant decrease in SBP with increased calcium intake. Previously, many of the same authors reported a significant inverse association between dietary calcium and SBP but not DBP among very young children, 3 to 6 years of age, enrolled in the Framingham Children's Study (Gillman et al., 1992). In general, it has been concluded that there is insufficient evidence to document a consistent relationship between calcium and blood pressure in children and adolescents (Simons-Morton and Obarzanek, 1997).

■ Magnesium

In the 1980s and 1990s, five observational studies of magnesium intake and blood pressure in children were reported (Staessen et al., 1983; Jenner et al., 1988; Knuiman et al., 1988; Wu et al., 1991; Gillman et al., 1992; Simons-Morton and Obarzanek, 1997). Three studies measured dietary intake and reported significant inverse associations between magnesium and DBP (Jenner et al., 1988; Simon et al., 1994) or SBP (Wu et al., 1991). No intervention studies on magnesium and blood pressure in children have been conducted. Simons-Morton and Obarzanek (1997) concluded that higher dietary magnesium might be associated with lower blood pressure in children and adolescents on the basis of the limited number of studies conducted, but conclusive data are still lacking.

■ Macronutrients and Fiber

Simons-Morton and Obarzanek (1997) identified two observational studies that explored the impact of multiple nutrients on blood pressure. An Australian study (Jenner et al., 1988) reported significant inverse associations between SBP and carbohydrates and polyunsaturated fats as well as a significant association between DBP and protein, carbohydrates, cholesterol and fiber. Ulbak et al. (2004) reported a significant association between protein intake and blood pressure in young Danish children. In this study, a daily increased intake of 9 g of dietary protein was associated with a 2 mmHg lowering in SBP and 3 mmHg decrease in DBP. Likewise, Simon et al. (1994) reported a significant inverse association between total dietary fiber and DBP. Other observational studies in adults have suggested an inverse association between fiber and blood pressure, but other confounding dietary and nondietary factors and limitations in dietary assessment methods limit meaningful conclusions (Sacks, 1993; He and Whelton, 1999).

Intervention studies with fiber have rarely cited blood pressure as the primary outcome measure and design limitations preclude causal associations (He and Whelton, 1999). Among the six intervention studies directly measuring blood pressure, dietary fiber, typically provided in cereal, was on average associated with a 1.6 mmHg reduction in SBP (95% CI 0.4-2.6 mmHg) and a 2.0 mmHg reduction in DBP (95% CI 1.1-2.9 mmHg) (He and Whelton, 1999). Fiber plays an important role as part of a healthy diet for adults and children (Williams, 1995). More studies controlling for type and amount of fiber (soluble vs. insoluble and food vs. supplement) and baseline blood pressure levels are badly needed.

Three studies have examined the effects of dietary fat on blood pressure (Stern et al., 1980; Vartiainen et al., 1986; Goldberg et al., 1992). One study, a two-school crossover study in boarding schools (Stern et al., 1980), indicated that higher intakes of polyunsaturated to saturated fat ratio did not reduce blood pressure. Stern et al. (1980) reported lower SBP among children who increased polyunsaturated fat intake to 20% of kilocalories, but practical limitations and questions of long-term safety remain unanswered. Simons-Morton and Obarzanek (1997) concluded that, from the small number of studies conducted, macronutrients and fiber might have an effect on blood pressure levels in children and adolescents.

Another finding further indicates that initial diet can influence blood pressure at birth. Breast fed infants exhibited significantly lower blood pressure than that of babies who were completely bottle-fed (Wilson et al., 1998; Adair et al., 2001). This relation requires further exploration.

■ Dietary Intervention Study in Children

In a study of more than 600 children with elevated low-density lipoprotein (LDL) cholesterol levels, the Dietary Intervention Study in Children (DISC) implemented a step II (National Cholesterol Education Program, 1993) type of diet to test the efficacy and safety of this approach (DISC Collaborative Research Group, 1995). Although not a primary outcome measure, blood pressure was measured and multiple 24-hour dietary recall reports were collected (Simons-Morton et al., 1997). The authors explored associations longitudinally between specific nutrients and blood pressure levels at baseline, year 1, and year 3. For SBP, inverse associations were identified with calcium ($p < 0.05$), magnesium, potassium, protein ($p < 0.01$), and fiber ($p < 0.05$). Direct associations were reported with total fat and mono-unsaturated fat ($p < 0.05$). For DBP, inverse associations were identified with calcium ($p < 0.01$), magnesium and potassium ($p < 0.05$), protein ($p < 0.01$), and carbohydrates and fiber ($p < 0.05$). Direct associations were identified with blood pressure and polyunsaturated fat ($p < 0.01$) and monounsaturated fat ($p < 0.05$). The authors concluded that among the children with elevated LDL cholesterol, dietary calcium, fiber, and fat seemed to influence blood pressure levels. The magnitude of the effects of these nutrients on blood pressure was significant but clinically small. The authors speculated that the nutrients with greatest favorable effects on blood pressure could be magnesium and calcium. Using regression coefficients that were significant from the longitudinal analysis, it was estimated that an increased intake of 65 mg/day of magnesium would be associated with 0.91 mmHg lower SBP and 0.72 mmHg lower DBP. The authors estimated that an increased intake of 331 mg/day of calcium would be associated with 0.93 mmHg lower DBP and 0.50 mmHg lower SBP (Simons-Morton et al., 1997). Direct interventions are needed to further test this association.

The DASH Diet: Potential Benefits for Children

Given the current evidence on individual nutrients and dietary factors, what would a potential diet to prevent hypertension in children look like? The DASH trials have demonstrated that a diet rich in fruits, vegetables, low-fat dairy products, and whole grains, and low in red meat, desserts, and saturated fats significantly lowers blood pressure in normotensive and hypertensive adults (Appel et al., 1997), with added benefits coming from reductions in sodium content (Sacks et al., 2001). The DASH studies have consistently shown that the recommended diet is effective in lowering blood pressure (Sacks et al., 2001), reducing isolated systolic hypertension (Moore et al., 2001) and lowering LDL cholesterol levels (Obarzanek et al., 2001).

Adapting the DASH Diet to Children

Despite the lack of research directly testing the efficacy, safety, and feasibility of implementing a DASH-type diet in children with normal to high blood pressure, there are numerous qualities of this type of eating pattern that could benefit younger individuals. As long as energy needs for growth are met, nutrient qualities inherent to the DASH diet would improve and enhance current dietary behaviors in children and adolescents.

To illustrate this approach, Table 11.1 compares the DASH diet recommended for adults with the U.S. Department of Agriculture (USDA) Food Guide Pyramid (USDA, 2005) servings and presents age-adjusted recommendations for children and adolescents (IOM, 2002). The adult serving sizes and frequencies appear on the right, with columns listing the age appropriate counterparts displayed on the left. For example, in the DASH diet 7 to 8 servings of whole grains are recommended for adults, compared to the USDA Food Guide Pyramid recommendations of 6 to 11 servings to achieve intake of 2000 calories per day. For middle and high school students, who on average need to meet approximately 2200 to 3000 calories, the DASH-type diet could include 9 to 11 servings of whole grains, compared to the Food Guide Pyramid recommendations of 6 to 11 servings, as in adults. For younger children in the 1300 to 1800 calorie range, the DASH-recommended servings of whole grains are adjusted to 6 to 7, similar to the Food Guide Pyramid recommendations of 6 servings per day.

Other food groups and accompanying serving sizes are presented accordingly. Also, to better illustrate the implementation of these recommendations across age groups, Tables 11.2 and 11.3 provide sample menus with respective nutrient analyses.

TABLE 11.1
Comparison of pediatric DASH vs. USDA Food Guide Pyramid dietary guidelines

Food Group	Preschool (Ages 2–6 Years) 1400–1600 Calories*		Elementary School (Ages 7–11 Years) 1600–2200 Calories*		Middle and High School (Ages 12–18 Years) 2000–2800 Calories		All Adults (Ages ≥19 Years) 2000 Calories	
	DASH	Pyramid	DASH	Pyramid	DASH	Pyramid	DASH	Pyramid
	Number of Daily Servings							
Grains	6	5	6	6	9–11	9	7–8	6

Examples:
1 slice whole-wheat bread or ½ whole-wheat pita; 1 cup raisin bran cereal or ½ cup cooked oatmeal; ½ cup whole-wheat pasta; brown or white rice; ½ small whole-grain bagel; 3 cups low-fat popcorn; 1 oz baked crackers, tortilla chips, or pretzels; 3 graham cracker squares, 2 flavored rice cakes, 9 animal crackers; 2 fat-free flavored fruit or fig bars

Vegetables	3	3	4	5	4–5	7	4–5	5

Examples:
6 oz vegetable juice; ½ cup any cooked vegetable (fresh or frozen); ½ cup mashed or one small potato (white or sweet potatoes); 5 baby carrots; 15 celery sticks; ½ chopped raw vegetables or 1 cup raw leafy vegetables

Fruits	2–3	3	4	3	4–5	4	4–5	4

Examples:
6 oz 100% fruit juice; ¼ cup dried fruit; ½ cup chopped raw fruit (fresh or frozen); ½ cup chopped cooked fruit (fresh or frozen)

Dairy†	2	2	3	3	3–4	3	2–3	3

Examples:
8 oz skim, 1%, 2% milk; 1-1/2 oz fat-free or low-fat cheese, yogurt, or frozen yogurt

Meats†	1–1½	1–1½	2	1–2	2	2–3	2	2	2

Examples:
3 oz cooked chicken breast, turkey breast, 90% lean ground beef, cuts of trimmed round, sirloin, or other lean red meats; 3 oz baked fish, including canned tuna; lean or extra-lean luncheon (low sodium) meat

Nuts, Seeds, and Dried Beans	½–1	*Part of meat group*	½–1	*Part of meat group*	1	*Part of meat group*	*4–5 per week*	*Part of meat group*

Examples:
2 tablespoons regular or reduced-fat peanut butter; 1/3 cup roasted almonds; 2 tablespoons sunflower seeds; ½ cup cooked black beans or fat-free "refried" beans; ½ cup lentils (e.g., in soup)

Fats and Oils	2	2–4	2–3	3–5	2–4	6–8	2–3	4–6

Examples:
1 teaspoon regular tub margarine or ½–1 tablespoon light tub margarine; 1 teaspoon oil; 1 tablespoon low-fat mayo; 2 tablespoons light salad dressing; ½ oz regular potato chips or 1 oz baked potato chips

Sweets	1–2	1–2	2–3	2	2	3–4	½–1	2

Examples:
1 tablespoon table sugar, jelly, or syrup; ½ oz jelly beans, licorice, or fruit chews; 1 popsicle or fudgesicle; 1/3 cup jello; ¼ cup sherbet or sorbet; 8 oz regular soda or non-carbonated sweetened beverages

DASH, Dietary Approaches to Stop Hypertension; USDA, U.S. Department of Agriculture.

*Suggested calorie levels for children are based on the *Institute of Medicine Dietary Reference Intakes for Macronutrients Report, 2002*, available at www.nap.edu/openbook/0309085373/html/R2.html, ISBN 0-309-08537-3 (hardcover). Energy needs are calculated by age, gender, and moderate activity level.

†The National Heart, Lung, and Blood Institute–prescribed DASH diet for an adult is based on a reference 2000 calories.

TABLE 11.2
Pediatric DASH sample menu for preschool children ages 2–6

Food Item	Amount	Servings
Breakfast		
Cooked cereal		
Oatmeal	½ cup cooked	1 grain
Raisins	2 tablespoons	½ fruit
2% milk	1 cup	1 dairy
Sugar	1 teaspoon	½ sweet
Orange juice, calcium-fortified	6 oz	1 fruit
Mid-morning Snack		
Animal crackers	9 pieces	1 grain
Banana	1 medium	1 fruit
Water	1 cup	
Lunch		
Sandwich		
Whole–wheat bread	2 slices	2 grains
Reduced-fat American cheese	1 slice or ¾ oz	½ dairy
Turkey breast deli meat	1 oz	$^1/_3$ meat
Low-fat mayo	1 tablespoon	1 fat
Baby carrots	6 medium	1 vegetable
100% vegetable or fruit juice blend	6 oz	1 vegetable
Afternoon Snack		
Graham crackers	3 squares	1 grain
with peanut butter	1 tablespoon	½ nuts
2% milk	1 cup	1 dairy
Dinner		
Hamburger		
90% lean ground beef	3 oz cooked	1 meat
Hamburger bun	1 medium	1 grain
Catsup	1 tablespoon	
Broccoli, cooked from frozen	½ cup	1 vegetable
with tub margarine	1 teaspoon	1 fat
Lemonade	1 cup	1 sweet

TABLE 11.2
Continued

Daily Totals	Menu Nutritional Analysis	Pediatric DASH Recommendations, Ages 2–6
Calories	1542	
Total fat	47 g (27% total calories)	
Saturated fats	15 g (9% total calories)	
Cholesterol	106 mg	
Protein	67 g	
Carbohydrate	227 g	
Sodium	2371 mg	
Fiber	19 g	
Grains	6	6
Vegetables	3	3
Fruit	2½	2–3
Dairy	2½	2
Meats	1⅓	1–1½
Nuts/seeds/beans	½	⅓-1
Fats and oils	2	2
Sweets	1	1–2

▪ SUMMARY

- Diet influences blood pressure throughout life and possibly even in utero.
- Relatively few studies have concentrated on the specific impact of certain nutrients on blood pressure in children but those that have most strongly advocate breast milk and prevention of weight gain as effective prevention strategies.
- Existing studies have most often focused on sodium intake, but limitations in study design and outcome measures have made it difficult to draw meaningful conclusions from these studies.
- Recent findings from the DASH trials provide compelling evidence that blood pressure can be reduced among normotensive and hypertensive adults.
- Despite the absence of direct evidence of a similar impact on children, there are numerous potential benefits from applying similar strategies to children.
- With close monitoring and ongoing follow-up, nonpharmacologic interventions including diet and physical activity, initiated during childhood, can offer lifelong benefits for children and their families.

TABLE 11.3
Pediatric DASH sample menus for children and adolescents ages 7–18

Food Item	Elementary School, Ages 7 to 11		Middle or High School, Ages 12 to 18	
	Amount	Servings	Amount	Servings
Breakfast				
Cereal: puffed oat circles with	1 cup	1 grain	2 cups	2 grains
Granulated sugar	None		½ tablespoon	½ sweet
Skim milk	1 cup	1 dairy	1 cup	1 dairy
Fresh sliced strawberries	½ cup	1 fruit	½ cup	1 fruit
Orange juice	6 oz	1 fruit	6 oz	1 fruit
Lunch				
Pizza (made with lean ground beef, low-fat cheese, and light salt)	6" diameter, thin crust	2 grains, 1 dairy	6" diameter, thin crust	2 grains, 1 dairy
Cola	1 cup	1 sweet	12 ounces	1–½ sweets
Low-fat frozen yogurt	None		1 cup	1 dairy
Afternoon Snack				
Apple	1 medium	1 fruit	1 medium	1 fruit
Granola bar	None		1	1 grain
Water	1 cup		1 cup	
Dinner				
Chicken vegetable stir-fry (made with low-sodium soy sauce and canola oil)	2 cups cooked	2 meats, 2 fats, 2 vegetables	2 cups cooked	2 meats, 2 fats, 2 vegetables
Steamed brown rice	½ cup	1 grain	1 cup	2 grains

	Menu, Ages 7 to 11		Menu, Ages 12 to 18	
Mixed vegetable salad with	2 cups	2 vegetables	2 cups	2 vegetables
Light salad dressing	2 tablespoons	1 fat	2 tablespoons	1 fat
Skim milk	1 cup	1 dairy	1 cup	1 dairy
Fudgesicle	1	1 sweet	1	1 sweet

Night Snack

Whole-wheat crackers, unsalted	14	2 grains	14	2 Grains
With peanut butter	1 tablespoon	½ nuts/seeds	2 tablespoons	1 nuts/seeds
Banana	1 medium	1 fruit	1 medium	1 fruit

Daily Totals

	Menu, Ages 7 to 11	Menu, Ages 12 to 18
Calories	2086	2760
Total fat	60 g	78 g
Saturated fats	15 g	21 g
Cholesterol	165 mg	174 mg
Protein	106 g	126 g
Carbohydrate	288 g	406 g
Sodium	2389 mg	2984 mg
Fiber	29 g	37 g

Sample Menu Servings vs. Pediatric DASH Dietary Guidelines

Food Item	Menu, Ages 7–11	DASH, Ages 7–11	Menu, Ages 12–18	DASH, Ages 12–18
Grains	6 grains	6 grains	9 grains	9–11 grains
Vegetables	4 vegetables	4 vegetables	4 vegetables	4–5 vegetables
Fruit	4 fruits	4 fruits	4 fruits	4–5 fruits
Dairy	3 dairy	3 dairy	4 dairy	3–4 dairy
Meats	2 meats	2 meats	2 meats	2–3 meats
Nuts/seeds/beans	½ nuts/seeds	½–1 nuts/seeds	1 nuts/seeds	1 nuts/seeds
Fats and oils	4 fats	2–3 fats	3 fats	2–4 fats
Sweets	2 sweets	2–3 sweets	3 ½ sweets	3–4 sweets

■ REFERENCES

Adair, L.S., C.W. Kuzawa, and J. Borja. 2001. Maternal Energy Stores and Diet Composition during Pregnancy Program Adolescent Blood Pressure. *Circulation* 104:1034–9.

Andersen, L.B., N. Wedderkopp, H.S. Hansen, A.R. Cooper, and K. Froberg. 2003. Biological Cardiovascular Risk Factors Cluster in Danish Children and Adolescents: The European Youth Heart Study. *Prev Med* 37:363–7.

Appel, L., T.J. Moore, E. Obarzanek, W.M. Vollmer, L.P. Svetkey, F.M. Sacks, G.A. Bray, T.M. Vogt, J.A. Cutler, M.M. Windhauser, P.H. Lin, and N. Karanja. 1997. A Clinical Trial of the Effects of Dietary Patterns on Blood Pressure. *N Engl J Med* 336:1117–24.

Armstrong, B. 1982. Water Sodium and Blood Pressure in Rural School Children. *Arch Environ Health* 37:236–45.

Arslanian, S., and C. Suprasongsin. 1996. Insulin Sensitivity, Lipids, and Body Composition in Childhood: Is Syndrome X" Present?" *J Clin Endocrinol Metab* 81:1058–62.

Barker, D.J., C. Osmond, J. Golding, D. Kuh, and M.E. Wadsworth. 1989. Growth in Utero, Blood Pressure in Childhood and Adult Life, and Mortality from Cardiovascular Disease. *BMJ* 298:564–7.

Berenson, G.S., S.R. Srinivasan, and T.A. Nicklas. 1998. Atherosclerosis: A Nutritional Disease of Childhood. *Am J Cardiol* 82:22T–29T.

Burke, V., R.A. Milligan, C. Thompson, A.C. Taggart, D.L. Dunbar, M.J. Spencer, A. Medland, M.P. Gracey, R. Vandongen, and L.J. Beilin. 1998. A Controlled Trial of Health Promotion Programs in 11–Year-Olds using Physical Activity "Enrichment" for Higher Risk Children. *J Pediatr* 132:840–8.

Calabrese, E.J., and R.W. Tuthill. 1985. The Massachusetts Blood Pressure Study, Part 3. Experimental Reduction of Sodium in Drinking Water: Effects on Blood Pressure. *Toxicol Ind Health* 1:19–34.

Campbell, D.M., M.H. Hall, D.J. Barker, J. Cross, A.W. Shiell, and K.M. Godfrey. 1996. Diet in Pregnancy and the Offspring's Blood Pressure 40 Years Later. *Br J Obstet Gynaecol* 103:273–80.

Cappuccio, F., and G. MacGregor. 1991. Does Potassium Intake Lower Blood Pressure? A Meta-Analysis of Published Trials. *J Hypertens* 9:465–73.

Chobanian, A.V., G.L. Bakris, H.R. Black, W.C. Cushman, L.A. Green, A.L. Izzo, D.W. Jones, B.J. Materson, S. Oparil, J.T. Wright, Jr., and E.J. Rocella. 2003. Seventh Report of the Joint National Committee on Prevention, Detection, Evaluation, and Treatment of High Blood Pressure. *Hypertension* 42:1206–52.

Clarke, W.R., R.F. Woolson, and R.M. Lauer. 1986. Changes in Ponderosity and Blood Pressure in Childhood: The Muscatine Study. *Am J Epidemiol* 124:195–206.

Connor, S.L., W.E. Connor, H. Henry, G. Sexton, and E.J. Keenan. 1984. The Effects of Familial Relationships, Age, Body Weight, and Diet on Blood Pressure and the 24 Hour Urinary Excretion of Sodium, Potassium, and Creatinine in Men, Women, and Children of Randomly Selected Families. *Circulation* 70:76–85.

Cooper, R., I. Soltero, K. Liu, D. Berkson, S. Levinson, and J. Stamler. 1980. The Association between Urinary Sodium Excretion and Blood Pressure in Children. *Circulation* 62:97–104.

Cooper, R., L. Van Horn, K. Liu, M. Trevisan, S. Nanas, H. Ueshima, E. Larbi, C.S. Yu, C. Sempos, D. LeGrady, and J. Stamler. 1984. A Randomized Trial on the Effect of Decreased Dietary Sodium Intake on Blood Pressure in Adolescents. *J Hypertens* 2:361–6.

DISC Collaborative Research Group. 1995. Efficacy and Safety of Lowering Dietary Intake of Total Fat, Saturated Fat, and Cholesterol in Children with Elevated LDL-cholesterol: The Dietary Intervention Study in Children (DISC). *JAMA* 273:1429–35.

Ellison, R.C., A.L. Capper, W.P. Stephenson, R.J. Goldberg, D.W. Hosmer, Jr., K.F. Humphrey, J.K. Ockene, W.J. Gamble, J.C. Witschi, and F.J. Stare. 1989. Effects on Blood

Pressure of a Decrease in Sodium Use in Institutional Food Preparation: The Exeter-Andover Project. *J Clin Epidemiol* 42:201–8.

Epstein, L.H., A. Valoski, R.R. Wing, and J. McCurley. 1990. Ten-Year Follow-Up of Behavioral, Family-Based Treatment for Obese Children. *JAMA* 264: 2519–23.

Falkner, B., S.R. Daniels, J.T. Flynn, S. Gidding, L.A. Green, J. Inglefinger, R.M. Lauer, B.Z. Morgenstern, R.J. Portman, R.J. Prineas, A.P. Rocchini, B. Rosner, A.R. Sinaiko, N. Stettler, E. Urbina, E.J. Roccella. 2004. The Fourth Report on the Diagnosis, Evaluation and Treatment of High Blood Pressure in Children and Adolescents. *Pediatrics* 114(2 Suppl):555–76.

Falkner, B., S.R. Daniels, M.J. Horan, J.M.H. Loggie, R.J. Prineas, B. Rosner, A.R. Sinaiko, E.J. Roccella, and D.E. Anderson. 1996. Update on the Task Force Report (1987) on High Blood Pressure in Children and Adolescents: A Working Group Report from the National High Blood Pressure Education Program. *Pediatrics* 98:649–58.

Falkner, B., and S. Michel. 1997. Blood Pressure Response to Sodium in Children and Adolescents. *Am J Clin Nutr* 65(suppl):618S–21S.

Faust, H.S. 1982. Effects of Drinking Water and Total Sodium Intake on Blood Pressure. *Am J Clin Nutr* 35:1459–67.

Fernandes, E., and B.W. McCrindle. 2000. Diagnosis and Treatment of Hypertension in Children and Adolescents. *Can J Cardiol* 16:801–11.

Folsom, A.R., G.L. Burke, C.L. Byers, R.G. Hutchinson, G. Heiss, J.M. Flack, D.R. Jacobs, Jr., D.B. Caan. 1991. Implications of Obesity for Cardiovascular Disease in Blacks: The CARDIA and ARIC Studies. *Am J Clin Nutr* 53:1604S–11S.

Fraser, G.E., R.L. Phillips, and R. Harris. 1983. Physical Fitness and Blood Pressure in School Children. *Circulation* 67:405–12.

Freedman, D.S., W.H. Dietz, S.R. Sunivasan, and G.S. Berensen. 1999. The Relation of Overweight to Cardiovascular Risk Factors among Children and Adolescents: The Bogalusa Heart Study. *Pediatrics* 103: 1175–82.

Geleijnse, J., D. Grobbee, and A. Hofman. 1990. Sodium and Potassium Intake and Blood Pressure Change in Childhood. *BMJ* 300:899–902.

Geleijnse, J.M., A. Hofman, J.C. Witteman, A.A. Hazebroek, H.A. Valkenburg, and D.E. Grobbee. 1997. Long-Term Effects of Neonatal Sodium Restriction on Blood Pressure. *Hypertension* 29:913–7.

Gidding, S.S., B.A. Dennison, L.L. Birch, S.R. Daniels, M.W. Gillman, A.H. Lichtenstein, K.T. Rattay, J. Steinberger, N. Stettler, and L. Van Horn. 2005. Dietary Recommendations for Children and Adolescents: A Guide for Practitioners: Consensus Statement From the American Heart Association. *Circulation* 112:2061–75.

Gillman, M.W., and R.C. Ellison. 1993. Childhood Prevention of Essential Hypertension. *Pediatr Clin North Am* 40:179–94.

Gillman, M.W., M.Y. Hood, L.L. Moore, U.S. Nguyen, M.R. Singer, and M.B. Andon. 1995. Effect of Calcium Supplementation on Blood Pressure in Children. *J Pediatr* 127:186–92.

Gillman, M.W., S.A. Oliveria, L.L. Moore, and R.C. Ellison. 1992. Inverse Association of Dietary Calcium with Systolic Blood Pressure in Young Children. *JAMA* 267:2340–3.

Gillum, R.F., P.J. Elmer, and R.J. Prineas. 1981. Changing Sodium Intake in Children. The Minneapolis Children's Blood Pressure Study. *Hypertension* 3:698–703.

Goldberg, R.J., R.C. Ellison, D.W. Hosmer, Jr., A.L. Capper, E. Puleo, W.J. Gamble, and J. Witschi. 1992. Effects of Alterations in Fatty Acid Intake on the Blood Pressure of Adolescents: The Exeter-Andover Project. *Am J Clin Nutr* 56:71–6.

Grimm, Jr., R.H., J.D. Neaton, P.J. Elmer, K.H. Svendsen, J. Levin, M. Segal, L. Holland, L.J. Witte, D.R. Clearman, P. Kofron, R.K. LaBounty, R. Crow, and R.J. Prineas. 1990. The Influence of Oral Potassium Chloride on Blood Pressure in Hypertensive Men on a Low-Sodium Diet. *N Engl J Med* 322:569–74.

Hansen, H.S., K. Froberg, N. Hyldebrandt, and J.R. Nielsen. 1991. A Controlled Study of

Eight Months of Physical Training and Reduction of Blood Pressure in Children: The Odense Schoolchild Study. *BMJ* 303:682–5.

He, J., and P. Whelton. 1999. Effect of Dietary Fiber and Protein Intake on Blood Pressure: A Review of the Epidemiologic Evidence. *Clin Exp Hypertens* 21:785–96.

Howe, P., L. Cobiac, and R. Smith. 1991. Lack of Effect of Short-Term Changes in Sodium Intake on Blood Pressure in Adolescent Schoolchildren. *J Hypertens* 9:191–86.

Howe, P., K. Juredini, and R. Smith. 1985. Sodium and Blood Pressure in Children—A Short-Term Dietary Intervention Study. *Proc Nutr Soc* 10:121–4.

Institute of Medicine Dietary Reference Intakes for Macronutrients Report, 2002 available at www.nap.edu/openbook/0309085373/html/R2.html or ISBN 0-309-08537-3 (hardcover).

Institute of Medicine. 2004. Dietary Reference Intakes: Water Potassium, Sodium, Chloride, and Sulfate. February 11.

Jenner, D.A., D.R. English, R. Vandongen, L.J. Beilin, B.K. Armstrong, M.R. Miller, and D. Dunbar. 1988. Diet and Blood Pressure in 9–Year-Old Australian Children. *Am J Clin Nutr* 47:1052–9.

Jones, R.D., R.P. Symonds, T. Habeshaw, E.R. Watson, J. Laurie, and D.W. Lamont. 1990. A Comparison of Remote Afterloading and Manually Inserted Caesium in the Treatment of Carcinoma of Cervix. *Clin Oncol* 2:193–8.

Karanja, N.M., E. Obarzanek, P.H. Lin, M.L. McCullough, K.M. Philips, J.F. Swain, C.M. Champagne, and K.P. Hoben. DASH Collaborative Research Group. 1999. Descriptive Characteristics of the Dietary Patterns used in the Dietary Approaches to Stop Hypertension Trial. *J Am Diet Assoc* 99(8 Suppl):S19–27.

Knuiman, J., J. Hautvast, K.F. Zwiauer, K. Widhalm, M. Desmet, G. DeBacker, R.R. Rahneva, V.S. Petrova, M. Dahl, J. Viikari, H. Rottka, N. Semmer, R. Kluthe, G. Dobos, D. Thiel, U. Laaser, A. Trichopoulou, L. Tzouvelekis, E. Greiner, I. Kamaras, L.S. Malatino, B. Stancanelli, E. Fossali, F. Sereni, F. Angelico, M. Delben, B. Cybulska, J. Charzewska, A. Cruz, I. Martins, F.J. Sanchez-Muniz, I. Goni, R. Tojo, E. Rey, and L. Westbom. 1988. Blood Pressure and Excretion of Sodium, Potassium, Calcium and Magnesium in 8– and 9–Year Old Boys from 19 European Centres. *Eur J Clin Nutr* 42:847–55.

Kuczmarski, R.J., J.J. Anderson, and G.G. Koch. 1994. Correlates of Blood Pressure in Seventh-Day Adventist (SDA) and Non-SDA Adolescents. *J Am Coll Nutr* 13:165–73.

Lauer, R.M., and W.R. Clarke. 1989. Childhood Risk Factors for High Adult Blood Pressure: The Muscatine Study. *Pediatrics* 84:633–41.

Lauer, R.M., W.R. Clarke, and R. Beaglehole. 1984. Level, Trend, and Variability of Blood Pressure during Childhood: The Muscatine Study. *Circulation* 69:242–9.

Lauer, R.M., W.E. Connor, P.E. Leaverton, M.A. Reiter, and W.R. Clarke. 1975. Coronary Heart Disease Risk Factors in School Children: The Muscatine Study. *J Pedratr* 86:697–706.

Law, C.M., M. de Swiet, C. Osmond, P.M. Fayers, D.J. Barker, A.M. Cruddas, and C.H. Fall. 1993. Initiation of Hypertension in Utero and its Amplification throughout Life. *BMJ* 306:24–7.

Leary, S.D., A.R. Ness, P.M. Emmett, G. Davey Smith, and J.E. Headley. ALSPAC study Team. 2005. Maternal Diet in Pregnancy and Offspring Blood Pressure. *Arch Dis Child* 90:492–3.

Liebman, M., L.F. Chopin, E. Carter, A.J. Clark, G.W. Disney, M. Hegsted, M.A. Kenney, Z.A. Kirmani, K.L. Koonce, M.K. Korslund, S.W. Moak, H. McCoy, S.F. Stallings, and T. Wakefield. 1986. Factors Related to Blood Pressure in a Biracial Adolescent Female Population. *Hypertension* 8:843–50.

Lin, P.H., M. Aikin, C. Champagne, S Craddick, F.M. Sacks, P. McCarron, M.M. Most-Windhauser, F. Rukenbrod, and L. Haworth. DASH-Sodium Collaborative Research Group. 2003. Food Group Sources of Nutrients in the Dietary Patterns of the DASH-Sodium Ttrial. *J Am Diet Assoc* 103:488–96.

Lobstein, T., L. Baur, and R. Uauy. IASO International Obesity Task Force. 2004. Obesity in Children and Young People: A Crisis in Public Health. *Obes Rev* 5(Suppl 1): 4–104.

Loos, R.J., R. Fagard, G. Beunen, C. Derom, and R. Vlietinck. 2001. Birth Weight and Blood Pressure in Young Adults: A Prospective Twin Study. *Circulation* 104:1633–8.

Luepker, R.V., C.L. Perry, S.M. McKinlay, P.R. Nader, G.S. Parcel, E.J. Stone, L.S. Webber, J.P. Elder, H.A. Feldman, C.C. Johnson, S.H. Kelder, and M. Wu. 1996. Outcomes of a Field Trial to Improve Children's Dietary Patterns and Physical Activity. The Child and Adolescent Trial for Cardiovascular Health. CATCH Collaborative Group. *JAMA* 275:768–76.

McGill, Jr., H.C., C.A. McMahan, E.E. Herderick, R.E. Tracy, G.T. Malcom, A.W. Zieske, and J.P. Strong. 2000. Effects of Coronary Heart Disease Risk Factors on Atherosclerosis of Selected Regions of the Aorta and Right Coronary Artery. PDAY Research Group. Pathobiological Determinants of Atherosclerosis in Youth. *Arterioscler Thromb Vasc Biol* 20:836–45.

Miller, J.Z., M.H. Weinberger, and J.C. Christian. 1987. Blood Pressure Response to Potassium Supplementation in Normotensive Adults and Children. *Hypertension* 10:437–42.

Miller, J.Z., M.H. Weinberger, S.A. Daugherty, N.S. Fineberg, J.C. Christian, and C.E. Grim. 1988. Blood Pressure Response to Dietary Sodium Restriction in Healthy Normotensive Children. *Am J Clin Nutr* 47:113–9.

Moore, T.J., P.R. Conlin, J. Ard, and L.P. Svetkey. 2001. DASH (Dietary Approaches to Stop Hypertension) Diet Is Effective Treatment for Stage 1 Isolated Systolic Hypertension. *Hypertension* 38:155–8.

Muntner, P., J. He, J.A. Cutler, R.P. Wildman, and P.K. Whelton. 2004. Trends in Blood Pressure among Children and Adolescents. *JAMA* 291:2107–13.

Must, A., J. Spadano, E.H. Coakley, A.E. Field, and W.H. Dietz. 1999. The Disease Burden Associated with Overweight and Obesity. *JAMA* 282:1523–9.

Nader, P.R., D.E. Sellers, C.C. Johnson, C.L Perry, E.J. Stone, K.C. Cook, J. Bebchuk, and R.V. Luepker. 1996. The Effect of Adult Participation in a School-Based Family Intervention to Improve Children's Diet and Physical Activity: The Child and Adolescent Trial for Cardiovascular Health. *Prev Med* 25:455–64.

Nader, P.R., E.J. Stone, L.A. Lytle, C.L. Perry, S.K. Osganian, S. Kelder, L.S. Webber, J.P. Elder, D. Montgomery, H.A. Feldman, M. Wu, C. Johnson, G.S. Parcel, and R.V. Luepker. 1999. Three-Year Maintenance of Improved Diet and Physical Activity: The CATCH Cohort. Child and Adolescent Trial for Cardiovascular Health. *Arch Pediatr Adolesc Med* 153:695–704.

National Cholesterol Education Program. 1993. Second Report of the Expert Panel on Detection, Evaluation, and Treatment of High Blood Cholesterol in Adults. Bethesda, MD: National Heart, Lung, and Blood Institute. NIH Publ. No. 93–3095.

[NHLBI] National Heart, Lung, and Blood Institute. 1977. Report of the Task Force on Blood Pressure Control in Children. *Pediatrics* 59:797–820.

[NHLBI] National Heart, Lung and Blood Institute. 1987. Report of the Second Task Force on Blood Pressure Control in Children. *Pediatics* 79:1–25.

NIH Publication No. 03-4082, Facts about the DASH Eating Plan, United States Department of Health and Human Services, National Institutes of Health, National Heart, Lung, and Blood Institute, Karanja NM et al. *J Am Diet Assoc* 8:S19–27, 1999. http://www.nhlbi.nih.gov/health/public/heart/hbp/dash/.

Obarzanek, E., F.M. Sacks, W.M. Vollmer, G.A. Bray, E.R. Miller, III, P.H.. Lin, N.M. Karanja, M.M. Most-Windhauser, T.J. Moore, J.F. Swain, C.W. Bales, and M.A. Proschan, DASH Research Group. 2001. Effects on Blood Lipids of a Blood Pressure-Lowering Diet: The Dietary Approaches to Stop Hypertension (DASH) Trial. *Am J Clin Nutr* 74:80–9.

Perry, C.L., R.V. Luepker, D.M. Murray, C. Kurth, R. Mullis, S. Crockett, and D.R. Jacobs, Jr. 1988. Parent Involvement with Children's Health Promotion: The Minnesota Home Team. *Am J Public Health* 78:1156–60.

Pomeranz, A., Z. Korzets, D. Vanunu, H. Krystal, and B. Wolach. 2000. Elevated Salt and Nitrate Levels in Drinking Water Cause an Increase of Blood Pressure in Schoolchildren. *Kidney Blood Press Res* 23:400–3.

Prineas, R., O. Gomez-Marin, and R. Gillum. 1985. Tracking of Blood Pressure in Children and Nonpharmacological Approaches to the Prevention of Hypertension. *Ann Behav Med* 7:25–30.

Raitakari, O.T., K.V. Porkka, L. Rasanen, T. Ronnemaa, and J.S. Viikari. 1994. Clustering and Six Year Cluster-Tracking of Serum Total Cholesterol, HDL-Cholesterol and Diastolic Blood Pressure in Children and Young Adults. The Cardiovascular Risk in Young Finns Study. *J Clin Epidemiol* 47:1085–93.

Reinehr, T. and W. Andler. 2004. Changes in the Atherogenic Risk Profile According to Degree of Weight Loss. *Arch Dis Child* 89:419–22.

Rocchini, A.P., V. Katch, J. Anderson, J. Hinderliter, D. Becque, M. Martin, and C. Marks. 1988. Blood Pressure in Obese Adolescents: Effect of Weight Loss. *Pediatrics* 82:16–23.

Rocchini, A.P., J. Key, D. Bondie, R. Chico, C. Moorehead, V. Katch, and M. Martin. 1989. The Effect of Weight Loss on the Sensitivity of Blood Pressure to Sodium in Obese Adolescents. *N Engl J Med* 321:580–5.

Roseboom, T.J., J.H. van der Meulen, A.C. Ravelli, G.A. van Montfrans, C. Osmond, D.J. Barker, and O.P. Bleker. 1999. Blood Pressure in Adults after Prenatal Exposure to Famine. *J Hypertens* 17:325–30.

Rosner, B., R. Prineas, S.R. Daniels, and J. Loggie. 2000. Blood Pressure Differences between Blacks and Whites in Relation to Body Size among US Children and Adolescents. *Am J Epidemiol* 151:1007–19.

Rosner, B., R.J. Prineas, J.M. Loggie, and S.R. Daniels. 1993. Blood Pressure Nomograms for Children and Adolescents, by Height, Sex, and Age, in the United States. *J Pediatr* 123:871–86.

Rouse, I.L., and L.J. Beilin. 1984. Vegetarian Diet and Blood Pressure. *J Hypertens* 2:231–40.

Sacks, F.M. 1993. Dietary Fiber and Cardiovascular Disease—Direct Protection or Indicator of a Healthy Lifestyle?" *Am J Prev Med* 9:259–60.

Sacks, F.M., E. Obarzanek, M.M. Windhauser, L.P. Svetkey, W.M. Vollmer, M. McCullough, N. Karanja, P.H. Lin, P. Steele, M.A. Proschan, M.A. Evans, L.J. Appel, G.A. Bray, T.M. Vogt and T.J. Moore, for the DASH Investigators. 1995. Rationale and Design of the Dietary Approaches to Stop Hypertension Trial (DASH). A Multicenter Controlled-Feeding Study of Dietary Patterns to Lower Blood Pressure. *Ann Epidemiol* 5:108–18.

Sacks, F.M., L.P. Svetkey, W.M. Vollmer, L.J. Appel, G.A. Bray, D. Harsha, E. Obarzanek, P.R. Conlin, E.R. Miller, III, D.G. Simons-Morton, N. Karanja, and P.H. Lin, DASH-Sodium Collaborative Research Group. 2001. Effects on Blood Pressure of Reduced Dietary Sodium and the Dietary Approaches to Stop Hypertension (DASH) Diet. *N Engl J Med* 344:3–10.

Simon, J.A., E. Obarzanek, S.R. Daniels, and M.M. Frederick. 1994. Dietary Cation Intake and Blood Pressure in Black Girls and White Girls. *Am J Epidemiol* 139:130–40.

Simons-Morton, D.G., S.A. Hunsberger, L. Van Horn, B.A. Barton, A.M. Robson, R.P. McMahon, L.E. Muhonen, P.O. Kwiterovich, N.L. Lasser, S.Y. Kimm, and M.R. Greenlick. 1997. Nutrient Intake and Blood Pressure in the Dietary Intervention Study in Children. *Hypertension* 29:930–6.

Simons-Morton, D.G., and E. Obarzanek. 1997. Diet and Blood Pressure in Children and Adolescents. *Pediatr Nephrol* 11:244–9.

Simons-Morton, D.G., G.S. Parcel, T. Baranowski, R. Forthofer, and N.M. O'Hara. 1991. Promoting Physical Activity and a Healthful Diet among Children: Results of a School-Based Intervention Study. *Am J Public Health* 81:986–91.

Sinaiko, A.R., R.P. Donahue, D.R. Jacobs, Jr., and R.J. Prineas. 1999. Relation of Weight and Rate of Increase in Weight during Childhood and Adolescence to Body Size, Blood Pressure, Fasting Insulin, and Lipids in Young Adults. The Minneapolis Children's Blood Pressure Study. *Circulation* 99:1471–6.

Sinaiko, A.R., O. Gomez-Marin, and R.J. Prineas. 1993. Effect of Low Sodium Diet or Potassium Supplementation on Adolescent Blood Pressure. *Hypertension* 21:989–94.

Sinaiko, A.R., O. Gomez-Marin, and R.J. Prineas. 1997. Relation of Fasting Insulin to Blood Pressure and Lipids in Adolescents and Parents. *Hypertension* 30:1554–9.

Singhal, A., T.J. Cole, and A. Lucas. 2001. Early Nutrition in Preterm Infants and Later Blood Pressure: Two Cohorts after Randomised Trials. *Lancet* 357:413–9.

Solomon, C.G., and J. Manson. 1997. Obesity and Mortality: A Review of the Epidemiologic Data. *Am J Clin Nutr* 66(Suppl):1044S–50S.

Sorof, J.M., G. Cardwell, K. Franco, and R.J. Portman. 2002. Ambulatory Blood Pressure and Left Ventricular Mass Index in Hypertensive Children. *Hypertension* 39:903–8.

Staessen, J., C. Bulpitt, R. Fagard, J.V. Joossens, P. Lijnen, and A. Amery. 1983. Four Urinary Cations and Blood Pressure. A Population Study in Two Belgian Towns. *Am J Epidemiol* 117:676–87.

Stanner, S.A., K. Bulmer, C. Andres, O.E. Lantseva, V. Borodina, V.V. Poteen, and J.S. Yudkin. 1997. Does Malnutrition in Utero Determine Diabetes and Coronary Heart Disease in Adulthood? Results from the Leningrad Siege Study, a Cross Sectional Study. *BMJ* 315:1342–8.

Stern, B., S. Heyden, D. Miller, G. Latham, A. Klimas, and K. Pilkington. 1980. Intervention Study in High School Students with Elevated Blood Pressures. Dietary Experiment with Polyunsaturated Fatty Acids. *Nutr Metab* 24.137–47.

Taittonen, L., M. Uhari, M. Nuutinen, J. Turtinen, T. Pokka, and H.K. Akerblom. 1996. Insulin and Blood Pressure among Healthy Children. Cardiovascular Risk in Young Finns. *Am J Hypertens* 9:194–9.

Tochikubo, O., O. Sasaki, S. Umemura, and Y. Kaneko. 1986. Management of Hypertension in High School Students by using New Salt Titrator Tape. *Hypertension* 8:1164–71.

Trevisan, M., R. Cooper, D. Ostrow, W. Miller, S. Sparks, Y. Leonas, A. Allen, M. Steinhauer, and J. Stamler. 1981. Dietary Sodium, Erythrocyte Sodium Concentration, Sodium Stimulated Lithium Efflux and Blood Pressure. *Clin Sci* 61(Suppl 7):29s–32s.

Tuthill, R.W., and E.J. Calabrese. 1985. The Massachusetts Blood Pressure Study, Part 4. Modest Sodium Supplementation and Blood Pressure Change in Boarding School Girls. *Toxicol Ind Health* 1:35–43.

Ulbak, J., L. Lauritzen, H.S. Hansen, and K.F. Michaelsen. 2004. Diet and Blood Pressure in 2.5-Y-Old Danish Children. *Am J Clin Nutr* 79:1095–102.

United States Department of Agriculture. 2005. Dietary Guidelines, available at www .healthierus.gov/dietaryguidelines/ or Home and Garden Bulletin 232, 5th edition (Stock Number 001-000-04719-1)

Vandongen, R., D.A. Jenner, C. Thompson, A.C. Taggart, E.E. Spickett, V. Burke, L.J. Beilin, R.A. Milligan, and D.L. Dunbar. 1995. A Controlled Evaluation of a Fitness and Nutrition Intervention Program on Cardiovascular Health in 10- to 12-Year-Old Children. *Prev Med* 24:9–22.

Vartiainen, E., P. Puska, P. Pietinen, A. Nissinen, U. Leino, and U. Uusitalo. 1986. Effects of Dietary Fat Modifications on Serum Lipids and Blood Pressure in Children. *Acta Paediatr Scand* 75:396–401.

Vollmer, W.M., F.M. Sacks, J. Ard, L.J. Appel, G.A. Bray, D.G. Simons-Morton, P.R. Conlin, L.P. Svetkey, T.P. Erlinger, T.J. Moore, and N. Karanja. DASH-Sodium Trial Collaborative Research Group. 2001. Effects of Diet & Sodium Intake on Blood Pressure: Subgroup Analysis of the DASH-Sodium Trial. *Ann Intern Med* 135:1019–28.

Watson, R., H. Langford, J. Abernethy, T. Barnes, and M. Watson. 1980. Urinary Electrolytes, Body Weight, and Blood Pressure: Pooled Cross-Sectional Results among Four Groups of Adolescent Females. *Hypertension* 2:193–8.

Webber, L.S., J.L. Cresanta, A.W. Voors, and G.S. Berenson. 1983. Tracking of Cardiovascular Disease Risk Factor Variables in School-Age Children. *J Chron Dis* 36:647–60.

Webber, L.S., S.K. Osganian, H.A. Feldman, M. Wu, T.L. McKenzie, M. Nichaman, L.A. Lytle, E. Edmundson, J. Cutler, P.R. Nader, and R.V. Luepker. 1996. Cardiovascular Risk Factors among Children after a 2 ½–Year Intervention—The CATCH Study. *Prev Med* 25:432–41.

Whelton, P.K., J. Buring, N.O. Borhani, J.D. Cohen, N. Cook, J.A. Cutler, J.E. Kiley, L.H. Kuller, S. Satterfield, F.M. Sacks, and J.O. Taylor, for the Trials of Hypertension Prevention (TOHP) Collaborative Research Group. 1995. The Effect of Potassium Supplementation in Persons with a High-Normal Blood Pressure. Results from Phase I of the Trials of Hypertension Prevention (TOHP). *Ann Epidemiol* 5:85–95.

Williams, C. 1995. Importance of Dietary Fiber in Childhood. *J Am Diet Assoc* 95:1040–9.

Wilson, A.C., J.S. Forsyth, S.A. Greene, L. Irvine, C. Hau, and P.W. Howie. 1998. Relation of Infant Diet to Childhood Health: Seven Year Follow Up of Cohort of Children in Dundee Infant Feeding Study. *BMJ* 316:21–5.

Wu, Y., R. Cai, B. Zhou, and X. Xu. 1991. Effects of Genetic Factors and Dietary Electrolytes on Blood Pressure of Rural Secondary School Students in Hanzhong. *Chin Med Sci J* 6:148–52.

Zhu, K.M., S.P. He, X.Q. Pan, X.R. Zheng, and Y.A. Gu. 1987. The Relation of Urinary Cations to Blood Pressure in Boys Aged Seven to Eight Years. *Am J Epidemiol* 126:658–63.

PART V

Obesity in Childhood and Adolescence

CHAPTER 12

The Epidemiology of Childhood Overweight and Obesity

Trudy L. Burns, Patricia A. Peyser, and Patricia A. Donohoue

Overweight refers to an excess of body weight and obesity refers to an excess of body fat. Although not infectious diseases, these conditions have reached epidemic proportions in the United States. In 1999 to 2000 (Ogden et al., 2002) an estimated 10.4% of children ages 2 to 5, 15.3% of children ages 6 to 11, and 15.5% of adolescents ages 12 to 19 years were overweight (body mass index [BMI] being at or above the age- and sex-specific 95th percentile defined by the Centers for Disease Control and Prevention [CDC] on the basis of nationally representative data obtained between 1971 and 1994). There were more than twice as many overweight children and more than three times as many overweight adolescents as there were in 1976 to 1980 (Fig. 12.1). The National Center for Health Statistics (NCHS) of the CDC has discouraged use of the term obesity when classifying children and adolescents; however, the two terms are used interchangeably in the chapters of this book.

Overweight and obesity are major public health problems in both developed and developing countries, and they are rapidly becoming the most important cause of adult chronic disease in the world (Visscher and Seidell, 2001). In the United States, obesity in adults is associated with higher morbidity from chronic conditions than that from poverty, smoking, or heavy drinking (Sturm and Wells, 2001), and with higher health care and medication costs than those related to smoking or heavy drinking (Sturm, 2002).

Overweight children and adolescents are more likely to have elevated blood pressure and serum lipid levels, orthopedic problems, sleep apnea, and psychological difficulties due to social stigmatization. They also have a higher prevalence

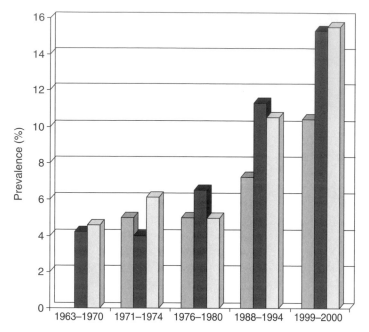

FIGURE 12.1

Prevalence of overweight (body mass index [BMI] ≥95th percentile based on 2000 Centers for Disease Control and Prevention [CDC] sex-specific BMI-for-age growth charts) for U.S. children and adolescents 2 to 5 (medium gray bars), 6 to 11 (black bars), and 12 to 19 (light gray bars) years of age, 1963 to 2000. Data for 1963 to 1965 are for children 6 to 11 years of age. Data for 1966 to 1970 are for adolescents 12 to 17 (not 12 to 19) years of age. Sources of data: CDC/National Center for Health Statistics (NCHS), National Health Examination Survey (NHES), and National Health and Nutrition Examination Survey (NHANES): NHES II (1963 to 1965), NHES III (1966 to 1970), NHANES I (1971 to 1974), NHANES II (1976 to 1980), NHANES III (1988 to 1994), and continuous NHANES 1999 and 2000 (Ogden et al., 2002).

of insulin resistance and type 2 diabetes (Goran et al., 2003; also see Chapter 15). In adults, obesity is associated with morbidity and mortality from a number of chronic medical conditions, including dyslipidemia; hypertension; cardiovascular diseases (CVD) such as coronary heart disease and ischemic stroke; type 2 diabetes; gallbladder, liver, musculoskeletal, and respiratory diseases; and some types of cancer (e.g., colon, prostate, endometrial, postmenopausal breast) (National Task Force on the Prevention and Treatment of Obesity, 2000; Visscher and Seidell, 2001; Calle et al., 2003). Obesity increases the risk for CVD indirectly through its association with hypertension, dyslipidemia, and insulin resistance (Melanson et al., 2001). There is also evidence to suggest that obesity is an independent risk factor for the development of CVD (Manson et al., 1995).

Among CVD risk factors, obesity is unique because of its social and cultural significance, in addition to its health significance.

Because overweight children and adolescents frequently become obese adults who are at increased risk for adverse health outcomes, there is increasing recognition that the prevalence of overweight children is an important public health concern (Dietz and Gortmaker, 2001; Kumanyika, 2001; Gillman et al., 2003). The problem of overweight children extends well beyond individual children to a world where overeating and physical inactivity are promoted, therefore, reducing the prevalence of overweight children must be a primary concern for nations worldwide. In December 2001, the U.S. Surgeon General issued a Call to Action (Table 12.1) to Prevent and Decrease Overweight and Obesity (www .surgeongeneral.gov/topics/obesity/).

This chapter describes the distribution of body size measures and discusses the current definition of overweight in children and adolescents. In addition, trends in the prevalence of overweight children and adolescents are described along with the familial aggregation of body size measures. Tracking of BMI into young adulthood and the association between BMI and CVD risk factors during childhood and young adult life, as well as implications for CVD morbidity and mortality in later adult life, are finally discussed.

■ DISTRIBUTION OF BODY SIZE MEASURES IN CHILDREN AND ADOLESCENTS

A number of cross-sectional health examination surveys that provide nationally representative data including body size measures in children and adolescents have been conducted by the NCHS. Each survey identified a stratified, multistage, probability sample of the civilian non-institutionalized U.S. population (Troiano et al., 1995). The National Health Examination Survey (NHES) Cycles II and III represent the earliest national data for height and weight among children and

TABLE 12.1
Principles of the U.S. Surgeon General's Call to Action to Prevent and Decrease Overweight and Obesity

---

- Promote the recognition of overweight and obesity as major public health problems
- Assist Americans in balancing healthful eating with regular physical activity to achieve and maintain a healthy or healthier body weight
- Identify effective and culturally appropriate interventions to prevent and treat overweight and obesity
- Encourage environmental changes that help prevent overweight and obesity
- Develop and enhance public–private partnerships to help implement this vision

---

Source: www.surgeongeneral.gov/topics/obesity/ December 2001.

adolescents. NHES II (conducted between 1963 and 1965) included children who were 6 to 11 years of age. NHES III (conducted between 1966 and 1970) included adolescents 12 to 17 years of age. The National Health and Nutrition Examination Surveys (NHANES) Cycles I (1971 to 1974), II (1976 to 1980), and III (1988 to 1994) and continuous NHANES (begun in 1999) included children and adolescents of all ages.

Sex-specific growth charts that contain a series of curved percentile lines showing the complete distribution of a body size measure across a range of ages or lengths and statures were first developed for U.S. children and adolescents in 1977 by the NCHS using data from NHES II and III and NHANES I. In 2000, the CDC released a revised set of growth charts (www.cdc.gov/growthcharts/). For children up to 3 years of age, the new sex-specific charts include weight-for-age, length-for-age, head circumference-for-age, and weight-for-length percentile curves. For children and adolescents 2 to 20 years of age, the new sex-specific charts include weight-for-age, stature-for-age, weight-for-stature, and, for the first time, body mass index-for-age (BMI = weight [kg] / height [m²] or BMI = 703 × weight [lbs] / height [in²]) percentile curves. For children 2 to 5 years of age, the BMI percentile curves (Fig. 12.2) are based on data from NHES II and III, and NHANES I, II, and III. For children and adolescents ≥6 years of age, NHANES III data were excluded from the computation of percentiles (Flegal et al., 2001) because of the increasing trends in overweight in this age group in NHANES III (Fig. 12.1), which would have produced higher percentile values than desirable in relation to current and future health.

For an individual child, the plotting of weight, stature, and BMI against the appropriate percentile grids (see, for example, Fig. 12.2A) can be used to identify a child who is growing well (pattern X) compared to a child who has growth difficulties (pattern Y or Z). For population and epidemiologic studies, growth charts can serve as a reference population and specific percentile points can be used to classify children and adolescents as overweight or underweight for their age and sex as discussed in the following section.

▪ DEFINITION OF OVERWEIGHT AND OBESITY IN CHILDREN AND ADOLESCENTS

A variety of measures including relative weight, weight-for-height indices, body circumferences, and skinfold thicknesses have been used to describe the prevalence of and trends in overweight and obesity among children and adolescents. The definitions of overweight and obesity have changed over time among researchers, and they differ for children and adolescents from those used for adults, as will be evident in the sections that follow.

Adiposity is the amount of fat in the body, expressed either as total body fat or as percent body fat. Children and adolescents are most accurately classified as obese using criteria based on measures of fatness or adiposity. However, such measures are not practical to obtain for epidemiologic studies nor in most clinical settings because complex laboratory procedures (e.g., underwater weighing, magnetic resonance imaging, computed tomography, dual-energy X-ray absorptiometry [DXA]) are required. Height and weight can be easily and quite precisely measured in the physician's office or at school. Body weight, while reasonably correlated with body fat, is also highly correlated with height. Weight adjusted for height, however, is a useful index for assessing overweight and it is also a reasonable indicator of body fatness, although stage of maturation, race, and sex have an impact on the association (Daniels et al., 1997; Pietrobelli et al., 1998).

Comparisons among various weight-for-height indices have identified the BMI, also called Quetelet's Index, as the most desirable index for both children and adults (Cole, 1991). The BMI is a single number that expresses the sum of the components that contribute to body weight—adipose tissue, lean body mass and bone. These components change at different ages and at different rates in boys and girls during growth and maturation, and therefore overweight criteria for children and adolescents that are based on BMI must be age- and sex-specific.

Body fat may be preferentially located in the abdomen (android obesity pattern) or surrounding the hips and thighs (gynoid obesity pattern). The android obesity pattern is more strongly associated with dyslipidemia, hypertension, and glucose intolerance (Kissebah and Krakower, 1994). Thus, even at the same level of overweight, an individual with a greater amount of visceral fat is more likely to have or develop serious health consequences associated with obesity.

Skinfold thicknesses and body circumferences can be measured to characterize fat distribution. The ratio of waist and hip circumferences is used as a surrogate index for the amount of visceral fat. The ratio of subscapular (on the trunk below the scapula) to triceps (on the upper arm) skinfolds provides a rough estimate of the ratio of truncal to peripheral fat. While BMI does not allow separation of the contributions of the fat and lean tissue to body weight, it is positively associated in children and adolescents with percent body fat as determined by DXA and underwater weighing, with correlation coefficients that range from 0.50 to 0.90 and are generally higher with DXA and for girls (Pietrobelli et al., 1998; Dietz and Bellizzi, 1999). The use of BMI as a measure of fatness requires the assumption that all individuals with a similar BMI have the same degree of fatness. However, the association between BMI and body fat appears to differ by race as well as by sex and stage of sexual maturation. In general, among individuals with equivalent BMIs, girls have higher body fat than boys, whites have higher body fat than blacks, and more mature individuals have lower body fat than less mature individuals (Daniels et al., 1997). In the clinical setting these may be important factors to consider, and a triceps skinfold thickness >95th percentile (see Barlow and Dietz, 1998, for reference percentiles) can be used to confirm that a child or adolescent with a high BMI also has excess body fat.

In U.S. adults, a BMI between 18.5 and 24.9 kg/m^2 is currently accepted as indicating a healthy weight, a BMI between 25.0 and 29.9 kg/m^2 indicates overweight, and a BMI $\geq$30 kg/m^2 indicates obesity (Visscher and Seidell, 2001). These

A

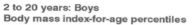

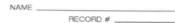

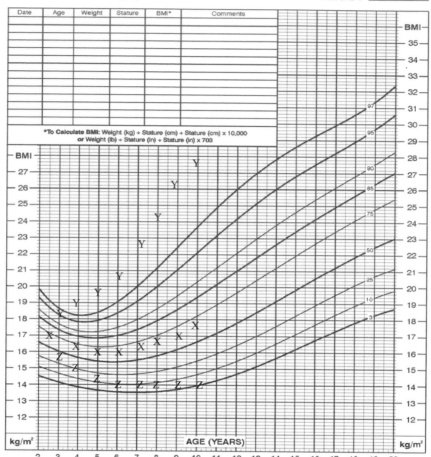

FIGURE 12.2

Body mass index (BMI)-for-age growth charts for boys (A) and girls (B) 2 to 20 years of age from the Centers for Disease Control and Prevention/National Center for Health Statistics. Panel A shows a boy who is growing well (pattern X) and two boys who have growth difficulties (patterns Y and Z).

Source: Developed by the National Center for Health Statistics in collaboration with the National Center for Chronic Disease Prevention and Health Promotion (2000); see http://www.cdc.gov/growthcharts.

238

B

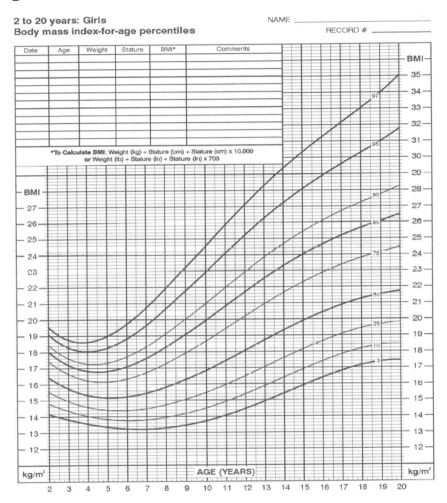

2 to 20 years: Girls
Body mass index-for-age percentiles

NAME _____

RECORD # _____

adult cut points are based on associations of BMI with chronic disease morbidity and mortality. Different BMI ranges have been proposed for populations within the Asia-Pacific region (www.idi.org.au/research.php Reports), because of differences in the observed associations of BMI with health-related risk factors in these populations.

Criteria used to identify underweight and overweight children and adolescents differ with age, and it is currently recommended (Himes and Dietz, 1994; Dietz and Bellizzi, 1999; Kuczmarski and Flegal, 2000) that they be based on percentiles from the 2000 CDC BMI-for-age growth charts (Fig. 12.2):

- Underweight: BMI <5th percentile. These children and adolescents should undergo an in-depth medical assessment.
- At risk of overweight: BMI between the 85th and 95th age- and sex-specific percentiles. These children and adolescents should undergo a second level of screening as long as their BMI is <30 kg/m² (see Table 13.3 in Chapter 13).
- Overweight: BMI ≥95th percentile, or BMI >30 kg/m², which ever is smaller. These children and adolescents should undergo an in-depth medical assessment (Barlow and Dietz, 1998).

There is no separate definition of obesity for children and adolescents, nor is the definition of overweight based on health outcomes or risk factors (Troiano and Flegal, 1998).

In U.S. children and adolescents, BMI declines and reaches a nadir between 4 and 8 years of age before beginning a gradual increase throughout adolescence and into adulthood. In boys (Fig. 12.2A), the increase after the nadir is nearly linear. In girls (Fig. 12.2B), there is a slight deceleration at about 16 years of age. The point at which BMI changes from decreasing to increasing is called the "adiposity rebound" (AR). It has been suggested that children whose AR begins at an earlier age are more likely to be obese as an adult and children whose AR begins at a later age are less likely (Rolland-Cachera et al., 1987; Whitaker et al., 1998). Dietz (2000) points out that children with higher BMIs also have an earlier AR (see, for example, the 90th percentile curve vs. the 10th percentile curve in Fig. 12.2) and it may simply be the BMI at the time of AR rather than the age when the AR occurs that is associated with adult obesity risk. However, Whitaker et al. (1998), using data from a retrospective cohort study that collected lifelong height and weight measurements, found that the odds of adult obesity (at 21 to 29 years of age) associated with an early AR are 6.0 times higher (95% CI 1.3–26.6) than the odds associated with a late AR, even after adjustment for parental BMI at the time the individual was 1.5 years of age and the individual's BMI at the time of AR.

International comparisons of the prevalence of childhood obesity have been a challenge because there has been a lack of consensus on the index to use, and there has been no internationally accepted standard definition of obesity for any index (Guillaume, 1999). Cole et al. (2000) proposed a standard to be used for international comparisons of overweight and obesity in children and adolescents (2 to 18 years of age). The standard is based on data from large national surveys conducted in six different countries; it was developed so that at age 18, a BMI at or above 25.0 kg/m² defines overweight, and a BMI at or above 30.0 kg/m² defines obesity, the accepted standard for adults.

It has been suggested that three critical periods exist for the development of obesity and its complications (Dietz, 1994; Whitaker and Dietz, 1998). The first is during gestation and early infancy, when intrauterine factors, especially those associated with maternal diabetes, appear to result in an increased risk of obesity in children and adolescents, and infant breastfeeding (Dietz, 2001; Gillman et al., 2001; Hediger et al., 2001) may be associated with a decrease in the risk of obesity. The second critical period is the period of AR, and the third is adolescence. Recommendations to health professionals for the identification and management of overweight children and adolescents are provided in two reports from expert committees (Himes and Dietz, 1994; Barlow and Dietz, 1998). Identification and management issues are also discussed in Chapters 13 and 14.

■ TRENDS IN PREVALENCE OF OVERWEIGHT CHILDREN AND ADOLESCENTS

When the overweight definition (BMI at or above the age- and sex-specific 95th percentile) is applied to data from U.S. national cross-sectional surveys (NHES II and III, NHANES I, II, III, and continuous NHANES), it is clear that the prevalence of overweight children and adolescents was relatively stable from the 1960s to 1980 (Fig. 12.1). However, from NHANES II (1976 to 1980) to NHANES III (1988 to 1994), the prevalence nearly doubled among both children and adolescents. Between those two surveys, the estimated prevalence of overweight children and adolescents increased from 5.0% to 7.2% for those 2 to 5 years of age, from 6.5% to 11.3% for those 6 to 11 years of age, and from 5.0% to 10.5% for those 12 to 19 years of age. The NHANES 1999 to 2000 estimates, which should be interpreted with caution because they are based on a smaller sample size than the multiyear NHANES estimates, suggest that since 1994, the prevalence has continued to increase to 10.4% for children 2 to 5, 15.3% for children 6 to 11, and 15.5% for adolescents 12 to 19 years of age (Ogden et al., 2002).

This increased prevalence is occurring regardless of age, sex, and race or ethnicity, regardless of whether the overweight definition is BMI ≥85th percentile or BMI ≥95th percentile, and it parallels the increased prevalence observed in adults (Troiano et al., 1995; Flegel et al., 2002; Kimm et al., 2002). Using a 95th percentile definition, the overweight prevalence estimates for non-Hispanic white (white), non-Hispanic black (black), and Mexican-American children and adolescents indicate that black girls between 6 and 19 years of age, and Mexican-American boys at all ages had the highest overweight prevalence during the period of NHANES 1999 to 2000 (Table 12.2) (Ogden et al., 2002). Girls and boys between 6 and 19 years of age had an overweight prevalence that was at least double the expected 5%.

Although American Indians living on reservations are not included in the NHANES surveys, a number of smaller surveys indicate that the obesity rates among American Indian children and adolescents are even higher than the NHANES rates for all races combined (Story et al., 1999). One of the goals of Healthy People 2010 (www.health.gov/healthypeople) is to "reduce the proportion of children and adolescents who are overweight or obese" to 5%. Given the prevalence estimates from NHANES 1999 to 2000 (Fig. 12.1), that goal will be very difficult to attain.

TABLE 12.2

Percentage of examined children and adolescents from the National
Health and Nutrition Examination Survey (1999–2000) who were
classified as overweight,* by sex, age, and race/ethnicity

Race/Ethnicity	Percent of Overweight Girls Age Group (Years)			Percent of Overweight Boys Age Group (Years)		
	2 to 5	6 to 11	12 to 19	2 to 5	6 to 11	12 to 19
White, non-Hispanic	11.5	11.6	12.4	8.8	12.0	12.8
Black, non-Hispanic	11.2	22.2	26.6	5.9	17.1	20.7
Mexican-American	9.2	19.6	19.4	13.0	27.3	27.5
Total	11.0	14.5	15.5	9.9	16.0	15.5

*Overweight = body mass index (kg/m^2) at or above age- and sex-specific 95th percentile CDC
growth charts.
Source: Adapted from Odgen et al. (2002).

Flegal and Troiano (2000) examined the change in the age- and sex-specific
BMI distributions from NHES II/III (1963 to 1970) to the BMI distributions from
NHANES III (1988 to 1994) for children and adolescents 6 to 17 years of age. For
each year of age, both the mean and median BMI and the overweight prevalence
were higher for NHANES III. Mean-difference plots were used to compare the age-
and sex-specific percentiles of the BMI distributions from the two surveys. In general, the plots showed that the BMI percentiles increased only slightly at the lower
end of the distribution. However, at the upper end of the distribution there was
an upward shift (by 2 to 6 kg/m^2 in NHANES III) accompanied by an increase in
the skewness of the overall distribution. This pattern suggests that the increases in
overweight represent a differential response to environmental change that may be
mediated by genetic susceptibility (Flegal and Troiano, 2000).

The prevalence of obesity is increasing in other developed and developing
countries of the world as well (World Health Organization, 1998; Martorell et al.,
2000; Friedrich, 2002). However, the prevalence of wasting (low weight-for-
stature), especially in the countries of Africa and Asia, is frequently still much
higher than the prevalence of obesity, and this can not be overlooked (de Onis
and Blossner, 2000).

As in the United States, the increased prevalence of obesity worldwide is
likely a response to environmental and societal changes, rather than to genetic
changes, or to the effects of immigration or emigration within a given population. In general, the increase is the most dramatic in countries where the standard of living has increased because of industrialization and globalization of
markets, and where food is more readily available and the need for physical la-
bor has decreased (Sorensen, 2000; Friedrich, 2002).

■ GENETIC FACTORS AND FAMILIAL
AGGREGATION OF BODY SIZE MEASURES

In rare instances human obesity may be associated with defects at a single genetic locus. Some of these include the Prader-Willi (Knoll et al., 1993) and Bardet-Biedl syndromes (Sheffield et al., 2001; Mykytyn et al., 2003), Alström syndrome (Michaud et al., 1996), and interstitial deletion of chromosome 18 (q12.2q21.1) (Wilson and Al Saadi, 1988). The mechanisms by which these genetic defects produce the obesity phenotype are unknown.

The importance of a heredity influence on human body size has been demonstrated in multiple studies of dizygotic and monozygotic twins, and of adopted individuals and their biologic siblings. Studies of twin pairs have demonstrated higher concordance for body size among monozygotic than dizygotic twins. In a study of 1974 monozygotic and 2097 dizygotic twin pairs, concordance for body size at six different degrees of overweight (15%, 20%, 25%, 30%, 35%, and 40% overweight) at approximately 20 years of age was 1.9- to 3.6-fold higher for monozygotic than dizygotic pairs (Stunkard et al., 1986). In a study of adult adoptees and their biologic full and half siblings, there was a significant correlation of BMI in biologic siblings across the entire distribution of body sizes. This correlation was much stronger for the full-siblings than for the half-siblings (Sorensen et al., 1989).

In several large unrelated populations, statistical evidence supporting the existence of recessive major gene effects on the determination of various body size measures has been identified. These include, for example, BMI in Muscatine, Iowa families (Moll et al., 1991), BMI in Caucasian and African-American families (Price, 1996), abdominal visceral fat in families from Québec (Bouchard et al., 1996), relative fat pattern in Utah pedigrees (Hasstedt et al., 1988), and obesity in American Pima Indians (Knowler et al., 1991).

The population of Muscatine, Iowa, has been studied for over 35 years with longitudinal follow-up of body size and relative fatness, cardiovascular risk factors, blood lipid levels, blood pressure, and other phenotypic features. In this population, there is a positive association between BMI and coronary risk factors among the school children and their family members (Burns et al., 1989), and there is increased familial cardiovascular mortality among persistently heavy school children (Burns et al., 1992). Both genetic and environmental factors appear to be involved in determining BMI variability in the Muscatine population (Moll et al., 1991); 35% of the variability in age- and sex-adjusted BMI is attributable to a single autosomal recessive locus with a major effect, and 42% of the variability is attributable to polygenic loci with small, additive effects on the determination of BMI.

Longitudinal studies have also demonstrated familial aggregation of obesity and cardiovascular risk in other communities. These include the Bogalusa Heart Study (Freedman et al., 1999; Srinivasan et al., 1999), the San Antonio Family Heart Study (Comuzzie et al., 1997; Burke et al., 1999), the HERITAGE

Family Study (Hong et al., 1998), the Québec Family Study (Rice et al., 1996), and studies of American Pima Indians (Norman et al., 1997).

■ TRACKING OF BODY MASS INDEX IN CHILDREN AND ADOLESCENTS

The major significance of childhood overweight is that it persists into adolescence and thereafter into adulthood, where it is associated with morbidity and mortality from chronic disease. There is a significant association between body size measures obtained during childhood and adolescence and those obtained between childhood and adulthood in the same individuals; a number of studies have shown that overweight children are more likely to become overweight adults (Rolland-Cachera et al., 1987; Clarke and Lauer, 1993; Whitaker et al., 1997, 1998; Guo and Chumlea, 1999; Guo et al., 2002).

Rolland-Cachera et al. (1987) tracked the development of adiposity in 164 healthy French subjects (85 boys and 79 girls) for whom height and weight measurements were obtained every 6 months from 1 month of age until adulthood (age 21 ± 2.5 years). Lean ($n = 44$), medium ($n = 75$) and fat ($n = 46$) subjects were defined at 1 year of age using the 25th and 75th BMI percentiles from a French reference population. At adulthood, 41%, 42%, and 41% of the lean, medium, and fat subjects, respectively, remained in their original BMI category. Forty-eight percent of the infants in the fat category changed to the medium category as adults, however, only 20% of the infants in the lean and medium categories changed to the fat category as adults. Therefore, the risk of being fat as an adult was more than twice as great for infants who were in the fat category at 1 year of age compared to infants in the lean or medium categories.

The predictive value of childhood BMI for overweight (BMI ≥25 kg/m^2) or obesity (BMI ≥30 kg/m^2) at 35 years of age was investigated by Guo et al. (2002) using data from the Fels Longitudinal Study. Annual height and weight data for 166 white males and 181 white females were available from 3 to 18 years of age and from 30 to 39 years of age. BMI measurements obtained at ages 3, 8, 13, and 18 years of age were used to represent early and late childhood, puberty, and post-puberty. Both men and women who were classified as overweight or obese at age 35 (mean of all available measurements between 30 and 39 years of age) had higher mean BMIs at ages 3, 8, 13, and 18 compared to those below the two BMI cut points. For children and adolescents with BMI at any age ≥95th percentile based on the 2000 CDC growth charts, the probability of being obese at age 35 ranged from 15% to 99%. Among boys ≤8 years of age, approximately 20% were obese as adults. Approximately 33% of the boys between 8 and 12 years of age were obese as adults, and 50% of the boys ≥13 years of age were obese. For girls of the same age, approximately 33%, 50%, and 67%, respectively, were obese as adults. The sensitivity and specificity of using a BMI ≥50th percentile at age 18 to predict overweight at age 35 were 0.83 and 0.72, respectively, for males, and 0.74 and 0.73, respectively, for females.

Between 1971 and 1981, the heights and weights of school children (predominantly of Northern European origin) were measured in six biennial Muscatine Study school surveys (Lauer and Clarke, 1989). Beginning in 1981, a representative sample of all school survey participants was measured between the ages of 21 to 25, 25 to 30, and 31 to 35 years, targeted to be near the 23rd, 28th, and 33rd birthdays. For 1355 young adults examined between the ages of 21 and 25, a total of 4248 childhood and adolescent measurements are available. Figure 12.3 shows the tracking of BMI measured at 9 to 10, 13 to 14, and 17 to 18 years of age into young adulthood (21 to 25 years of age) for females (Fig. 12.3A) and males (Fig. 12.3B). Childhood and adolescent BMI measurements were classified as being $\geq$ 85th percentile or between the 25th and 75th percentiles based on the 2000 CDC growth charts. Young adults were classified as normal ($18.5 \leq BMI < 25.0$), overweight ($25.0 \leq BMI < 30.0$) or obese ($BMI \geq 30.0$). There were approximately 300 males and 300 females for whom BMI measurements were available at age 9 to 10 and between 21 and 25 years of age (500 at age 13 to 14, and 300 at age 17 to 18). Regardless of the childhood age group or sex, less than 5% of those whose BMI was between the 25th and 75th age- and sex specific percentiles during childhood and adolescence were obese as young adults, and less than 30% were overweight (Fig. 12.3). In contrast, 29% to 40% of females and 34% to 58% of males whose BMI was $\geq$85th percentile during childhood and adolescence were overweight as young adults, and an additional 41% to 49% of females and 34% to 40% of males were obese. The relative risk of a BMI $\geq$25.0 at age 21 to 25 in those with a childhood or adolescent BMI $\geq$85th percentile relative to those with a childhood or adolescent BMI between the 25th and 75th percentiles was 3.7 (95% CI 2.7–5.1), 6.8 (4.7–9.7), and 5.9 (4.0–8.8) for females with childhood measurements at ages 9 to 10, 13 to 14, and 17 to 18, respectively, all with $p < 0.0001$. The corresponding relative risks for males were 3.0 (95% CI 2.2–4.2), 2.8 (2.2–3.4), and 3.7 (2.8–4.8), all with $p < 0.0001$.

Whitaker et al. (1997) investigated the association between obesity (BMI $\geq$27.8 kg/m^2 for men and $\geq$27.3 kg/m^2 for women) in young adulthood (21 to 29 years of age) and obesity at various times throughout childhood and adolescence (BMI $\geq$85th percentile from NHANES I and II), along with parental obesity (BMI $\geq$27.8 kg/m^2 for fathers and $\geq$27.3 kg/m^2 for mothers). Childhood obesity at 1 to 2 years of age was not significantly associated with adult obesity. However, for every other age interval, the odds of being an obese adult were significantly higher for obese children and adolescents relative to non-obese children and adolescents (3 to 5 years of age, odds ratio [OR] = 4.1; 6 to 9 years of age, OR = 10.3; 10 to 14 years of age, OR = 28.3; and 15 to 17 years of age, OR = 20.3). In children less than 3 years of age, the parents' obesity status was the strongest predictor of young adult obesity. The effect of parental obesity was most pronounced for children less than 10 years of age, for example, the probability

A

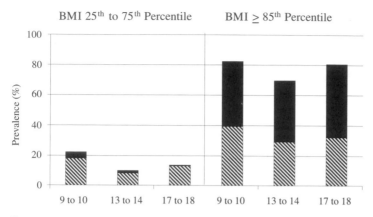

B

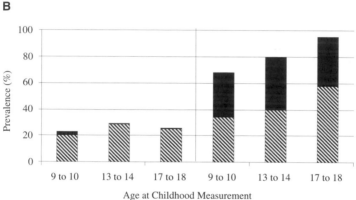

Age at Childhood Measurement

FIGURE 12.3

Prevalence of overweight ($25.0 \leq$ BMI < 30.0 kg/m² [gray bars]) and obesity (BMI ≥ 30.0 kg/m² [black bars]) in Muscatine Study young adult (21 to 25 years of age) females (A) and males (B) whose BMI was available from childhood at ages 9 to 10, 13 to 14, or 17 to 18. Childhood BMI was classified as being between the 25th and 75th age- and sex-specific percentiles (left side of figure) or $\geq$85th percentile (right side of figure) based on the 2000 Centers for Disease Control and Prevention growth charts.

that a child 3 to 5 years of age was obese as a young adult increased from 24% if neither parent was obese when the child was 3 to 5 years of age to 62% if at least one parent was obese. Thus, clinicians should consider parental obesity when monitoring the growth patterns of children.

The dramatic increase in the prevalence of overweight children and adolescents (Fig. 12.1), combined with the significant tracking of BMI from adolescence into adulthood, suggests that the next generation of adults will include a larger proportion of individuals who are at risk for obesity-related health conditions. Prevention efforts in children and adolescents must be focused on those who are not yet overweight. However, because up to 15% are already overweight (Fig. 12.1), intervention strategies must also be targeted at those individuals, with the goal of preventing obesity in adulthood (see Chapters 13 and 14).

■ RELATIONSHIP BETWEEN CHILDHOOD OVERWEIGHT, CARDIOVASCULAR RISK FACTORS, AND ADULT CARDIOVASCULAR MORBIDITY AND MORTALITY

The major health complications of childhood overweight are not usually manifest for several decades. Overweight children and adolescents are nonetheless at a substantially increased risk for adverse levels of several CVD risk factors including lipids, lipoproteins, insulin, and blood pressure levels. The association between BMI and concurrent CVD risk factor levels was investigated in 9167 children and adolescents who were 5 to 17 (mean 11.9) years of age at their last Bogolusa Heart Study school survey examination (Freedman et al., 1999). Over weight was defined as >95th age- and sex-specific percentile based on data from NHES II and III, and NHANES I, II, and III. Low-density lipoprotein (LDL) cholesterol or triglyceride levels >130 mg/dL (3.4 mmol/L) were classified as high; high-density lipoprotein (HDL) cholesterol levels <35 mg/dL (0.9 mmol/L) were classified as low; and insulin levels greater than the age-, sex-, and race (36% black)-specific 95th percentile were classified as high. Children were classified as having high systolic or diastolic blood pressure on the basis of age-, sex-, race-, and height-adjusted values >95th percentile. Fifty-nine percent of overweight children and adolescents had at least one CVD risk factor, whereas 27% had two or more risk factors. For non-overweight children and adolescents, 27% had at least one risk factor and only 5% had two or more risk factors. Ninety percent of the 80 children and adolescents who had elevated insulin and triglyceride levels were also overweight (Freedman et al., 1999).

Between 1971 and 1996, investigators for the Muscatine Study conducted 37,285 examinations of 17,269 children and adolescents between the ages of 5 and 18 years. The association between BMI and concurrent CVD risk factor levels is described in Table 12.3 for examinations conducted at ages 6, 11, and 16. For girls at each age, there was a slight, but not significant increased risk of upper-decile age-, sex-, and survey year—specific total cholesterol levels for those whose BMI was over the 85th percentile based on 2000 CDC growth charts relative to those whose BMI was between the 25th and 75th percentiles. For boys, there was a significantly increased risk at ages 11 and 16. At each age, and for both girls and boys, the risk of upper-decile triglyceride and systolic and diastolic blood pressure levels was consistently and significantly higher for children and adolescents with high BMIs. So, the association between BMI and triglycerides and blood pressures is evident in children as young as 6 years of age.

TABLE 12.3

Odds of having a risk factor level in the highest age-, sex-, and survey year-specific decile for Muscatine Study school children at ages 6, 11, and 16, for those whose concurrent body mass index was ≥85th age-, sex-, and survey year-specific percentile relative to those whose body mass index was between the 25th and 75th percentiles.*

Risk Factor	6 Years of Age		11 Years of Age		16 Years of Age	
	Girls	Boys	Girls	Boys	Girls	Boys
Total cholesterol	1.1 (0.6–2.0) p > 0.70 n = 593 198 mg/dL	1.5 (0.9–2.6) p > 0.10 n = 633 193 mg/dL	1.2 (0.8–2.0) p > 0.40 n = 743 204 mg/dL	2.0 (1.2–3.2) p < 0.01 n = 777 204 mg/dL	1.2 (0.6–2.4) p > 0.50 n = 477 210 mg/dL	3.1 (1.6,–5.7) p < 0.001 n = 434 188 mg/dL
Triglycerides	2.3 (1.4–3.9) p < 0.0025 n = 592 110 mg/dL)	1.8 (1.0–3.0) p < 0.05 n = 633 103 mg/dL	3.2 (2.0–5.0) p < 0.0001 n = 743 144 mg/dL	4.0 (2.5–6.5) p < 0.0001 n = 777 142 mg/dL	4.5 (2.5–8.2) p < 0.0001 n = 477 137 mg/dL	2.6 (1.4–4.9) p < 0.005 n = 434 141 mg/dL
Systolic blood pressure	2.7 (1.8–4.0) p < 0.0001 n = 1017 114 mmHg	2.9 (2.0–4.2) p < 0.0001 n = 1090 116 mmHg	3.2 (2.1–4.8) p < 0.0001 n = 1073 130 mmHg	4.0 (2.7–6.1) p < 0.0001 n = 1115 126 mmHg	4.4 (2.6–7.3) p < 0.0001 n = 658 132 mmHg	3.0 (1.8–5.0) p < 0.0001 n = 606 142 mmHg
Diastolic blood pressure	2.2 (1.5–3.4) p < 0.0005 n = 1010 80 mmHg	2.3 (1.5–3.4) p < 0.0001 n = 1087 80 mmHg	2.3 (1.6–3.4) p < 0.0001 n = 1068 84 mmHg	2.5 (1.7–3.7) p < 0.0001 n = 1109 82 mmHg	2.9 (1.7–4.9) p < 0.0001 n = 658 90 mmHg	2.1 (1.2–3.5) p < 0.01 n = 606 90 mmHg

*Percentiles based on the CDC growth charts. Values given are as follows: odds ratio (95% confidence interval); p value; number included in the analysis (BMI 25th to 75th or ≥85th percentile); median value of the risk factor for children and adolescents in the upper decile. The median BMI for children with BMI ≥85th percentile was 18.3, 23.2, and 28.0 for girls age 6, 11, and16, respectively, and 18.1, 22.7, and 26.8 for boys ages 6, 11, and 16, respectively.

Prospective data from both the Muscatine Study (Lauer and Clarke, 1989; Lauer et al., 1989) and the Bogolusa Heart Study (Srinivasan et al., 1996; Freedman et al., 2001) show that overweight acquired in adolescence persists into young adulthood when it is frequently associated with CVD risk factors, such as adverse blood pressure and lipid levels. Overweight adolescents (13 to 17 years of age with BMI >75th percentile) who remain overweight young adults are 8.5 times more likely to have hypertension as young adults (27 to 31 years of age) than lean adolescents (25th < BMI < 50th percentile) who remain lean young adults. They also are 2.4 times more likely to have total cholesterol values >240 mg/dL (6.2 mmol/L), 3.0 times more likely to have LDL cholesterol values >160 mg/dL (4.1 mmol/L), and 8.0 times more likely to have HDL cholesterol levels <35 mg/dL (0.9 mmol/L) (Srinivasan et al., 1996).

The best criterion by which to judge the health consequences of excess body weight during childhood and adolescence is to examine in those same children and adolescents the risk of adult morbidity and mortality. Because of the length of time involved, such investigations are rare. In one long-term investigation, lean (25th < BMI < 50th percentile) and overweight (BMI > 75th percentile) participants from the Harvard Growth Study (ages 13 to 18 in 1922 to 1935) were followed up in 1988 to obtain morbidity and mortality information (Must et al., 1992). Overweight adolescent boys had increased risks of death from all causes, from coronary heart disease and from atherosclerotic cerebrovascular disease as adults when compared to their lean peers; there was no increased risk for overweight adolescent girls. Adolescent boys and girls who were overweight had an increased risk of morbidity as adults from both coronary heart disease and atherosclerosis. Adolescent weight status was a more powerful predictor than adult weight. The ongoing Muscatine Study is examining early indicators (coronary artery calcium and carotid artery intimal-medial thickening) of the atherosclerotic process in school survey participants from the 1970s (see Chapters 4 and 5).

The development of atherosclerosis and hypertension is a lifelong process. Numerous investigations have found that overweight children and adolescents are at increased risk for adverse CVD risk factor levels in young adult life, in part because excess body size persists into young adulthood. These adverse risk factor levels are, in turn, associated with an increased risk of CVD morbidity and mortality in later adult life. Therefore, the treatment and management of overweight children and adolescents should be high on the list of public health priorities.

■ SUMMARY

- Childhood overweight and obesity is a serious public health problem.
- Obesity is the most prevalent nutritional disorder in children and adolescents.
- The prevalence of overweight among U.S. children and adolescents, especially among African-Americans, Mexican-Americans, and American

Indians, has shown a dramatic increase since 1980. Preventive measures are warranted, especially for high-risk youth, and they may need to be targeted specifically to reduce the disparities in higher-risk populations.

• Fifty-nine percent of children and adolescents with a BMI-for-age above the 95th percentile have at least one CVD risk factor, while 27% have two or more risk factors.

• Overweight children are likely to become overweight adults.

• Tracking of BMI throughout childhood and adolescence would help parents and health professionals identify those who are tending toward or consistently at BMI levels associated with increased health risks and who are likely to be at increased risk for CVD morbidity and mortality in adulthood.

• Prevention of obesity in children and adolescents should be a useful public health strategy for preventing CVD in later adult life.

▥ REFERENCES

Barlow, S.E., and W.H. Dietz. 1998. Obesity Evaluation and Treatment: Expert Committee Recommendations. *Pediatrics* 102:e29.

Bouchard, C., T. Rice, S. Lemieux, J-P. Després, L. Pérusse, and D.C. Rao. 1996. Major Gene for Abdominal Visceral Fat Area in the Québec Family Study. *Int J Obes* 20:420–7.

Burke, J.P., K. Williams, S.P. Gaskill, H.P. Hazuda, S.M. Haffner, and M.P. Stern. 1999. Rapid Rise in the Incidence of Type 2 Diabetes From 1987 to 1996—Results from the San Antonio Heart Study. *Arch Intern Med* 159:1450–6.

Burns, T.L., P.P. Moll, and R.M. Lauer. 1989. The Relation between Ponderosity and Coronary Risk Factors in Children and their Relatives. *Am J Epidemiol* 129:973–87.

Burns, T.L., P.P. Moll, and R.M. Lauer. 1992. Increased Familial Cardiovascular Mortality in Obese Schoolchildren: The Muscatine Ponderosity Family Study. *Pediatrics* 89:262–8.

Calle, E.E., C. Rodriquez, K. Walker-Thurmond, and M.J. Thun. 2003. Overweight, Obesity, and Mortality from Cancer in a Prospectively Studied Cohort of U.S. Adults. *N Engl J Med* 348:1625–38.

Clarke, W.R., and R.M. Lauer. 1993. Does Childhood Obesity Track into Adulthood?" *Crit Rev Food Sci Nutr* 33:423–30.

Cole, T.J. 1991. Weight-Stature Indices to Measure Underweight, Overweight, and Obesity. In: *Anthropometric Assessment of Nutritional Status*. Edited by J.H. Himes. New York: Wiley-Liss, pp. 83–111.

Cole, T.J., M.C. Bellizzi, K.M. Flegal, and W.H. Dietz. 2000. Establishing a Standard Definition for Childhood Overweight and Obesity Worldwide: International Survey. *BMJ* 320:1–6.

Comuzzie, A.G., J.E. Hixson, L. Almasy, B.D. Mitchell, M.C. Mahaney, T.D. Dyer, M.P. Stern, J.W. MacCluer, and J. Blangero. 1997. A Major Quantitative Trait Locus Determining Serum Leptin Levels and Fat Mass Is Located on Human Chromosome 2. *Nat Genet* 15:273–6.

Daniels, S.R., P.R. Khoury, and J.A. Morrison. 1997. The Utility of Body Mass Index as a Measure of Body Fatness in Children and Adolescents: Differences by Race and Gender. *Pediatrics* 99:804–7.

de Onis, M., and M. Blossner. 2000. Prevalence and Trends of Overweight among Preschool Children in Developing Countries. *Am J Clin Nutr* 72:1032–9.

Dietz, W.H. 1994. Critical Periods in Childhood for the Development of Obesity. *Am J Clin Nutr* 59:955–9.

Dietz, W.H. 2000. Adiposity Rebound: Reality or Epiphenomenon?" *Lancet* 356:2027–8.

Dietz, W.H. 2001. Breastfeeding May Help Prevent Childhood Overweight. *JAMA* 285:2506–7.

Dietz, W.H., and M.C. Bellizzi. 1999. Introduction: the Use of BMI to Assess Obesity in Children. *Am J Clin Nutr* 70:123S–5S.

Dietz, W.H., and S.L. Gortmaker. 2001. Preventing Obesity in Children and Adolescents. *Annu Rev Public Health* 22:337–53.

Flegel, K.M., M.D. Carroll, C.L. Ogden, and C.L. Johnson. 2002. Prevalence and Trends in Obesity among US Adults, 1999–2000. *JAMA* 288:1723–7.

Flegal, K.M., C.L. Ogden, R. Wei, R.J. Kuczmarski, and C.L. Johnson. 2001. Prevalence of Overweight in US Children: Comparison of US Growth Charts from the Centers for Disease Control and Prevention with Other Reference Values for Body Mass Index. *Am J Clin Nutr* 73:1086–93.

Flegal, K.M, and R.P. Troiano. 2000. Changes in the Distribution of Body Mass Index of Adults and Children in the US Population. *Int J Obes Relat Metab Disord* 24:807–18.

Freedman, D.S., W.H. Dietz, S.R. Srinivasan, and G.S. Berenson. 1999. The Relation of Overweight to Cardiovascular Risk Factors among Children and Adolescents: The Bogalusa Heart Study. *Pediatrics* 103:1175–82.

Freedman, D., L. Khan, W.H. Dietz, S.R. Srinivasan, and G.S. Berenson. 2001. Relationship of Childhood Obesity to Coronary Heart Disease Risk Factors in Adulthood: The Bogalusa Heart Study. *Pediatrics* 108:712–8.

Friedrich, M.J. 2002. Epidemic of Obesity Expands its Spread to Developing Countries. *JAMA* 287:1382–6.

Gillman, M.W., S. Rifas-Shiman, C.S. Berkey, A.E. Field, and G.A. Colditz. 2003. Maternal Gestational Diabetes, Birth Weight, and Adolescent Obesity. *Pediatrics* 111:e221–6.

Gillman, M.W., S.L. Rifas-Shiman, C.A. Camargo, C.S. Berkey, A.L. Frazier, H.R.H. Rockett, A.E. Field and G.A. Colditz. 2001. Risk of Overweight among Adolescents Who Were Breastfed as Infants. *JAMA* 285:2461–7.

Goran, M.I., G.D.C. Ball, and M.L. Cruz. 2003. Obesity and Risk of Type 2 Diabetes and Cardiovascular Disease in Children and Adolescents. *J Clin Endocrinol Metab* 88:1417–27.

Guillaume, M. 1999. Defining Obesity in Childhood: Current Practice. *Am J Clin Nutr* 70:126S–30S.

Guo, S.S., and W.C. Chumlea. 1999. Tracking of Body Mass Index in Children in Relation to Overweight in Adulthood. *Am J Clin Nutr* 70:145S–8S.

Guo, S.S., W. Wu, W.C. Chumlea, and A.F. Roche. 2002. Predicting Overweight and Obesity in Adulthood from Body Mass Index Values in Childhood and Adolescence. *Am J Clin Nutr* 76:653–8.

Hasstedt S.J., M.E. Ramirez, H. Kuida, and R.R. Williams. 1988. Recessive Inheritance of a Relative Fat Pattern. *Am J Hum Genet* 45:917–25.

Hediger, M.L., M.D. Overpeck, R.J. Kuczmarski, and W.J. Ruan. 2001. Association between Infant Breastfeeding and Overweight in Young Children. *JAMA* 285:2453–60.

Himes, J.H., and W.H. Dietz. 1994. Guidelines for Overweight in Adolescent Preventive Services: Recommendations from an Expert Committee. *Am J Clin Nutr* 59:307–16.

Hong, Y., T. Rice, J. Gagnon, J-P. Despres, A. Nadeau, L. Perusse, C. Bouchard, A.S. Leon, J.S. Skinner, J.H. Wilmore, and D.C. Rao. 1998. Familial Clustering of Insulin and Abdominal Visceral Fat: The HERITAGE Family Study. *J Clin Endocrin Metab* 83:4239–45.

Kimm, S.Y.S., B.A. Barton, E. Obarzanck, R.P. McMahon, S.S. Kronsberg, M.A. Waclawiw, J.A. Morrison, G.B. Schreiber, Z.I. Sabry, and S.R. Daniels. 2002. Obesity Development during Adolescence in a Biracial Cohort: The NHLBI Growth and Health Study. *Pediatrics* 110:e54–8.

Kissebah, A.H., and G.R. Krakower. 1994. Regional Adiposity and Morbidity. *Physiol Rev* 74:761–811.

Knoll, J.H., D. Sinnett, J. Wagstaff, K. Glatt, A.S. Wilcox, P.M. Whiting, P. Wingrove, J,M, Sikela, and M. Lalande. 1993. FISH Ordering of Reference Markers and of the Gene for the Alpha 5 Subunit of the Gamma-Aminobutyric Acid Receptor (GABRA5) within the Angelman and Prader-Willi Syndrome Chromosomal Regions. *Hum Mol Genet* 2:183–9.

Knowler, W.C., D.J. Pettitt, M.F. Saad, M.A. Charles, R.G. Nelson, B.V. Howard, C. Bogardus, and P.H. Bennett. 1991. Obesity in the Pima Indians: Its Magnitude and Relationship with Diabetes. *Am J Clin Nutr* 53:1543S–51S.

Kuczmarski, R.J., and K.M. Flegal. 2000. Criteria for Definition of Overweight in Transition: Background and Recommendations for the United States. *Am J Clin Nutr* 72:1074–81.

Kumanyika, S.K. 2001. Minisymposium on Obesity: Overview and Some Strategic Considerations. *Annu Rev Public Health* 22:293–308.

Lauer, R.M., and W.R. Clarke. 1989. Childhood Risk Factors for High Adult Blood Pressure: The Muscatine Study. *Pediatrics* 84:633–41.

Lauer, R.M., J.H. Lee, and W.R. Clarke. 1989. Predicting Adult Cholesterol Levels from Measurements in Childhood and Adolescence: The Muscatine Study. *Bull N Y Acad Med* 65:1127–42.

Manson, J.E., W.C. Willett, M.J. Stampfer, G.A. Colditz, D.J. Hunter, S.E. Hankinson, C.H. Hennekens, and F.E. Speizer. 1995. Body Weight and Mortality among Women. *N Engl J Med* 333:677–85.

Martorell, R., L. Kettel Khan, M.L. Hughes, and L.M. Grummer-Strawn. 2000. Overweight and Obesity in Preschool Children from Developing Countries. *Int J Obes Rel Metab Dis* 24:959–67.

Melanson, K.J., K.J. McInnis, J.M. Rippe, G. Blackburn, and P.F. Wilson. 2001. Obesity and Cardiovascular Disease Risk: Research Update. *Cardiol Rev* 9:202–7.

Michaud, J.L., E. Heon, F. Guilbert, J. Weill, B. Puech, L. Benson, J.F. Smallhorn, C.T. Shuman, J.R. Buncie, A.V. Levin, R. Weksberg, and G.M. Breviere. 1996. Natural History of Alstrom Syndrome in Early Childhood: Onset with Dilated Cardiomyopathy. *J Pediatr* 128:225–9.

Moll P.P., T.L. Burns, and R.M. Lauer. 1991. The Genetic and Environmental Sources of Body Mass Index Variability: The Muscatine Ponderosity Family Study. *Am J Hum Genet* 49:1243–55.

Must, A., P.F. Jacques, G.E. Dallal, C.J. Bajema, and W.H. Dietz. 1992. Long-Term Morbidity and Mortality of Overweight Adolescents. A Follow-up of the Harvard Growth Study of 1922 to 1935. *N Engl J Med* 327:1350–5.

Mykytyn, K., D.Y. Nishimura, C.C. Searby, G. Beck, K. Bugge, H.L. Haines, A.S. Cormier, G.F. Cox, A.B. Fulton, R. Carmi, A. Iannaccone, S.G. Jacobson, R.G. Weleber, A.F. Wright, R. Riise, R.C.M. Hennekam, G. Luleci, S. Berker-Karauzum, L.G. Biesecker, E.M. Stone, and V.C. Sheffield. 2003. Evaluation of Complex Inheritance Involving the Most Common Bardet-Biedl Syndrome Locus (*BBS1*). *Am J Hum Genet* 72:429–37.

National Task Force on the Prevention and Treatment of Obesity. 2000. Overweight, Obesity and Health Risk. *Arch Intern Med* 160: 898–904.

Norman, R.A., D.B. Thompsom, T. Foroud, W.T. Garvey, P.H. Bennett, C. Bogardus, and E. Ravussin. 1997. Genome Wide Search for Genes Influencing Percent Body Fat in Pima Indians: Suggestive Linkage at Chromosome 11q21–q22. *Am J Hum Genet* 60:166–73.

Ogden, C.L., K.M. Flegal, M.D. Carroll, and C.L. Johnson. 2002. Prevalence and Trends in Overweight among US Children and Adolescents, 1999–2000. *JAMA* 288:1728–32.

Pietrobelli, A., M.S. Faith, D.B. Allison, D. Gallagher, G. Chiumello, and S.B. Heymsfield. 1998. Body Mass Index as a Measure of Adiposity among Children and Adolescents: A Validation Study. *J Pediatr* 132:204–10.

Price, R.A. 1996. Within Birth Cohort Segregation Analyses Support Recessive Inheritance of Body Mass Index in White and African-American Families. *Int J Obes* 20:1044–7.

Rice, T., A. Nadeau, L. Perusse, C. Bouchard, and D.C. Rao. 1996. Familial Correlations in the Québec Family Study: Cross-Trait Familial Resemblance for Body Fat with Plasma Glucose and Insulin. *Diabetologia* 39:1357–64.

Rolland-Cachera, M-F., M. Deheeger, M. Guilloud-Bataille, P. Avons, E. Patois, and M. Sempe. 1987. Tracking the Development of Adiposity from One Month of Age to Adulthood. *Ann Hum Biol* 14:219–29.

Sheffield, V.C., D. Nishimura, and E.M. Stone. 2001. The Molecular Genetics of Bardet-Biedl Syndrome. *Curr Opin Genet Dev* 11:317–21.

Sorensen, T., R.A. Price, A.J. Stunkard, and F. Schulsinger. 1989. Genetics of Obesity in Adult Adoptees and their Biological Siblings. *BMJ* 298:87–90.

Sorensen, T.L.A. 2000. The Changing Lifestyle in the World. *Diabetes Care* 23:B1–4.

Srinivasan, S.R., W. Bao, W.A. Wattigney, and G.S. Berenson. 1996. Adolescent Overweight Is Associated with Adult Overweight and Related Multiple Cardiovascular Risk Factors: The Bogolusa Heart Study. *Metabolism* 45:235–40.

Srinivasan, S.R., L. Myers, and G.S. Berenson. 1999. Temporal Association between Obesity and Hyperinsulinemia in Children, Adolescents, and Young Adults: The Bogalusa Heart Study. *Metabolism* 48:928–34.

Story, M., M. Evans, R.R. Fabsitz, T.E. Clay, B. Holy Rock, and B. Broussard. 1999. The Epidemic of Obesity in American Indian Communities and the Need for Childhood Obesity-Prevention Programs. *Am J Clin Nutr* 69(Suppl):747S–54S.

Stunkard, A.J., T.T. Foch, and Z. Hrubec. 1986. A Twin Study of Human Obesity. *JAMA* 256:51–4.

Sturm, R. 2002. The Effects of Obesity, Smoking, and Drinking on Medical Problems and Costs. *Health Affairs* 21.245—53.

Sturm, R., and K.B. Wells. 2001. Does Obesity Contribute as much to Morbidity as Poverty or Smoking? *Public Health* 115:229–35.

Troiano, R.P., and K.M. Flegal. 1998. Overweight Children and Adolescents: Description, Epidemiology, and Demographics. *Pediatrics* 101:497–504.

Troiano, R.P., K.M. Flegal, R.J. Kuczmarski, S.M. Campbell, and C.L. Johnson. 1995. Overweight Prevalence and Trends for Children and Adolescents. *Arch Pediatr Adolesc Med* 149:1085–91.

Visscher, T.L.S., and J.C. Seidell. 2001. The Public Health Impact of Obesity. *Annu Rev Public Health* 22:355–75.

Whitaker, R.C., and W.H. Dietz. 1998. Role of the Prenatal Environment in the Development of Obesity. *J Pediatr* 132:768–76.

Whitaker, R.C., M.S. Pepe, J.A. Wright, K.D. Seidel, and W.H. Dietz. 1998. Early Adiposity Rebound and the Risk of Adult Obesity. *Pediatrics* 101:e5.

Whitaker, R.C., J.A. Wright, M.S. Pepe, K.D. Seidel, and W.H. Dietz. 1997. Predicting Obesity in Young Adulthood from Childhood and Parental Obesity. *N Engl J Med* 337:869–73.

Wilson, G.N., and A.A. Al Saadi. 1988. Obesity and Abnormal Behaviour Associated with Interstitial Deletion of Chromosome 18 (q12.2q21.1). *J Med Genet* 26:62–3.

World Health Organization. 1998. Report of a WHO Consultation on Obesity 3–5 June 1997. *Obesity: Preventing and Managing the Global Epidemic.* Geneva: World Health Organization.

CHAPTER 13

Identification and Management of Obese Children and Adolescents

Andrew M. Tershakovec and Robert I. Berkowitz

The prevalence of obesity in children is increasing dramatically (Troiano et al., 1995; Ogden et al., 2002). The most recent national data collected in 1999 and 2000 show that 15% of 6- to19-year old children were overweight (body mass index [BMI] at or above the 95th percentile), while 10% of 2- to 5-year-olds were overweight. This represents a 35% to 48% increase from the data that were collected between 1988 and 1994. Even greater increases occurred among Mexican-American and non-Hispanic black children (Ogden et al., 2002). Given the dramatic increase in the prevalence of obesity, the pediatric care community needs to attain effective skills and experience in addressing this growing public health problem. This chapter focuses on the approach to identifying the obese child and subsequent interventions to prevent or treat obesity.

ASSESSING THE OBESE CHILD

The assessment and subsequent intervention for an obese child must be comprehensive and multidisciplinary. The assessment should focus on the following issues: anthropometric assessment, dietary intake, the child's environment, medical issues, and psychosocial issues.

Anthropometric Assessment

Obesity refers to excess body fat. Real body composition assessment by means of accurate body composition assessment methods, such as underwater weighing or dual energy X-ray absorptiometry, are not easily accessible for practicing physicians, nor are they practical for widespread use as a screening instrument. Therefore, other methods, which estimate or act as a proxy measure for adiposity, are used.

The regular National Center for Health Statistics (NCHS) growth curves can be utilized to determine a child's age- and sex-specific weight and height percentiles. One of the most commonly used measures to assess relative weight is the body mass index [BMI = weight (kg)/height (m²)]. In adults, a BMI above 25 defines overweight, and above 30 defines obesity. In addition, the First Federal Obesity Clinical Guidelines also use the waist measurement along with the BMI to set priorities for clinical intervention in adults (National Heart, Lung and Blood Institute [NHLBI], 1998). Unfortunately, these guidelines cannot be applied to children, as BMI changes with age in children. Therefore, we are not able to set a particular BMI cut point to define obesity in children. The new NCHS growth charts (available at the Centers for Disease and Prevention [CDC] Web site) include sex-specific age vs. BMI charts, which allow assessment of BMI percentile. According to the guidelines provided with the growth charts, a child with a BMI between the 85th and 95th percentile is at risk for being overweight, while those at or above the 95th percentile are overweight. Although the adult guidelines differentiate between obese and overweight, no such differential is made for children. Also, it must be emphasized that BMI is a screening instrument, which requires further confirmation.

The ultimate question is whether the child has excess adipose tissue. Skinfold thickness measurements do specifically provide some measure of adiposity, however, these measurements are difficult to complete accurately, especially with very obese individuals. In fact, the skinfolds of very obese individuals may be too big to measure with existing calipers. In general, a triceps skinfold thickness >85th percentile is considered overweight, and >95th percentile indicates obesity. Equations have been developed that estimate body composition based on skinfold thickness measurements (Slaughter et al., 1988; Zemel et al., 1997). If they are to be used, however, it is important to make sure that the specific equation has been validated for use with the age, sex, and ethnic group of interest.

Assessing Dietary Intake

Obesity is caused by an energy imbalance, in which the individual expends less energy than he or she takes in. A chronic, small energy imbalance can have a profound effect on weight gain. For example, a 100 kcal/day positive energy balance would induce a weight gain of approximately 10 pounds per year, or

100 pounds over 10 years. The fact that such a small chronic difference in energy balance can have such a dramatic effect on body weight makes therapeutic attempts at treating obesity frustratingly difficult.

Data suggest that obese children tend to eat higher-fat diets (Maffeis et al., 1996). The higher caloric density of fat and of high-fat food may support a higher caloric intake. The body also expends less energy metabolizing and storing fat. Recent information also suggests that humans have a preference for high-caloric density foods (Rolls et al., 1999). It is postulated that as humans evolved in an environment where food was relatively scarce, a preference for high-caloric density foods created a survival advantage. In our current environment, where most people have easy access to an abundance of high-caloric density foods, this preference for high-density foods may be supporting the increasing prevalence of obesity.

Misinterpretation of the public health efforts to lower the fat intake of the American diet may also have contributed to the problem of obesity. One byproduct of this campaign has been the adoption by many people of the attitude that since high-fat foods are "bad" for you, low-fat foods must be good for you. This attitude may be appropriate for foods of high nutrient density, such as low-fat milk and meats, but not for low nutrient density foods, such as cookies and cakes. Thus, following such a broad-based low-fat diet, including high-calorie, low-fat products, may actually increase caloric intake. However, following a low-fat, low-caloric density diet does seem to have utility in weight management. A survey of obese adults who were successful at maintaining an average of 13.6 kg of weight loss for at least 1 year demonstrated that these persons almost universally followed a low-fat diet (Shick et al., 1998).

Recently there has been interest in and promotion of lower-carbohydrate diets. It is proposed that eating a diet high in high-glycemic index foods induces a high insulin response, which sets off a cascade that promotes excessive food intake. The data supporting this theory are very limited, especially relating to children (Ludwig et al., 1999). Clearly, this approach needs to be studied before it is implemented in children, especially given the described long-term success with weight loss and maintenance described above with a low-fat and low-caloric density diet.

Assessment of the caloric intake and caloric needs of children and adolescents and of the impact of caloric intake on excessive weight gain is difficult. Surveys suggest that obese adolescents may underreport caloric intake by 40% to 60% (Bandini et al., 1990). Thus, diet recalls or other methods to assess the caloric intake of obese individuals must be taken with a grain of salt. Furthermore, standardized resting energy expenditure prediction equations, which calculate energy requirements of obese children, tend to overestimate the true caloric needs of obese children and adolescents (Maffeis et al., 1993). Actually measuring resting energy expenditure may help provide the individual with more useful nutritional advice.

There is increasing evidence that parenting style can also influence dietary behavior. The best predictor of children's ability to regulate their own caloric intake is parental control during meals. For example, children whose mother imposed more control on them during meals (through statements like "clean off your plate" or "just take another bite") were less able to appropriately self-control their caloric intake (Johnson and Birch, 1994). It has been suggested that when external control is imposed on children during meals, they lose the natural ability to control their own intake. These children are then at risk for eating inappropriately in response to external cues, having lost their natural internal control mechanisms. Thus the child's food environment and control associated with feeding should be assessed.

Assessing the Environment

Several environmental factors have been associated with a greater risk of obesity in children, including socioeconomic factors, parental education, and family size. A large national survey of 6- to 11-year-old children showed that rates of obesity were higher in the fall and winter, in metropolitan areas, and in the North east and Midwest United States (Dietz and Gortmaker, 1984). These results suggest that the regions and seasons that allow and support more outdoor activities are also associated with less obesity; children playing outdoors are more active than children playing indoors.

Television, computers, and video games have profoundly changed the environment of children. Television watching is associated with less physical activity, even in children as young as 3 to 4 years of age (DuRant et al., 1994). A relation between television watching and obesity has been clearly described in older children, including a clear dose response (Dietz and Gortmaker, 1985; Gortmaker et al., 1996; Andersen et al., 1998). For example, 10- to 15-year-old children were 5.5 times as likely to be overweight if they watched more than 5 hours of television per day, compared to those who watched less than 2 hours per day. Although excessive use of computers and video games has not been extensively studied, a similar effect is likely.

In addition to TV watching, other factors also seem to play a role in decreased physical activity. Children who watch more television ask their parents more frequently to buy food. The mothers of children who watch more television subsequently buy their children the requested foods more frequently (Taras et al., 1989). This pattern suggests that the food-oriented advertising aimed at children encourages them to ask their parents for the advertised foods. In turn, the more the children ask for these foods, the more the parents buy the foods. Thus television watching seems to alter the behavior of both children and parents.

In assessment of the obese child, an evaluation of the child's environment should also be included, such as the child's schedule, after-school care, hobbies, opportunities for spontaneous play (e.g., playing outside with friends) and/or organized activities, and concerns about safety in the neighborhood. It is also important to note the schedule and setting for eating, the person(s) who supervises food and eating, and the child's sedentary activities (including television and videos, video games, computer time, and telephone use).

■ Assessing the Health Consequences of Obesity

Obesity in adults is associated with an increased risk for mortality, coronary heart disease, hypertension, lipid disorders, type 2 diabetes, orthopedic problems, stroke, gall bladder disease, sleep apnea, and some cancers (Lee et al., 1993; Giovannucci et al., 1995; Manson et al., 1995; NHLBI, 1998). Medical problems associated with obesity usually occur in adults, but they can also develop or begin to develop in obese children (Gidding et al., 1996). Although acute medical problems that require immediate intervention are rare in obese children, the practitioner should screen all obese children for these acute issues and consider implementing interventions that have potential for long-term prevention.

Assessment of an obese child should include a routine history and physical examination. Certain syndromes (e.g., Prader-Willi syndrome) are associated with an increased rate of obesity. However, identifiable syndromes associated with obesity are very rare. For example, the genetic and other syndromes associated with childhood obesity listed in Table 13.1 represent less than 1% of the cases of obesity in children (Dietz and Robinson, 1993). As part of the assessment of an obese child, the signs of such conditions should nonetheless be reviewed. Practitioners should also be familiar with the secondary medical problems associated with obesity (Table 13.2).

TABLE 13.1
Conditions associated with childhood obesity

Endocrine Causes

Cushing syndrome
Hypothyroidism
Hyperinsulinemia
Growth hormone deficiency
Hypothalamic dysfunction
Prader-Willi syndrome
Stein-Leventhal syndrome (polycystic ovary)
Pseudohypoparathyroidism type I

Genetic Syndromes

Turner syndrome
Laurence-Moon Biedl syndrome
Alstrom-Hallgren syndrome

Other Syndromes

Cohen syndrome
Carpenter syndrome

Source: Adapted from Dietz and Robinson (1993) and Curran and Barness (2000).

TABLE 13.2
Assessment of medical conditions related to obesity and its treatment

Findings	Potential Conditions
History	
Developmental delay	Genetic
Poor linear growth	Hypothyroidism, Cushing syndrome, Prader-Willi syndrome, genetic disorder
Headaches	Pseudotumor cerebri
Nighttime breathing difficulty	Sleep apnea, obesity hypoventilation syndrome
Daytime somnolence	Sleep apnea, obesity hypoventilation syndrome
Abdominal pain	Gall bladder disease
Hip or knee pain	Slipped capital femoral epiphysis
Oligomenorrhea or amenorrhea	Polycystic ovary syndrome
Excessive urination	Type 2 diabetes
Family History	
Obesity	
Type 2 diabetes	
Cardiovascular disease	
Hypertension	
Dyslipidemia	
Gall bladder disease	
Social and Psychologic History	
Tobacco, alcohol, drug use	
Depression	
Eating disorder	
Social isolation, depression	Lowered self-esteem
Increased family conflicts	
School performance	
Physical Examination	
Height, weight, and body mass index	Short height–hypothyroidism, Prader-Willi syndrome, genetic disorder
Excessive and rapid weight loss, arrhythmia, muscle spasm	Inadequate nutrition, provision of imbalanced diet
Blood pressure	Risk of cardiovascular disease; Cushing syndrome
Dysmorphic features	Genetic disorders, including Prader-Willi syndrome
Acanthosis nigricans	Insulin resistance, type 2 diabetes
Hirsutism	Polycystic ovary syndrome; Cushing syndrome
Violaceous striae	Cushing syndrome
Optic disks	Pseudomotor cerebri
Tonsils	Sleep apnea
Abdominal pain, vomiting	Gall bladder disease
Hepatomegaly	Steatohepatitis
Undescended testicle	Prader-Willi syndrome
Limited hip range of motion	Slipped capital femoral epiphysis
Lower leg bowing	Blount disease

Source: Adapted from Barlow and Dietz (1998).

Family history of cardiovascular disease has been used to identify children at risk for premature heart disease. Given the clustering of obesity within families it would seem appropriate to use a similar strategy with obesity and related comorbidities and to institute anticipatory health promotion efforts for children of obese or overweight parents. This may be especially important for children with a positive family history of type 2 diabetes.

The specific signs and symptoms associated with obesity or the treatment of obesity are listed in Table 13.2. All of these should be considered when assessing an obese child. Further assessment should be dependent on specific physical findings or history (e.g., large tonsils and loud, irregular snoring potentially suggestive of sleep apnea; poor growth, potentially associated with a syndrome or endocrinologic issues). In addition, screening for dyslipidemia and insulin resistance should be considered. Because of the association between dyslipidemia and obesity, the clustering of cardiovascular (CVD) risk factors in obese individuals, and the relatively poor predictive value of family history to predict child hyperlipidemia, lipid profile screening should be considered as part of the initial evaluation of the obese child. Similarly, fasting glucose and insulin level or formal glucose tolerance testing should be considered for those with acanthosis nigricans, the significantly obese, those with a positive family history of type 2 diabetes, or for certain ethnic groups (such as African-Americans) (American Diabetes Association, 2000). Families will commonly state that their child's obesity is related to endocrinologic causes, but thyroid function testing or other screening without specific indications has a very low yield.

Measurement of resting metabolic rate should be considered. Because the resting energy expenditure prediction equations are relatively inaccurate for obese children and adolescents, actual measurement will enable more appropriate dietary counseling. This method is especially important in assessment of obesity because of inaccuracies in diet recall. In addition, many families feel their child's obesity is linked to a low metabolic rate, thus lifestyle intervention is futile. Concrete assessment of metabolic rate allows a factual discussion of this possibility.

Assessing Cardiovascular Disease Risk Factors

Obesity, abdominal fat, and visceral fat have been shown to be associated with CVD risk factors, including dyslipidemia, increased blood pressure, and hyperinsulinemia, in children and adults (Freedman et al., 1987, 1989; Landin et al., 1989; Boyko et al., 1996; Caprio et al., 1996; Daniels et al., 1998). Most commonly, obesity is associated with elevations in triglyceride level and decreases in high-density lipoprotein cholesterol (HDL-C). Even relatively small changes in weight in adults (10% of body weight) have been associated with improvement in CVD risk factors (Van Gaal et al., 1997; Wadden et al., 1999). Although the data are more limited for children, it appears that changes in overweight status have similar effects on CVD risk in children (Epstein et al., 1989).

In addition, the list of CVD risk factors associated with obesity includes such things as low anti-oxidant intake or status, small low-density lipoprotein cholesterol (LDL-C) size, altered hemostatic and fibrinolytic factors, and altered sympathetic nervous system tone (Sowers et al., 1982; Ohrvall et al., 1993; Ferguson et al., 1998). Weight loss has been associated with short term improvement in many of these factors, such as blood pressure, lipoprotein profile, hemostatic activity, norepinephrine level, total body fat, and visceral abdominal fat (Reisin et al., 1983; Becque et al., 1988; Rocchini et al., 1988, 1992; Torigoe et al., 1997). The degree of weight loss needed to induce significant change in these factors has not yet been defined.

Assessing Type 2 Diabetes Mellitus

Although type 2 diabetes used to be a relatively rare problem in children, it is now becoming more common (see Chapter 15). This trend forecasts an epidemic of adults developing obesity and diabetes-related comorbidities. In addition, experience with diabetic adults suggests that weight management and/or weight maintenance after weight loss may be more difficult for persons with type 2 diabetes. Thus preventive and therapeutic efforts to manage obesity and type 2 diabetes need to begin in childhood.

Assessing Other Medical Factors

Other factors that may be primarily or secondarily related to obesity are listed in Table 13.2. As previously noted, assessment for these factors should be guided by the history and physical examination findings. In addition to the well-publicized factors known for some time to be associated with obesity, other factors, such as the association between abnormal liver function tests, nonalcoholic steatohepatitis, and obesity, have also been described (Moran et al., 1983). Preliminary information indicates that liver function test abnormalities may respond to treatment with vitamin E, suggesting a potential oxidant or anti-oxidant role in the process. Adults with obesity-related steatohepatitis have developed cirrhosis and in some instances have gone on to develop liver failure and undergo liver transplant.

Assessing Psychological Factors

Although overweight and obese children and adolescents do not have greater levels of psychological problems than their non-obese counterparts, it is important to screen for psychosocial and psychiatric disorders. If left untreated, such disorders may impede weight loss progress. History taking will often identify the most common undiagnosed difficulties.

The most common psychological problem is depression, with symptoms of low energy, poor self-esteem, irritability, and difficulty in concentration;

overeating and sleeping too much may be present as well. The Child Depression Inventory (Kovacs, 1992) is a self-administered questionnaire that has been validated for use with children and adolescents to screen for depression. Although overweight children are not more prone to suffer from depression, they are vulnerable to disparagement about their body. It is thus important for all staff to be sensitive to the needs of the overweight patient.

Other types of difficulties to screen for include anxiety, sleep problems, drug or alcohol problems, academic or learning problems, conduct disorder, and oppositional disorder. If left untreated, these disorders may impair the child's ability to lose weight. This effect has not been confirmed, however, because these populations have not been well studied in terms of response to weight loss treatment. With the new age of pharmacologic interventions, patients with seizure disorders and major psychiatric syndromes (schizophrenia, bipolar disorder, and pervasive developmental disorders) are often treated with new antiseizure and antipsychotic medications that frequently have a side effect of weight gain. Thus close collaboration with a neurologist or psychiatrist is required to develop a weight management program adapted to the special needs of these patients.

Significant life-stressors, elicited on review of the family history, can determine the timing of weight management treatment. A significant loss or death in the family, for example, may cause serious distress for the child or adolescent, such that other forms of counseling may be needed prior to attempting weight loss counseling. Major family problems or parental psychopathology also need to be recognized and may often impact efforts at treatment. Appropriate guidance and referral of the parent to other resources will be a major support for the child. For example, if a parent has a major problem with alcohol or depression, this will have enormous consequences on family life. Helping the parent to obtain treatment will often have a positive impact on the child.

Although it is unusual to observe anorexia nervosa or bulimia nervosa among obese adolescents, screening for these disorders is important prior to initiating weight loss attempts. Any history of vomiting or purging (use of laxatives or emetics) or exercising to extremes in order to lose weight is a sign for further psychological evaluation.

Binge eating disorder (BED) is a relatively newly defined eating problem that can have features similar to bulimia nervosa, except there is no history of vomiting or other forms of purging. BED is characterized by overeating while feeling a sense of being out of control with one's eating. In this disorder, binge eating occurs on at least 2 days a week for at least 6 months. BED is associated with distress and depression and has been reported to occur in up to 30% of obese adolescents seeking treatment (Berkowitz et al., 1993). In addition to standard weight loss treatment, cognitive behavioral therapy may be helpful for this disorder.

The presence of serious psychiatric or psychosocial difficulties may require a delay in weight loss treatment while other, more pressing needs are addressed. In these circumstances it is important to encourage children and their families to return for treatment at a more stable time.

■ RECOMMENDATIONS FOR ASSESSMENT AND GOALS OF THERAPY

The Expert Panel on Clinical Guidelines for Overweight in Adolescent Preventive Services was convened as an advisory group to two national health initiatives (Himes and Dietz, 1994); a summary of their recommendations is provided in Table 13.3. In 1997, the Maternal and Child Health Bureau convened the Expert Committee on Obesity Evaluation and Treatment (Barlow and Dietz, 1998), which largely confirmed the previous recommendations listed in Table 13.3, with the following exception: the 1997 committee defined a rapid increase in BMI as an increase of 3 to 4 kg/m² in 1 year. In addition, the 1997 panel developed guidelines for medical, family, and psychosocial screening and physical examinations (Table 13.4), including a listing of medical conditions associated with obesity (Table 13.2). The 1997 panel suggested the following indications for referral to a pediatric obesity treatment specialist: pseudotumor cerebri, sleep apnea, obesity hypoventilation

TABLE 13.3
Diagnostic tests to consider in assessment of overweight children and adolescents

Guidelines for Preventive Adolescent Services

Use body mass index (BMI) to define overweight.

BMI ≥95th percentile or BMI >30 kg/m² defines overweight adolescents who should receive an in-depth medical assessment.

Adolescents with a BMI between the 85th and 95th percentiles or >30 kg/m² should be referred to second-level screening.

Second-level Screening

Review family history of cardiovascular disease or diabetes mellitus and parental history of hypercholesterolemia or obesity.

Blood pressure assessment

Total cholesterol screening (elevated ≥200 mg/dL [5.2 mmol/L])

Assess recent weight changes, and determine if there has been a rapid increase in weight (BMI increase in last year ≥2 kg/m²).

Assess adolescent's concern about current weight status or emotional or psychological manifestations thought to be related to overweight or perceptions of overweight.

Adolescents with positive second-level screening should complete an in-depth medical assessment.

Suggestions for in-depth medical assessments:
  Physical examination, including assessment of sexual maturation
  Anthropometry to assess triceps and subscapular skinfolds
  Lipoprotein fractions (total cholesterol, HDL-C, triglyceride, and calculated LDL-C)

Source: Adapted from Himes and Dietz (1994).

TABLE 13.4
Goals of therapy for overweight children and adolescents

Behavior

Develop awareness of current eating habits, activity, and parenting behavior

Identify problem behaviors

Modify current behavior

Continue to be aware of behavior and recognize changes that occur as child grows, gains independence, etc.

Medical

Improvement or resolution of secondary complications of obesity

Weight

Weight *maintenance* is the goal in the following situations:
    2- to 7-year-old children
        BMI 85th to 95th percentile
        BMI ≥95th percentile without complications of obesity
    >7-year-old children
        BMI 85th to 95th percentile without complications of obesity
Weight *loss* is the goal in the following situations:
    2- to 7-year-old children
        BMI ≥95th percentile with complications of obesity
    >7-year-old children
        BMI 85th to 95th percentile with complications of obesity
        BMI ≥95th percentile

Source: Adapted from Barlow and Dietz (1998).

syndrome, orthopedic problems, massive overweight in children or adolescents, and severe overweight in children less than 2 years of age.

    The Expert Panel (1994) recommended that the child and family's readiness to make changes be assessed. Families of young children may be able to make changes in diet and physical activity by altering the child's environment, without direct cooperation of the child. However, attempts to impose changes when the older child or adolescent is resistant or not interested or when the family is not willing or able to be supportive will probably be futile. In this environment, such attempts may create family problems, discourage future attempts at weight control, and damage the child's self-esteem. Similarly, a psychosocial screen of the family is useful to identify issues that may impede initiation of a behavior modification program. Significant psychological problems and eating disorders in particular may need to be addressed initially and adequately before weight management is instituted. Many parents of obese children have difficulties with setting limits and with parenting skills. These issues should be assessed prior to initiating therapy.

The 1997 committee also defined the goals of therapy (Table 13.4). The committee recommended that therapy be started early, that the child and family be informed of the medical complications of obesity, that all caregivers in the program be included, and that small, gradual, but long-term changes be made. The chronicity of the risk of obesity needs to be emphasized to all families. Practice of a healthy lifestyle is a lifelong issue for the obese child.

■ TREATMENT

In planning treatment of the obese child, it is important to complete the assessment and then prioritize the intervention. Significant medical issues, such as sleep apnea, significant hypertension, or slipped capital femoral epiphysis, require immediate intervention. Other issues, such as hyperlipidemia or Blount's disease, may require further assessment and intervention, but in a less urgent manner. Although it is important to address the comorbidities associated with obesity, it is even more important to remember that obesity is the primary process. The success of treatment for these comorbidities will likely be compromised if the primary process (e.g., obesity) is not addressed.

It is also important to establish realistic goals for weight management. Relatively small changes in weight (5% to 10%) may significantly improve health risk factors (Goldstein, 1992). The weight loss goals of the child and family may nonetheless be significantly greater. Experience with overweight adults suggests that the goals of persons in weight loss programs are frequently unrealistic (Foster et al., 1997, 2001).

■ Behavior Modification

An integral part of behavior modification is the inclusion of parents in the intervention. Behavioral approaches developed from notions that behaviors are learned or conditioned and that the social environment reinforces the development and maintenance of normal and abnormal behaviors. Thus, the focus of behavior modification is to develop new learning and new habits, in part to help people learn to cope with a "toxic environment" (Brownell, 2002) filled with high-fat, energy-dense foods and a sedentary lifestyle. The following is a brief description of the components of behavior modification procedures used for weight management programs for both children and adults, developed by a number of investigators (Epstein et al., 1980, 1988, 1990; Wadden et al., 1990) over the last few decades.

Behavioral programs for children and adolescents include the following topics: (1) understanding the causes of obesity; (2) the need for healthy nutrition (low-fat, nutritionally balanced eating plan); (3) use of a menu plan based on the Food Guide Pyramid; (4) the need for self-monitoring of calories and physical activity (daily diaries); (5) stimulus-control procedures; (6) coping with high-risk social or psychological situations that trigger excess eating; (7) increasing physical activity; and (8) minimizing inactivity (such as TV watching or computer use). Adolescents are required to turn in their food-intake and exercise records (daily diaries) and take mini-tests each session. Adolescents and parents receive manuals with lessons and homework assignments for each meeting. Parents are taught how to assist their children and reinforce new habits, more directly so for younger children. Children and adolescents usually have group meetings separate from their parents, who join other parents in a behavioral group meeting that occurs at the same time. Some of the essential features of a behavioral approach are discussed below.

Self-monitoring

Self-monitoring and, for younger children, monitoring by parents of eating and activity behaviors provide direct feedback about these behaviors. This in turn enables goal setting and habit change. During the first week, an overview of topics such as thinking positively about weight control, healthy eating behavior, exercise, and the use of food records (self-monitoring) is given. Starting at week 1, for example, adolescents begin recording their food intake in their diaries and turn these in before the group meetings. The group leader reviews the diaries and writes a brief note of encouragement, with possible solutions for any problems noted. The entire group discusses what they have learned from their diaries and participants begin to learn to modify their behavior. Children and teens are taught to measure their foods so that they can more accurately assess quantities and the caloric content of commonly eaten foods. They quickly come to realize that large portions of high-fat foods are associated with excess calories and that moderate sized, low-fat portions are associated with weight loss.

Physical Activity

Increasing participants' physical activity level is also a primary goal of the behavioral program, through focus on increasing lifestyle activities. Often the goal is an additional 30 minutes or more of walking (or other moderate activity) four or more times a week. Participants record their physical activity in their daily diaries. All subjects are encouraged to reduce the amount of time they spend watching TV, using home computers, and taking part in other sedentary behaviors.

Stimulus Control

Children and parents are encouraged to limit the number of places where they eat and thus minimize the conditioning of eating while doing other activities. They are instructed to eat only in the kitchen or dining room when at home. Further efforts at stimulus control include limiting the types of activities in which the adolescents engage while eating (such as TV watching). Families are encouraged to store foods out of site and to minimize the amount of junk foods (soda, candy, and sweets in general) in the home. Adolescents are instructed in methods of slowing their eating and to leave a small amount of food on their plate.

High-Risk Situations

Children and adolescents also get help in coping with "high-risk" eating situations, such as convenience stores, school lunchrooms, and fast-food restaurants. They are encouraged to plan ahead for parties where there may be many high-fat foods and treats so they can socialize but adhere to their nutritional program. They are also instructed in the benefits of positive self-talk, even in the face of a lapse. They are taught cognitive restructuring to cope with automatic negative thoughts about themselves.

Long-term weight management is the topic of meetings later in the program, which focus on weight loss maintenance. Children and adolescents are encouraged to set goals, focus on continuing the new health habits they have developed, and obtain continued support from family and friends.

Parents' Program

The parents' group sessions cover the same topics, at the same weeks, as those reviewed in the children's meeting. Parents are encouraged to support and reinforce their children's habit changes and to model healthy eating and activity habits themselves. Parents are instructed to assist their children in four principal ways:

1. Limit the number of high-fat, high-sugar foods that parents bring into the home. By purchasing less high-fat foods at the grocery store, they facilitate their child's adherence to a healthy diet.
2. Model the eating and activity habits that their child is to adopt. This includes eating slowly, storing foods out of sight, increasing physical activity (and decreasing sedentary activity), and reducing consumption of high-fat and high—sugar content foods. Parents who are overweight are encouraged to reduce their weight (if they have no medical contraindications to weight loss, as determined by their family physician). In doing so, parents will increase the likelihood of their modeling appropriate behaviors.
3. Support their child in making appropriate lifestyle changes. This includes on-the-spot verbal reinforcement (e.g., "It's great to see you going out to play basketball") and contracting (developing an agreement between the parent(s) and child in which goals are set and rewards earned by meeting goals).
4. Learn communication skills to use with their children, such as praising them generously for appropriate behavior change, and not criticizing them when

they engage in undesired behaviors (e.g., eating a high-fat snack). Parents are encouraged during weekly meetings to discuss any concerns about their child's eating and exercise habits.

■ Nutritional Management

Epstein and colleagues (1980, 1990) have conducted the most comprehensive and well-documented long-term weight management programs for children. In their program, 8- to 12-year-old children were enrolled in group therapy in which diet, exercise, and behavior management information was provided. In general, dietary modification in weight management programs includes easy-to-follow dietary programs (Haddock et al., 1994). The traffic light diet used by Epstein and Squires (1988) is an example of such a program. Foods are designated as green-, yellow-, or red-light foods, based on their caloric density. Children are given guidelines on caloric intake and limits on the number of red-light foods they are allowed to eat per week. An accompanying behavioral modification program encourages compliance with all aspects of the program via contracting and self-monitoring. The goal of this nutrition intervention is to provide an easy method of identifying and limiting the intake of calorically dense foods. In general, this program also results in participants eating a lower-fat diet.

In a meta-analysis of treatment for child and adolescent obesity, the utility of different components of the programs was evaluated (Haddock et al., 1994). The researchers demonstrated that programs that were comprehensive in nature (e.g., included behavior modification procedures, dietary change, and exercise) produced better results, and that inclusion of behavior modification techniques in particular was important. In this analysis, the components of the dietary modification were separately evaluated. Surprisingly, programs that included the recommended components of dietary modification (diet easily understood by the child, caloric intake tailored to the child's needs, diet focused on decreasing fat and caloric intake, dietary component supervised by a dietary expert) were less or no more effective than programs without these components. In addition, the efficacy of parental involvement was not confirmed in this analysis. The reasons for the lack of improved outcome when the programs included recommended dietary components or parental participation are unknown and should be studied more fully, particularly since the previously described results support the importance of parental involvement.

A protein-modified fast has also been used to induce a relatively rapid weight loss in severely obese individuals. Although the experience is relatively limited in children, one study involving 12 obese adolescents who followed a diet providing 880 kcal/day and 2.5 g protein per kg ideal body weight has been reported. These participants decreased their percent overweight from 54% to 25% over 3 months and were able to maintain their relative weight over the next 9 months (Stallings et al., 1998). Such programs must be carried out with careful supervision to ensure that participants are eating a complete and appropriately balanced diet and to monitor for possible complications. For example, persons undergoing such rapid weight loss may be at risk for cholelithiasis (Thomas, 1995). Although it seems that immediate weight loss can be induced with such programs, anecdotal reports of poor long-term weight maintenance after the transition to a regular diet are common.

Recently much interest has been expressed in the use of low-carbohydrate diets for weight management. High-glycemic index diets are thought to promote overeating and increased weight gain and to worsen blood lipid levels (Morris and Zemel, 1999; Ludwig et al., 1999). This finding is consistent with the recently described association between consumption of sugar-sweetened drinks and obesity and excess weight gain in children (Ludwig et al., 2001). Preliminary data also suggest that a ketogenic diet or a low glycemic index can induce greater weight loss over 3 to 4 months for obese adolescents (Spieth et al., 2000; Sondike et al., 2003). However, the longer-term efficacy and safety of such diets have not been studied in children or adults.

■ Drug Therapy for Obesity

Experience with drug therapy to help induce weight loss is limited in children and adolescents. In adults it has been demonstrated that drug therapy is significantly more effective when used with an active lifestyle modification program (Wadden et al., 2001). Thus drug therapy should not be looked upon as a simple cure all, but only as a potential adjunct to an active weight management program. In addition, because subjects treated with weight loss medications regain most of the lost weight when the medication is stopped, the long-term effect of drug therapy for a growing child or adolescent must be considered. In general, the unexpected cardiac valvulopathy thought to be associated with the use of fenfluramine and phentermine (Jick et al., 1998; Khan et al., 1998; Wadden et al., 1998; Weissman et al., 1998; Seghatol and Rigolin, 2002) has made practitioners especially cautious in using medications for weight loss. Thus, a careful risk–benefit analysis by a clinician expert in weight management drug therapy should be undertaken before considering drug therapy for obese children or adolescents.

Of the two most recently introduced weight loss medications, sibutramine and orlistat, sibutramine has been approved for use in adolescents 16 years of age and older. These two medications work through very different mechanisms. Sibutramine works centrally as a norepinephrine, serotonin, and dopamine reuptake inhibitor. Obese adolescents receiving sibutramine and participating in a group behavior weight control program in a randomized, double-blinded, placebo-controlled trial reduced their BMI 8.5% over 6 months, compared to a 4.0% BMI reduction in the placebo-behavior weight control group. The most common side effects were changes in pulse or blood pressure (Berkowitz et al., 2003).

Orlistat works as a reversible inhibitor of gastric and pancreatic lipases, inducing fat malabsorption. In a 3-month open label trial, severely obese adolescents (mean BMI 44.1) participating in a multidisciplinary weight loss program, lost 3.8% of initial weight. Gastrointestinal side effects were the most common adverse events (McDuffie et al., 2002).

■ Reimbursement for Pediatric Weight Management Services

Many insurance companies will not cover pediatric weight management services (Tershakovec et al., 1999). Even in instances where the child has an obesity-associated comorbidity, it is common for treatment of the secondary problem to be covered, but not the primary problem (obesity). Although efforts are still needed to improve outcome with weight management, long-term moderate success in the treatment of childhood obesity has been demonstrated (Epstein et al., 1990). Medical care providers should actively lobby insurance companies to cover these important prevention and therapeutic programs.

■ SUMMARY

- The prevalence of overweight is rising rapidly in children and adolescents. The increases are especially rapid in certain ethnic groups, such as Mexican-Americans and African-Americans.
- Obesity-related health consequences, such as high blood pressure and type 2 diabetes, are becoming more common in children and adolescents.
- The etiology of obesity in children is multifactorial. A comprehensive evaluation, including an assessment of the obese child's family medical and psychosocial history, home and school environment, dietary intake, and physical and leisure activities, should be undertaken. The medical assessment should include appropriate psychosocial and medical screening.
- Weight management should be multifactorial and include components to support behavior modification, dietary change, and increased physical activity. Intervention should also take into account the child's and family's environment and their personal commitment to and resources for changing behavior.
- Many special diets or weight loss regimens have not been adequately tested for safety and efficacy. Without supporting information, such interventions should not be used in children and adolescents. Very aggressive weight loss interventions should only be considered in special circumstances where the risk outweighs the benefit and other less invasive interventions have failed.

■ REFERENCES

American Diabetes Association. 2000. Type 2 Diabetes in Children and Adolescents. *Pediatrics* 105:671–80.

Andersen, R.E., C.J. Crespo, S.J. Bartlett, L.J. Cheskin, and M. Pratt. 1998. Relationship of Physical Activity and Television Watching with Body Weight and Level of Fatness among Children. *JAMA* 279:938–42.

Bandini, L.G., D.A. Schoeller, H.N. Cyr, and W.H. Dietz. 1990. Validity of Reported Energy Intake in Obese and Nonobese Adolescents. *Am J Clin Nutr* 52:421–5.

Barlow, S.E., and W.H. Dietz. 1998. Obesity Evaluation and Treatment: Expert Committee Recommendations. *Pediatrics* 102:E29.

Becque, M.D., V.L. Katch, A.P. Rocchini, C.R. Marks, and C. Moorehead. 1988. Coronary Risk Incidence of Obese Adolescents: Reduction by Exercise Plus Diet Intervention. *Pediatrics* 81:605–12.

Berkowitz, R., A.J. Stunkard, and V.A. Stalings. 1993. Binge-Eating Disorder in Obese Adolescent Girls. *Ann N Y Acad Sci* 699:200–6.

Berkowitz, R.I., T.A. Wadden, A.M. Tershakovec, and J. Cronquist. 2003. Behavior Therapy and Sibutramine for the Treatment of Adolescent Obesity: A Randomized, Placebo Controlled Trial. *JAMA* 289(14):1805–12.

Boyko, E.J., D.L. Leonetti, R.W. Bergstrom, L. Newell-Morris, and W.Y. Fujimoto. 1996. Visceral Adiposity, Fasting Plasma Insulin, and Lipid and Lipoprotein Levels in Japanese Americans. *Int J Obes* 20:801–8

Brownell, K.D. 2002. The Environment and Obesity. In: *Eating Disorders and Obesity*, 2nd ed. Edited by C.G. Fairburn and K.D. Brownell. New York & London: Guilford Press, pp. 433–8.

Caprio, S., L.D. Hyman, S. McCarthy, R. Lange, M. Bronson, and W.V. Tamborlane. 1996. Fat Distribution and Cardiovascular Risk Factors in Obese Adolescent Girls: Importance of the Intraabdominal Fat Depot. *Am J Clin Nutr* 64:12–7.

Centers for Disease Control and Prevention. Clinical Growth Charts. Available at: HYPERLINK http://www.cdc.gov/nchs/about/major/nhanes/growthcharts/clinical_charts .htm —www.cdc.gov/nchs/about/major/nhanes/growthcharts/clinical_charts.htm

Curran, J.S., and L.A. Barness. 2000. Obesity. In: *Textbook of Pediatrics*, 16th ed. Edited by R.E. Behrman, R.M. Kliegman, and H.B. Jenson. Philadelphia: W.B. Saunders, pp. 172–6.

Daniels, S.R., J.A. Morrison, D.L. Sprecher, P.R. Khoury, and T.R. Kimball. 1998. Association of Body Fat Distribution and Cardiovascular Risk Factors in Children and Adolescents. *Pediatr Res* 43:90A.

Dietz, W.H., and S.L. Gortmaker. 1984. Factors within the Physical Environment Associated with Childhood Obesity. *Am J Clin Nutr* 39:619–24.

Dietz, W.H., and S.L. Gortmaker. 1985. Do We Fatten Our Children at the Television Set? Obesity and Television Viewing in Children and Adolescents. *Pediatrics* 75:807–12.

Dietz, W.H., and T.N. Robinson. 1993. Assessment and Treatment of Childhood Obesity. *Pediatr Rev* 14:337–44.

DuRant, R.H., T. Baranowski, M. Johnson, and W.O. Thompson. 1994. The Relationship among Television Watching, Physical Activity, and Body Composition of Young Children. *Pediatrics* 94:449–55.

Epstein, L.H., L.H. Kuller, R.R. Wing, A. Valoski, and J. McCurley. 1989. The Effect of Weight Control on Lipid Changes in Obese Children. *Am J Dis Child* 143:454–7.

Epstein, L.H., and S. Squires. 1988. *The Stoplight Diet for Children: An Eight-Week Program for Parents and Children*. Boston: Little, Brown.

Epstein, L.H., A. Valoski, R.R. Wing, and T.A. McCurley. 1990. Ten-Year Follow-up of Behavioral, Family-Based Treatment for Obese Children. *JAMA* 264:2519–23.

Epstein, L.H., R.R. Wing, L. Steranchak, B. Dickson, and J. Michelson. 1980. Comparison of Family-Based Behavior Modification and Nutrition Education for Childhood Obesity. *J Pediatr Psychol* 5:25–36.

Ferguson, M.A., B. Gutin, S. Owens, M. Litaker, R.P. Tracy, and J. Allison. 1998. Fat Distribution and Hemostatic Measures in Obese Children. *Am J Clin Nutr* 67:1136–40.

Foster, G.D., T.A. Wadden, S. Phelan, D.B. Sarwer, and R.S. Sanderson. 2001. Obese Patients' Perceptions of Treatment Outcomes and the Factors that Influence Them. *Arch Intern Med* 161:2133–9.

Foster, G.D., T.A. Wadden, R.A. Vogt, and G. Brewer. 1997. What is a Reasonable Weight Loss? Patients' Expectations and Evaluations of Obesity Treatment Outcomes. *J Consult Clin Psychol* 65:79–85.

Freedman, D.S., S.R. Srinivasan, G.L. Burke, C.L. Shear, C.G. Smoak, D.W. Harsha, L.K.S. Webber, and G.S. Berenson. 1989. Relation of Body Fat Distribution to Hyperinsulinemia in Children and Adolescents: The Bogalusa Heart Study. *Am J Clin Nutr* 50:930–9.

Freedman, D.S., S.R. Srinivasan, D.W. Harsha, L.K.S. Webber, and G.S. Berenson. 1987. Relation of Body Fat Patterning to Lipid and Lipoprotein Concentrations in Children and Adolescents: The Bogalusa Heart Study. *Am J Clin Nutr* 46:403–10.

Gidding, S.S., R.L. Leibel, S. Daniels, M. Rosenbaum, L. Van Horn, and G.R. Marx. 1996. Understanding Obesity in Youth. A Statement for Healthcare Professionals from the Committee on Atherosclerosis and Hypertension in the Young of the Council on Cardiovascular Disease in the Young and the Nutrition Committee, American Heart Association. *Circulation* 94:3383–7.

Giovannucci, E., A. Ascherio, E.B. Rimm, G.A. Colditz, M.J. Stempfer, and W.C. Willett. 1995. Physical Activity, Obesity, and Risk for Colon Cancer and Adenoma in Men. *Ann Intern Med* 122:327–34.

Goldstein, D.J. 1992. Beneficial Health Effects of Modest Weight Loss. *Int J Obes* 16:397–415.

Gortmaker, S.L., A. Must, A.M. Sobol, K. Peterson, G.A. Colditz, and W.H. Dietz. 1996. Television Viewing as a Cause of Increasing Obesity among Children in the United States, 1986–1990. *Arch Pediatr Adolesc Med* 150:356–62.

Haddock, C.K., W.R. Shadish, R.C. Klesges, and R.J. Stein. 1994. Treatments for Childhood and Adolescent Obesity. *Ann Behav Med* 16:235–44.

Himes, J.H., and W.H. Dietz. 1994. Guidelines for Overweight in Adolescent Preventive Services: Recommendations from an Expert Committee. *Am J Clin Nutr* 59:307–16.

Jick, H, C. Vasilakis, L.A. Weinrauch, C.R. Meier, S.S. Jick, and L.E. Derby. 1998. A Population-Based Study of Appetite-Suppressant Drugs and the Risk of Cardiac-Valve Regurgitation. *N Engl J Med* 339: 719–24.

Johnson, S.L., and L.L. Birch. 1994. Parents' and Children's Adiposity and Eating Style. *Pediatrics* 94:653–61.

Khan, M.A., C.A. Herzog, J.V. St. Peter, G.G. Hartley, R. Madlon-Kay, C.D. Dick, R.W. Asinger, and J.T. Vessey. 1998. The Prevalence of Cardiac Valvular Insufficiency Assessed by Transthoracic Echocardiography in Obese Patients Treated with Appetite-Suppressant Drugs. *N Engl J Med* 339:713–8.

Kovacs, M. 1992. *Child Depression Inventory Manual.* Toronto: Multi-Health Systems, Inc.

Landin, K., M. Krotkiewski, and U. Smith. 1989. Importance of Obesity for the Metabolic Abnormalities Associated with Abdominal Fat Distribution. *Metabolism* 38:572–6.

Lee, I.M., J.E. Manson, C.H. Hennekens, and R.S. Paffenbarger. 1993. Body Weight and Mortality. A 27–Year Follow-Up of Middle-Aged Men. *JAMA* 270:2823–8.

Ludwig, D.S., J.A. Majzoub, A. Al-Zahrani, G.E. Dallal, I. Blanco, and S.B. Roberts. 1999. High Glycemic Index Foods, Overeating, and Obesity. *Pediatrics* 103:1–6.

Ludwig, D.S., K.E. Peterson, and S.L. Gortmaker. 2001. Relation between Consumption of Sugar-Sweetened Drinks and Childhood Obesity: A Prospective, Observational Analysis. *Lancet* 357:490–1.

Maffeis, C., L. Pinelli, and Y. Schutz. 1996. Fat Intake and Adiposity in 8- to 11-Year-Old Obese Children. *Int J Obes* 20:170–4.

Maffeis, C., Y. Schutz, R. Micciolo, L. Zoccante, and L. Pinelli. 1993. Resting Metabolic Rate in Six- to Ten-Year-Old Obese and Nonobese Children. *J Pediatr* 122:556–62.

Manson, J.A., W.C. Willett, M.J. Stampfer, G.A. Colditz, D.J. Hunter, S.E. Hankinson, C.H. Hennekens, and F.E. Speizer. 1995. Body Weight and Mortality among Women. *N Engl J Med* 333:667–85.

McDuffie, J.R., K.A. Calis, G.I. Uwaifo, N.G. Sebring, E.M. Fallon, V.S. Hubbard, and J.A. Yanovski. 2002. Three-Month Tolerability of Orlistat in Adolescents with Obesity-Related Comorbid Conditions. *Obes Res* 10: 642–50.

Moran, J.R., F.K. Ghishan, S.A. Halter, and H.L. Greene. 1983. Steatohepatitis in Obese Children: A Cause of Chronic Liver Dysfunction. *Am J Gastroenterol* 78:374–7.

Morris, K.L., and M.B. Zemel. 1999. Glycemic Index, Cardiovascular Disease, and Obesity. *Nutr Rev* 57:273–6.

National Heart, Lung and Blood Institute. 1998. Statement on First Federal Obesity Clinical Guidelines. NIH Publication 984083. Bethesda, MD.

Ogden, C.L., K.M. Flegal, M.D. Carroll, and C.L. Johnson. 2002. Prevalence and Trends in Overweight among US Children and Adolescents. *JAMA* 288:1728–32.

Ohrvall, M., S. Tengblad, and B. Vessby. 1993. Lower Tocopherol Serum Levels in Subjects with Abdominal Adiposity. *J Intern Med* 234:53–60.

Reisin, E., E.D. Frohlich, F.H. Messerli, G.R. Dreslinski, F.G. Dunn, M.M. Jones, and H.M. Batson. 1983. Cardiovascular Changes after Weight Reduction in Obesity Hypertension. *Ann Intern Med* 98:315–9.

Rocchini, A.P., V. Katch, J. Anderson, J. Hinderliter, D. Becque, M. Martin, and C. Marks. 1988. Blood Pressure in Obese Adolescents Effect on Weight Loss. *Pediatrics* 82:16–23.

Rocchini, A.P., C. Moorehead, V. Katch, J. Key, and K.M. Finta. 1992. Forearm Resistance Vessel Abnormalities and Insulin Resistance in Obese Adolescents. *Hypertension* 19:615–20.

Rolls, B.J, E.A. Bell, V.H. Castellanos, C.L. Pelkman, and M.L. Thowart. 1999. Energy Density but not Fat Content of Foods Affected Energy Intake in Lean and Obese Women. *Am J Clin Nutr* 69:863–71.

Seghatol, F.F., and V.H. Rigolin. 2002. Appetite Suppressants and Valvular Heart Disease. *Curr Opin Cardiol* 17: 486–92.

Shick, S.M., R.R. Wing, M.L. Klem, T. McGuire, J.O. Hill, and H. Seagle. 1998. Persons Successful at Long-Term Weight Loss and Maintenance Continue to Consume a Low-Energy, Low-Fat Diet. *J Am Diet Assoc* 98:408–13.

Slaughter, M., T.G. Lohman, and R.A. Boileau. 1988. Skinfold Equations for Estimation of Body Fatness in Children and Youth. *Hum Biol* 60:709–23.

Sondike, S.B., N. Cooperman, and M.S. Jacobson. 2003. Effects of a Low-Carbohydrate Diet on Weight Loss and Cardiovascular Risk Factors in Overweight Adolescents. *J Pediatr* 142:253–8.

Sowers, J.R., L.A. Whitfield, R.A. Catania, A. Stern, M.L. Tuck, L. Dornfeld, and M. Maxwell. 1982. Role of the Sympathetic Nervous System in Blood Pressure Maintenance in Obesity. *J Clin Endocrinol Metab* 54:1181–6.

Spieth, L.E., J.D. Harnish, C.M. Lenders, L.B. Raezer, M.A. Pereira, S.J. Hangen, and D.S. Ludwig. 2000. A Low-Glycemic Index Diet in the Treatment of Pediatric Obesity. *Arch Pediatr Adoles Med* 154, 947–51.

Stallings, V.A., E.H. Archibald, P.B. Pencharz, J.E. Harrison, and L.E. Bell. 1998. One-Year Follow-Up of Weight, Total Body Potassium, and Total Body Nitrogen in Obese Adolescents Treated with the Protein-Sparing Modified Fast. *Am J Clin Nutr* 48:91–4.

Taras, H.L., J.F. Sallis, T.L. Patterson, and P.R. Nader. 1989. Television's Influence on Children's Diet and Physical Activity. *Behav Pediatr* 10:176–80.

Tershakovec, A.M., M.H. Watson, W.J. Wenner, and A.L. Marx. 1999. Insurance Reimbursement for the Treatment of Obesity in Children. *J Pediatr* 134:573–8.

Thomas, P.R. (ed.). 1995. *Weighing the Options—Criteria for Evaluating Weight-Management Programs.* Washington, DC: National Academy Press, pp. 102–17.

Torigoe, K., O. Numata, M. Matsunaga, Y. Tanaka, C. Imai, and H. Yamazaki. 1997. Effect of Weight Loss on Body Fat Distribution in Obese Children. *Acta Paediatr Jpn* 39:28–33.

Troiano, R.P., K.M. Flegal, R.J. Kuczmarski, S.M. Campbell, and C.L. Johnson. 1995. Overweight Prevalence and Trends for Children and Adolescents. *Arch Pediatr Adolesc Med* 149:1085–91.

Van Gaal, L.F., M.A. Wauters, and I.H. De Leeuw. 1997. The Beneficial Effects of Modest Weight Loss on Cardiovascular Risk Factors. *Int J Obes* 21(Suppl. 1):S5–S9.

Wadden, T.A., D.A. Anderson, and G.D. Foster. 1999. Two-Year Changes in Lipids and Lipoproteins Associated with Maintenance of a 5% to 10% Reduction in Initial Weight: Some Findings and Questions. *Obes Res* 7:170–8.

Wadden, T.A., R.I. Berkowitz, D.B. Sarwer, R. Prus-Wisniewski, and C. Steinberg. 2001. Benefits of Lifestyle Modification in the Pharmacologic Treatment of Obesity: A Randomized Trial. *Arch Intern Med* 161: 218–27.

Wadden, T.A., R.I. Berkowitz, F. Silvestry, R.A. Vogt, M.G. St. John-Sutton, A.J. Stunkard, G.D. Foster, and J.L. Aber. 1998. The Fen-Phen Finale: A Study of Weight Loss and Valvular Heart Disease. *Obes Res* 6: 278–84.

Wadden, T.A., A.J. Stunkard, L. Rich, C.J. Rubin ,G. Sweidel, and S. McKinney. 1990. Obesity in Black Adolescent Girls: A Controlled Clinical Trial of Treatment by Diet, Behavior Modification, and Parental Support. *Pediatrics* 85:345–52.

Weissman, N.J., J.F. Tighe, Jr., J.S. Gottdiener, and J.T. Gwynne. 1998. An Assessment of Heart-Valve Abnormalities in Obese Patients Taking Dexfenfluramine, Sustained-Release Dexfenfluramine, or Placebo. Sustained-Release Dexfenfluramine Study Group. *N Engl J Med* 339:725–32.

Zemel, B.S., E.M. Riley, and V.A. Stallings. 1997. Evaluation of Methodology for Nutritional Assessment in Children: Anthropometry, Body Composition, and Energy Expenditure. *Annu Rev Nutr* 17:211–35.

CHAPTER 14

The Need for Physical Activity among Children and Adolescents for Prevention and Treatment of Obesity

Brian E. Saelens

Physical activity in childhood exerts both immediate and long-term effects on health, particularly for children already at risk for incurring negative weight-related consequences. Numerous mechanisms exist by which physical activity likely benefits children and adults, including but not limited to better cardiovascular fitness, weight control, and insulin sensitivity. High levels of physical activity in childhood could convey long-term benefit into adulthood regardless of the level of physical activity retained into adulthood. Children's physical activity can also have a more immediate benefit to health in childhood, with better tracking of positive health into adulthood and thus transmission of long-term benefits. In an attempt to convey to health practitioners information about the current status of knowledge about children's physical activity, this chapter provides an overview of evidence regarding the impact of physical activity on children's health. It also discusses the prevalence and correlates of physical activity among children, as well as interventions and recommendations for activity. Given the increasing prevalence of childhood obesity, physical activity benefits and interventions are considered with particular relevance for overweight children.

EFFECTS OF PHYSICAL ACTIVITY IN CHILDHOOD

Physical activity is important for all children and adolescents to prevent obesity and its consequences. Physical activity improves the health of children with already unfavorable health risk profiles (e.g., obese children). Increasing physical activity is critical to the treatment and prevention of overweight and obesity in children for better weight control (Epstein and Goldfield, 1999) and improved cardiovascular fitness (Gutin et al., 2002). An increase in physical activity also appears to reduce problems characteristic of insulin resistance among obese children, particularly if the physical activity is high intensity or vigorous (Kang et al., 2002). Some investigators have found positive associations between physical activity and insulin sensitivity among healthy non-overweight children, although these associations appear stronger among children with some current marker of health risk (e.g., higher than average blood pressure) (Schmitz et al., 2002). Identification of the cardiovascular effects of high visceral or intra-abdominal fat accumulation among children (Goran and Gower, 1999) has prompted investigation into the effects of physical activity on body fat distribution. Intra-abdominal fat accumulation is lower among more active adults (Hunter et al., 1996; Kanaley et al., 2001; Reichman et al., 2002) and interventions to increase physical activity appear to decrease intra-abdominal fat in adults (Irwin et al., 2003), perhaps even without absolute weight changes (Thomas et al., 2000). Whether the level of physical activity in children is related to their visceral fat accumulation has received little research attention (see Roemmich et al. (2000) for an exception). The little evidence that does exist suggests that obese children, rather than lean children, may derive the most significant benefit of reduced visceral fat accumulation from physical activity and training interventions (Table 14.1), perhaps because of the lower absolute magnitude of visceral fat in lean children.

With these known positive effects of physical activity on children's long-term health and the immediate benefits for an increasing childhood population at risk for cardiovascular disease secondary to the rising obesity prevalence (Ogden et al., 2002), it is useful to examine the current physical activity levels of U.S. children, the current recommendations for children's physical activity, and the correlates of and interventions for children's physical activity.

PREVALENCE OF PHYSICAL ACTIVITY

It is estimated that less than one-third of U.S. adolescents engage in more than 30 minutes of moderate intensity activity on most days of the week, and this fraction is even lower among African-American youth (U.S. Department of Health and Human Services [USDHHS], 2000). A higher percentage of high school students, approximately 65%, meet the recommendation for vigorous

TABLE 14.1

Effects of physical activity and training interventions on children's
visceral or intra-abdominal fat accumulation

Reference	Sample	Physical Activity Intervention	Impact on Visceral Fat
Eliakim et al. (1997)	15- to 17-year-old nonoverweight adolescent females ($n = 44$) randomly assigned to PA intervention or non-PA control	5 times per week sessions of mostly aerobic PA for 5 weeks	No significant differences between PA intervention and control adolescents at postintervention
Gutin et al. (2002)	13- to 16-year-old obese adolescents ($n = 80$) randomly assigned to LSE alone, LSE + moderate-intensity PA, or LSE + high-intensity PA	5 times per week sessions of moderate or high-intensity aerobic PA only offered to adolescents assigned to their respective conditions	Combined across PA intensity conditions, adolescents provided LSE + PA interventions decreased average visceral fat significantly more than adolescents provided LSE alone from baseline to postintervention
Owens et al. (1999)	7- to 11-year-old obese children ($n = 74$) randomly assigned to PA intervention or non-PA control	5 times per week 40-minute sessions of mostly aerobic PA offered for 4 months	Intervention children had a significantly smaller increase (+0.5%) in average visceral fat than control children (+8.1%) from baseline to postintervention
Treuth et al. (1998)	7- to 10-year-old obese girls ($n = 11$)	3 times per week 20-minute sessions of strength training for 5 months	Maintenance of intra-abdominal fat from baseline to postintervention, despite children's average increase in total fat mass and age

LSE, lifestyle education; PA, physical activity.

physical activity of 3 or more days per week for 20+ minutes (USDHHS, 2000). These estimates are generally derived from self-report measures on nationally representative samples. Physical activity self-reports are often highly inaccurate, particularly among children. Indeed, the proportion of children meeting physical activity recommendations differs markedly depending on whether self-report or more objective measures of physical activity are used. While a review of methods for assessing physical activity among children is beyond the scope of this chapter, it is an important consideration in evaluating the prevalence of and interventions for children's physical activity (Sallis and Saelens, 2000; Sirard and Pate, 2001).

The use of accelerometers and heart rate monitoring are more objective methods of assessing physical activity. Recent investigation with accelerometers found that most children are physically active for more than 30 minutes each day. Younger children generally reach the level of more than 60 minutes of moderate physical activity on most days, although there is a precipitous decline with age in childhood. Approximately 30% of high school students are not engaging in at least 60 minutes of moderate-intensity physical activity on most days of the week (Pate et al., 2002). However, the most alarming finding from the objective measurement of physical activity is the extremely low prevalence of children engaging in 3 or more days per week of 20+ minutes of continuous vigorous physical activity. In one study, less than 3% of children met this vigorous physical activity level as evaluated by an accelerometer, with little variation by age or sex (Pate et al., 2002). Others have found similar low rates of vigorous activity among children when using objective measures to obtain estimates of children's physical activity (Strauss et al., 2001). A review of heart-rate monitoring studies found that children had elevated heart rates, which were consistent with moderate-intensity physical activity, at daily levels of 60+ minutes. Also consistent with the accelerometer findings on vigorous physical activity, average minutes per day of higher heart rate reserve values (heart rate reserve >60%, a proxy for vigorous physical activity) were less than 15 minutes per day (Epstein et al., 2001).

▪ Age

Cross-sectional research suggests reduced rates of physical activity in childhood through the latter part of adolescence (USDHHS, 1996; Caspersen et al., 2000). More recent longitudinal data provide further evidence of this decline, at least among girls (Strauss et al., 2001; Kimm et al., 2002). In a large cohort of black and white girls, Kimm and colleagues observed a significant decline of more than 80% in physical activity from age 9 to 10 years to age 18 to 19 years. The most striking finding was that by age 16, 56% of black girls and 31% of white girls reported no habitual physical activity outside of school (Kimm et al., 2002). These declines were evidenced in another longitudinal study including both boys and girls followed from early to late adolescence (Aaron et al., 2002). In an attempt to evaluate the source of decreased overall physical activity, this latter study examined separately the number of physical activities that adolescents reported doing and the time spent on each physical activity. These investigators found that the decrease in the number of physical activities engaged in, not the amount of time spent in specific physical activities, was primarily responsible for the overall decline in total physical activity (Aaron et al., 2002). Results from a study using objective measures of physical activity concur with the self-reported decline in physical activity with age, but the most dramatic decreases in physical activity were found in middle childhood, rather than in adolescence (Trost et al., 2002). Regardless, by the end of childhood, the average child has decreased his or her physical activity from an earlier higher level.

■ Sex

Overall, girls tend to report lower rates of physical activity than boys (USDHHS, 1996; Gordon-Larsen et al., 1999), although sex differences tend to fluctuate by physical activity type and by age. The largest sex differences in reported sustained physical activity (e.g., frequency of bouts of physical activity) and vigorous physical activity appear in middle to late adolescence, with at least some convergence among the sexes in sustained rates of physical activity by early adulthood (Caspersen et al., 2000). Girls and women consistently report lower rates of strengthening exercise than men (Caspersen et al., 2000). Objectively measured physical activity findings generally converge with self-report data, with boys engaging in more overall physical activity and particularly with higher vigorous intensity than girls (Trost et al., 2002). It is noteworthy that the magnitude of these sex differences was smaller when measured objectively than the sex differences found with self-report of physical activity.

In summary, U.S. children appear to be more active than U.S. adults on average and few younger children report being completely inactive. Younger children engage in more physical activity than adolescents and boys are more active on average than girls (Caspersen et al., 2000). Many children, however, are not engaging often in vigorous-intensity physical activity, which appears especially important for maintaining and improving cardiovascular fitness. Cardiovascular fitness may be more closely related to health indices than levels of overall physical activity among children (Katzmarzyk et al., 1999), although measurement reliability may be attenuating relations observed between physical activity levels and health indices. Measurement issues may also be contributing to the inconsistent evidence of whether obese and non-obese children differ in their levels of physical activity (Sallis et al., 2000). To date, recommendations for children's physical activity are not based on weight or other health status effects, but will likely continue to evolve as knowledge increases about the effects of physical activity.

■ RECOMMENDATIONS FOR PHYSICAL ACTIVITY

It is telling that the first recommendation to health care providers from a recent committee targeting the cardiovascular health of children is to assess and encourage children's physical activity (Williams et al., 2002). This recommendation is similar to the first behavioral prescription of the 2000 *dietary* guidelines for Americans, to be physically active each day (U.S. Department of Agriculture and U.S. Department of Health and Human Services, 2000). Also noteworthy in the former document is that there is no specific recommendation for the amount of physical activity in which children would ideally engage. This is likely not so much an oversight as a general lack of consensus on the amount and type of physical activity that is optimal for children's immediate and long-term health. Given the growing epidemic of childhood (Ogden et al., 2002) and adult (Flegal et al., 2002) obesity, the documented effects of adult physical activity on adult health, and signs of decreasing opportunities for physical activity (e.g., fewer physical education offerings in schools), public health guidelines are increasing their focus on physical activity in children.

Recommendations for the amount of physical activity in which children should engage for health benefits have largely been derived from recommendations for physical activity in adults (Pate et al., 1995), in part because of the existing longitudinal literature that has established inverse dose—response relationships between adults' levels of physical activity and chronic disease (Blair et al., 1996; USDHHS, 1996). It is clear that adults derive direct cardiovascular and overall health benefits from engaging in physical activity (USDHHS, 1996). There is a history of fluctuation in the type, amount, and duration of physical activity recommended for adults, but research appears to be coming closer to building a consensus around physical activity prescriptions and specific disease likelihood for adults.

There remains no consensus on recommendations for children's physical activity, likely because of the current lack of longitudinal data on children's physical activity and long-term health. An expert consensus conference suggested that children engage in developmentally appropriate 60+ minutes of at least moderate intensity physical activity each day, with an additional recommendation for children to engage in muscular strength- and flexibility-related activities at least twice per week (Pate et al., 1998; Cavill et al., 2001). These guidelines suggest initially lower levels of physical activity for children currently engaged in little activity (Cavill et al., 2001). As seen in Table 14.2, objectives from *Healthy People 2010* (USDHHS, 2000) for children's physical activity suggest a different recommended amount, frequency, and duration of physical activity. Some have challenged the empirical arguments used to establish specific guidelines of physical activity for children, contending that in addition to the inconsistent or current lack of evidence on the relation between children's physical activity and health, there is little evidence of the form of these relationships (e.g., linear, hyperbolic) that would suggest a specific threshold for physical activity levels (Twisk, 2001). Few argue, however, that children are getting too much physical activity or that all children are being active enough. Many indicators associated with children's participation in physical activity suggest a need for children to adopt more active lifestyles.

TABLE 14.2

Selected physical activity guidelines and operational definitions

Source	Guideline	Operational Definition
HP 2010, goal 22.6	Engage in moderate physical activity for at least 30 minutes per day on 5 or more days per week.	On 5 or more days during the week, physical activity at an intensity of three or more METS observed during 30 or more 1-minute periods
HP 2010, goal 22.7	Engage in vigorous physical activity that promotes development and maintenance of cardiorespiratory fitness, 3 or more days per week for 20 or more minutes	On 3 or more days during the week, physical activity at an intensity of six or more METS observed during 20 or more continuous minutes
United Kingdom Expert Consensus Group	Participate in physical activity of at least moderate intensity for an average of 1 hour per day	On 5 or more days during the week, physical activity at an intensity of three or more METS observed during 60 or more 1-minute periods

HP 2010: *Healthy People 2010*; METS, measure of activity intensity, ratio of activity metabolic rate to resting metabolic rate.
Source: Adapted from *Ann Epidemiol* 12:303–8. Pate et al. Compliance with Physical Activity Guidelines: Prevalence in a Population of Children and Youth. Copyright © 2002, with permission from Elsevier.

In concert with recommendations for increasing children's physical activity, there have been recent calls to reduce the time children spend in sedentary behaviors, including television watching. One *Healthy People 2010* objective is to reduce adolescents' television watching to less than 2 hours per day (USDHHS, 2000), a standard met by approximately one-half of the adolescent population. The American Academy of Pediatrics has extended this recommendation to all children, with an additional recommendation to discourage television watching altogether for children under 2 years of age (American Academy of Pediatrics: Committee on Public Education, 2001). The evidence for the positive relationship between sedentary activity time and obesity appears more consistent among adults, but there is growing evidence linking children's higher sedentary activity time and obesity (Saelens, 2003). Sedentary activity time may be interfering with children's physical activity, particularly moderate-intensity physical activity (Strauss et al., 2001). Both clinic-based and school-based interventions, as well as activity choice laboratory studies, indicate that targeting reductions in time spent in even a subset of sedentary behaviors can translate into more physical activity and lower obesity rates (Saelens, 2003). Reducing children's time spent in sedentary behaviors may be an important component of increasing their physical activity.

While far from a consensus recommendation, given the rising rates of obesity and the more well-documented positive effects of physical activity in adulthood, children should try to engage in at least 60 minutes of at least moderate-intensity physical activity on most days of the week. It appears that integration of at least some vigorous physical activity adds some unique benefits to being active frequently enough. This level of physical activity may have to be increased for children already at risk for weight-related comorbidities and may not be adequate for weight loss among already overweight children.

CORRELATES OF PHYSICAL ACTIVITY

One strategy to begin addressing ways to increase children's physical activity or to target specific low-activity children for intervention is to examine the factors related to higher or lower physical activity. A review examined the consistency with which various possible correlates of children's physical activity were found to be associated with children's physical activity, including psychosocial and environmental correlates (Sallis et al., 2000).

Psychosocial Correlates

Psychosocial correlates of children's physical activity include attitudes, cognitions, preferences, cultural, and social influences on physical activity. For example, the level of barriers (e.g., lack of time) that children perceive to being active is one of the strongest negative correlates of their physical activity. Consistent positive correlates among younger children include prior physical activity and current intention to be active (Sallis et al., 2000). Among adolescents, achievement orientation, perceived competence in physical activity, current intention to be active, and support from parents and others appear to be reliable psychosocial correlates of physical activity (Sallis et al., 2000).

Environmental Correlates

Although to date environmental variables have been much less frequently studied than demographic (e.g., age, sex) and psychosocial variables, these factors are beginning to receive more attention as possible determinants of children's physical activity. For younger children, access to physical activity facilities and programs and the amount of time spent outdoors are positively related to physical activity. Similarly for adolescents, opportunities to exercise appear related to more physical activity (Sallis et al., 2000).

■ PHYSICAL ACTIVITY INTERVENTIONS

Some of the strategies and interventions proposed to increase children's physical activity stem from the psychosocial correlates of children's physical activity. For example, interventions based on social cognitive theory attempt to help children overcome barriers to physical activity by altering their cognitions about physical activity and the consequences of engaging in active behaviors. There has been considerable interest in identifying comprehensive interventions that are most efficacious at increasing and sustaining increases in children's physical activity, for the purpose of both obesity prevention and intervention.

■ Physical Activity Interventions for Prevention of Obesity

Many interventions for physical activity among youth have been framed in part as obesity prevention interventions. Some investigators have compiled and reviewed physical activity intervention programs for children (Stone et al., 1998; Sallis and Owen, 1999). Of the few childhood obesity prevention programs that have been evaluated, conclusions are tentative on whether physical activity alone, without dietary intervention, can prevent the development of obesity in childhood (Campbell et al., 2001).

A review of some completed and planned studies on physical activity is informative about the direction in which interventionists believe programs should be headed and how the most impact can be obtained. In general, authors of intervention programs have documented improvements in knowledge and attitudes about physical activity, as well as increases in children's physical activity, at least within the context in which children were being targeted. School has been the primary context in which physical activity interventions for children are delivered, perhaps because of the precipitous drop in the number of children attending (USDHHS, 1996) and being active in physical education classes. Children also spend a considerable part of their day in school and most U.S. children attend school, making it an opportune context in which to have a large impact. It is perhaps also recognized that school settings are more readily controllable and modifiable than the many environments outside school to which children are exposed (e.g., home, neighborhood). Further, there is no evidence indicating that when children are less active in school they compensate by increasing their physical activity later in the day outside of school (Dale et al., 2000).

Many studies have examined the impact of non-physical education class curriculum-based interventions to increase children's physical activity or decrease sedentary behavior, either with or without a concurrent dietary intervention. These have included skills-based instruction (e.g., self-monitoring, goal setting) in classes to help children learn the skills that will help them be more active (Gortmaker et al., 1999; Robinson, 1999). Complete curricula have been published and are readily available for some of these interventions (e.g., Cheung et al., 2001; also see www.sparkpe.org). Other trials have specifically targeted improving the curriculum of physical education classes and the amount and intensity of physical activity within physical education classes, with some success relative to children provided no intervention (Luepker et al., 1996; Sallis et al., 1997). Evidence that improvements in children's physical activity are sustained after intervention cessation is less promising, and there is little evidence that interventions for increasing physical activity in school have effects outside of school (Stone et al., 1998).

There has been a significant decrease in the percentage of students participating in daily school physical education, from estimates of over 40% in 1991 to less than 30% only 8 years later in 1999 (USDHHS, 2000). Even among those students in physical education classes, only about one-third spend 50% or more of their time being active during the class. In an attempt to increase physical activity throughout the school day, another program integrates short bouts of physical activity into the classroom setting, with classroom teachers leading the brief activity sessions (Stewart et al., 2002).

Other attempts have sought to promote physical activity in non-school contexts. The adolescent version of the program Patient-centered Assessment and Counseling for Exercise plus Nutrition (PACE+) introduces physical activity intervention initially in the primary-care office, with skills-based instruction and contact through phone and mail thereafter. There is preliminary evidence of efficacy of this integrative office- and home-based intervention for increasing physical activity, specifically among adolescents choosing to target increases in moderate-intensity physical activity (Patrick et al., 2001). A larger trial examining the efficacy of the PACE+ intervention for adolescents' physical activity and dietary modification is under way.

■ Physical Activity Components of Interventions to Prevent Pediatric Obesity

There is adequate evidence that the inclusion of a physical activity component in pediatric-obesity interventions improves children's weight outcomes more than dietary modification alone (Epstein and Goldfield, 1999). As detailed in Table 14.1, physical activity interventions alone may reduce visceral fat accumulation among obese children and have other positive effects on health, but there is little evidence that physical activity intervention without dietary modification results in whole body fat reduction or long-term weight control among obese children (Epstein et al., 1998; Jelalian and Saelens, 1999). There is no consensus on the specific strategies or types of physical activity that lead most readily to increases in obese children's physical activity within the context of a pediatric obesity intervention (Epstein and Goldfield, 1999), but numerous strategies have been employed to increase children's levels of physical activity within these interventions. Many of these strategies are listed in Table 14.3.

■ Environmental Approaches

Most prior trials to increase children's physical activity have focused on teaching behavioral skills. This is perhaps due to the curriculum focus of school settings, the translation of adult physical activity interventions, or the reliance on social cognitive and other cognitive-behavioral theories that are an attempt to directly target individuals' cognition and behavioral precedents and consequences. More recent approaches to understanding health behaviors have begun to consider factors outside the individual that may be influencing such behaviors, with a growing interest in the impact of environments on physical activity (King et al. 2002; Sallis and Owen, 2002). The contrast between behavior skills approaches and environmental approaches to change children's physical activity is presented in Table 14.3.

Stemming from the transportation and urban planning literatures, investigators have speculated that neighborhood design could be affecting physical activity by discouraging or encouraging walking and cycling trips (Handy et al., 2002; Saelens et al., 2003). Proximity to recreation and physical activity facilities appears related to higher physical activity (Sallis et al., 1990). Empirical work examining environmental influences on children's physical activity is just beginning to emerge. In one study, the likelihood of children being active during

TABLE 14.3
Examples of skills-based strategies and environmental change strategies for increasing children's physical activity

Skills-based Strategies	Environmental Change Strategies
Pre-plan to increase physical activity	Increase physical activity facilities
Set goals around frequency, duration, and intensity of physical activity	Increase access to existing physical activity facilities
Self-monitor and track physical activity	Remove sedentary activity options
Make rewards contingent on increasing physical activity	Change policies (e.g., school gym class time, curriculum) regarding physical activity
Practice problem solving to overcome barriers to greater physical activity	Increase adult supervision in physical activity settings
	Change media and other cueing materials (e.g., posters) to promote physical activity
	Decrease access to sedentary activities
	Have others model increased physical activity

unstructured time at school appears to be related in part to the presence or absence of space for physical activity (and equipment availability) and presence or absence of adult supervision (Sallis et al., 2001). More than 40% of the variance in girls' and boys' physical activity before school, during lunch, and after school on school grounds was explained by the environmental and supervision variables. Others have proposed examining the neighborhood environment and its impact on children walking and/or biking to and from school, as an opportunity to increase a type of physical activity that can be readily incorporated into the daily routine of children (Tudor-Locke et al., 2001).

Attempts have been made to extend physical activity interventions beyond physical education classes within the school setting. Shifting away from a behavior change skills- or instruction-only-based program, Sallis and colleagues developed an intervention targeting environmental and policy changes within middle schools around eating and physical activity. The physical activity intervention included improving the availability of physical activity equipment, distribution of newsletters, flyers, and bulletins about physical activity, and increasing supervision within activity contexts (e.g., playgrounds) during non-structured parts of the school day, including before and after school and after lunch. Schools provided this intervention evidenced higher amounts of physical activity among their boys at post-intervention, with greater increases of activity for boys both in and out of physical education classes relative to schools not receiving the intervention. There was no intervention vs. control school difference in girls' physical activity (Sallis et al., 2003).

With an increased focus on environmental factors, investigators are beginning to expand their examination of the contexts or behavior settings in which children's physical activity occurs or could occur. Community-based interventions for increasing children's physical activity have rarely been evaluated and have a history of poor participant retention and modest efficacy for increasing children's physical activity (Stone et al., 1998). Recent intervention and evaluation attempts are trying to address these shortcomings. The Trial of Activity for Adolescent Girls (TAAG) is a large multicenter trial attempting to increase physical activity among adolescent girls. The trial is designed to test the effectiveness of an integrated school- and community-based intervention to prevent declines in levels of physical activity and cardiopulmonary fitness among girls in early adolescence. Pending results, it is likely that future interventions will attempt to increase children's physical activity across various contexts.

Clearly, further investigation is required to identify the most potent environmental factors influencing children's physical activity and to test modification of these factors in intervention trials. Environmental approaches have the potential to affect populations, rather than simply individuals targeted for intervention. In addition, environmental modifications that require less effort to sustain than skills- or curriculum-based physical activity interventions for children may be more likely to result in sustained higher levels of physical activity. Further investigation also has the potential to identify the optimal combination of skills-based training and environmental change to increase children's physical activity.

Identifying Mediators

Many studies have compared multicomponent physical activity interventions for children to no or minimal intervention conditions. Few studies have actually examined mediators through which interventions for increasing children's physical activity are proposed to operate (Lewis et al., 2002). For example, social cognitive theory would suggest that increasing self-efficacy and perceived competence for physical activity would increase physical activity. Interventions designed on social cognitive principles should evaluate both children's change in physical activity and change in self-efficacy and then evaluate the relation between these changes. Investigations of mediators of intervention success are rare within childhood physical activity intervention trials but warrant further consideration (Lewis et al., 2002).

SUMMARY

- There is growing concern that U.S. children are entering adulthood with considerably more chronic disease risk factors than ever before, including higher rates of obesity and type 2 diabetes.
- On average, children with such risk factors appear to benefit from increasing their physical activity.
- Whereas the evidence is less clear for healthy children, and the exact nature of the physical activity-to-health risk relation is less well understood than for adults, the average U.S. child would likely benefit from increasing his/her physical activity level, particularly in adolescence.
- School-based interventions have met with some success in increasing children's physical activity, but this efficacy needs to translate into more sustained improvements in children's physical activity in the long term and across different settings.

REFERENCES

Aaron, D.J., K.L. Storti, R.J. Robertson, A.M. Kriska, and R.E. LaPorte. 2002. Longitudinal Study of the Number and Choice of Leisure Time Physical Activities from Mid to Late Adolescence: Implications for School Curricula and Community Recreation Programs. *Arch Pediatr Adolesc Med* 156:1075–80.

American Academy of Pediatrics: Committee on Public Education. 2001. Children, Adolescents, and Television (RE0043). *Pediatrics* 107:423–6.

Blair, S.N., J.B. Kampert, H.W. Kohl, III, C.E. Barlow, C.A. Macera, R.S. Paffenbarger, and L.W. Gibbons. 1996. Influences of Cardiorespiratory Fitness and Other Precursors on

Cardiovascular Disease and All-Cause Mortality in Men and Women. *JAMA* 276:205–10.

Campbell, K., E. Waters, S. O'Meara, and C. Summerbell. 2001. Interventions for Preventing Obesity in Childhood. A Systematic Review. *Obes Rev* 2:149–57.

Caspersen, C.J., M.A. Pereira, and K.M. Curran. 2000. Changes in Physical Activity Patterns in the United States, by Sex and Cross-Sectional Age. *Med Sci Sports Exer* 32:1601–9.

Cavill, N., S. Biddle, and J.F. Sallis. 2001. Health Enhancing Physical Activity for Young People: Statement of the United Kingdom Expert Consensus Conference. *Pediatr Exer Sci* 13:12–25.

Cheung, L.W.Y., S.L. Gortmaker, and H. Dart. 2001. *Eat Well & Keep Moving: An Interdisciplinary Curriculum for Teaching Upper Elementary School Nutrition and Physical Activity.* Champaign, IL: Human Kinetics.

Dale, D., C.B. Corbin, and K.S. Dale. 2000. Restricting Opportunities to be Active During School Time: Do Children Compensate by Increasing Physical Activity Levels After School? *Res Quart Exer Sport* 71:240–8.

Eliakim, A., G.S. Burke, and D.M. Cooper. 1997. Fitness, Fatness, and the Effect of Training Assessed by Magnetic Resonance Imaging and Skinfold-Thickness Measurements in Healthy Adolescent Females. *Am J Clin Nutr* 66:223–31.

Epstein, L.H., and G.S. Goldfield. 1999. Physical Activity in the Treatment of Childhood Overweight and Obesity: Current Evidence and Research Issues. *Med Sci Sports Exer* 31:S553–9.

Epstein, L.H., M.D. Myers, H.A. Raynor, and B.E. Saelens. 1998. Treatment of Pediatric Obesity. *Pediatrics* 101:554–70.

Epstein, L.H., R.A. Paluch, L.E. Kalakanis, G.S. Goldfield, F.J. Cerny, and J.N. Roemmich. 2001. *How Much Activity Do Youth Get? A Quantitative Review of Heart-Rate Measured Activity. Pediatrics.* Available at: http://www.pediatrics.org/cgi/content/full/108/3/e44.

Flegal, K.M., M.D. Carroll, C.L. Ogden, and C.L. Johnson. 2002. Prevalence and Trends in Obesity among US Adults, 1999–2000. *JAMA* 288:1723–27.

Goran, M.I., and B.A. Gower. 1999. Relation between Visceral Fat and Disease Risk in Children and Adolescents. *Am J Clin Nutr* 70:149S–56S.

Gordon-Larsen, P., R.G. McMurray, and B.M. Popkin. 1999. Adolescent Physical Activity and Inactivity Vary by Ethnicity: The National Longitudinal Study of Adolescent Health. *J Pediatr* 135:301–6.

Gortmaker, S.L., K. Peterson, J. Wiecha, A.M. Sobol, S. Dixit, M.K. Fox, and N. Laird. 1999. Reducing Obesity Via a School-Based Interdisciplinary Intervention among Youth: Planet Health. *Arch Pediatr Adoles Med* 153:409–18.

Gutin, B., P. Barbeau, S. Owens, C.R. Lemmon, M. Bauman, J. Allison, H-S. Kang, and M.S. Litaker. 2002. Effects of Exercise Intensity on Cardiovascular Fitness, Total Body Composition, and Visceral Adiposity of Obese Adolescents. *Am J Clin Nutr* 75:818–26.

Handy, S.L., M.G. Boarnet, R. Ewing, and R.E. Killingsworth. 2002. How the Built Environment Affects Physical Activity: Views from Urban Planning. *Am J Prev Med* 23(2S):64–73.

Hunter, G.R., T. Kekes-Szabo, M.S. Treuth, M.J. Williams, M. Goran, and C. Pichon. 1996. Intra-Abdominal Adipose Tissue, Physical Activity and Cardiovascular Risk in Pre- and Post-Menopausal Women. *Int J Obes* 20:860–5.

Irwin, M.L., Y. Yasui, C.M. Ulrich, D. Bowen, R.E. Rudolph, R.S. Schwartz, M. Yakawa, E. Aiello, J.D. Potter, and A. McTiernan. 2003. Effect of Exercise on Total and Intra-Abdominal Body Fat in Postmenopausal Women. *JAMA* 289:323–30.

Jelalian, E., and B.E. Saelens. 1999. Empirically Supported Treatments in Pediatric Psychology: Pediatric Obesity. *J Pediatr Psychol* 24:223–48.

Kanaley, J.A., C. Sames, L. Swisher, A.G. Swick, L.L. Ploutz-Snyder, C.M. Steppan, K.S. Sagendorf, D. Feiglin, E.B. Jaynes, R.A. Meyer, and R.S. Weinstock. 2001. Abdominal Fat

Distribution in Pre- and Postmenopausal Women: The Impact of Physical Activity, Age, and Menopausal Status. *Metabolism* 50:976–82.

Kang, H-S., B. Gutin, P. Barbeau, S. Owens, C.R. Lemmon, J. Allison, M.S. Litaker, and N-A. Le. 2002. Physical Training Improves Insulin Resistance Syndrome Markers in Obese Adolescents. *Med Sci Sports Exer* 34:1920–7.

Katzmarzyk, P.T., R.M Malina, and C. Bouchard. 1999. Physical Activity, Physical Fitness, and Coronary Heart Disease Risk Factors in Youth: The Quebec Family Study. *Prev Med* 29:555–62.

Kimm, S.Y.S., N.W. Glynn, A.M. Kriska, B.A. Barton, S.S. Kronsberg, S.R. Daniels, P.B. Crawford, Z.I. Sabry, and K. Liu. 2002. Decline in Physical Activity in Black Girls and White Girls during Adolescence. *N Engl J Med* 347:709–15.

King, A.C., D. Stokols, E. Talen, G.S. Brassington, and R.E. Killingsworth. 2002. Theoretical Approaches to the Promotion of Physical Activity. *Am J Prev Med* 23(2S):15–25.

Lewis, B.A., B.H. Marcus, R.R. Pate, and A.L. Dunn. 2002. Psychosocial Mediators of Physical Activity Behavior among Adults and Children. *Am J Prev Med* 23(2S):26–35.

Luepker, R.V., C.L. Perry, S.M. McKinlay, P.R. Nader, G.S. Parcel, E.J. Stone, L.S. Webber, J.P. Elder, H.A. Feldman, C.C. Johnson, S.H. Kelder, and M. Wu. 1996. Outcomes of a Field Trial to Improve Children's Dietary Patterns and Physical Activity: The Child and Adolescent Trial for Cardiovascular Health (CATCH). *JAMA* 275:768–76.

Ogden, C.L., K.M. Flegal, M.D. Carroll, and C.L. Johnson. 2002. Prevalence and Trends in Overweight among US Children and Adolescents, 1999—2000. *JAMA* 288:1728–32.

Owens, S., B. Gutin, J. Allison, S. Riggs, M. Ferguson, M. Litaker, and W. Thompson. 1999. Effect of Physical Training on Total and Visceral Fat in Obese Children. *Med Sci Sports Exer* 31:143–8.

Pate, R.R., P.S. Freedson, J.F. Sallis, W.C. Taylor, J. Sirard, S.G. Trost, and M. Dowda. 2002. Compliance with Physical Activity Guidelines: Prevalence in a Population of Children and Youth. *Ann Epidemiol* 12:303–8.

Pate, R.R., M. Pratt, S.N. Blair, W.L. Haskell, C.A. Macera, C. Bouchard, D. Buchner, W. Ettinger, G.W. Heath, A.C. King, A. Kriska, A.S. Leon, B.H. Marcus, J. Morris, R.S. Paffenbarger, K. Patrick, M.L. Polluck, J.M. Rippe, J. Sallis, and J.H. Wilmore. 1995. Physical Activity and Public Health: A Recommendation from the Centers for Disease Control and Prevention and the American College of Sports Medicine. *JAMA* 273:402–7.

Pate, R., S. Trost, and C. Williams. 1998. Critique of Existing Guidelines for Physical Activity in Young People. In: *Young and Active? Young People and Health-Enhancing Physical Activity—Evidence and Implications.* Edited by S. Biddle, J. Sallis and N. Cavill. London: Health Education Authority, pp. 162–73.

Patrick, K., J.F. Sallis, J.J. Prochaska, D.D. Lydston, K.J. Calfas, M.F. Zabinski, D.E. Wilfley, B.J. Long, S. Thompson, J. Rupp, B.E. Saelens, and D.R. Brown. 2001. A Multi-Component Program for Nutrition and Physical Activity Change in Primary Care: PACE+ for Adolescents. *Arch Pediatr Adolesc Med* 155:940–6.

Reichman, S.E., R.E. Schoen, J.L. Weissfeld, F.L. Thaete, and A.M. Kriska. 2002. Association of Physical Activity and Visceral Adipose Tissue in Older Women and Men. *Obes Res* 10:1065–73.

Robinson, T.N. 1999. Reducing Children's Television Viewing to Prevent Obesity: A Randomized Controlled Trial. *JAMA* 282:1561–7.

Roemmich, J.N., P.A. Clark, K. Walter, J. Patrie, A. Weltman, and A.D. Rogol. 2000. Pubertal Alterations in Growth and Body Composition. V. Energy Expenditure, Adiposity, and Fat Distribution. *Am J Physiol—* 279:E1426–36.

Saelens, B.E. 2003. Helping Individuals Reduce Sedentary Behavior. In: *Obesity: Etiology, Assessment, Treatment and Prevention.* Edited by R.E. Andersen. Champaign, IL: Human Kinetics, pp. 217–38.

Saelens, B.E., J.F. Sallis, and L.D. Frank. 2003. Environmental Correlates of Walking and Cycling: Findings from the Transportation, Urban Design, and Planning Literature. *Ann Behav Med* 25:80–91.

Sallis, J.F., T.L. Conway, J.J. Prochaska, T.L. McKenzie, S.J. Marshall, and M. Brown. 2001. The Association of School Environments with Youth Physical Activity. *Am J Public Health* 91:618–20.

Sallis, J.F., M.F. Hovell, C.R. Hofstetter, J.P. Elder, M. Hackley, C.J. Caspersen, and K.E. Powell. 1990. Distance between Homes and Exercise Facilities Related to Frequency of Exercise among San Diego Residents. *Public Health Rep* 105:179–85.

Sallis, J.F., T.L. McKenzie, J.E. Alcaraz, B. Kolody, N. Faucette, and M.F. Hovell. 1997. The Effects of a 2–Year Physical Education Program (SPARK) on Physical Activity and Fitness in Elementary School Students. School, Play and Active Recreation for Kids. *Am J Public Health* 87:1328–34.

Sallis, J.F., T.L. McKenzie, T.L. Conway, J.P. Elder, J.J. Prochaska, M. Brown, M.M. Zive, S.J. Marshall, and J.E. Alcaraz. 2003. Environmental and Policy Interventions for Eating and Physical Activity on Middle School Campuses. *Am J Prev Med* 24:209–17.

Sallis, J.F., and N. Owen. 1999. *Physical Activity and Behavioral Medicine.* Thousand Oaks, CA: Sage.

Sallis, J.F., and N. Owen. 2002. Ecological Models of Health Behavior. In: *Health Behavior and Health Education: Theory, Research, and Practice.* Edited by K. Glanz, B.K. Rimer, and F.M. Lewis. San Francisco: Jossey-Bass, pp. 462–84.

Sallis, J.F., J.J. Prochaska, and W.C. Taylor. 2000. A Review of Correlates of Physical Activity of Children and Adolescents. *Med Sci Sports Exer* 32:963–75.

Sallis, J.F., and B.E. Saelens. 2000. Assessment of Physical Activity by Self-Report: Status, Limitations, and Future Directions. *Res Quart Exer Sport* 71(2 Suppl):S1–14.

Schmitz, K.H., D.R. Jacobs, Jr., C-P. Hong, J. Steinberger, A. Moran, and A.R. Sinaiko. 2002. Association of Physical Activity with Insulin Sensitivity in Children. *Int J Obes* 26:1310–6.

Sirard, J.R., and R.R. Pate. 2001. Physical Activity Assessment in Children and Adolescents. *Sports Med* 31:439–54.

Stewart, J.A., H.W. Kohl, J.A. Doyle, G.R. Fontaine, D. Kibbe, and B. Moore. 2002. Evaluation of Exercise Levels and Energy Expenditures Achieved during Participation in the Take 10! In-Class Physical Activity Program. *Med Sci Sports Exer* 34:S300.

Stone, E.J., T.L. McKenzie, G.J. Welk, and M.L. Booth. 1998. Effects of Physical Activity Interventions in Youth: Review and Synthesis. *Am J Prev Med* 15:298–315.

Strauss, R.S., D. Rodzilsky, G. Burack, and M. Colin. 2001. Psychosocial Correlates of Physical Activity in Healthy Children. *Arch Pediatr Adoles Med* 155:897–902.

Thomas, E.L., A.E. Brynes, J. McCarthy, A.P. Goldstone, J.V. Hajnal, N. Saeed, G. Frost, and J.D. Bell. 2000. Preferential Loss of Visceral Fat Following Aerobic Exercise, Measured by Magnetic Resonance Imaging. *Lipids* 35:769–76.

Treuth, M.S., G.R. Hunter, R. Figueroa-Colon, and M.I. Goran. 1998. Effects of Strength Training on Intra-Abdominal Adipose Tissue in Obese Prepubertal Girls. *Med Sci Sports Exer* 30:1738–43.

Trost, S.G., R.R. Pate, J.F. Sallis, P.S. Freedson, W.C. Taylor, M. Dowda, and J. Sirard. 2002. Age and Gender Differences in Objectively Measured Physical Activity in Youth. *Med Sci Sports Exer* 34:350–5.

Tudor-Locke, C., B.E. Ainsworth, and B.M. Popkin. 2001. Active Commuting to School: An Overlooked Source of Children's Physical Activity? *Sports Med* 31:309–13.

Twisk, J.W.R. 2001. Physical Activity Guidelines for Children and Adolescents: A Critical Review. *Sports Med* 31:617–27.

U.S. Department of Agriculture and U.S. Department of Health and Human Services. 2000. *Dietary Guidelines for Americans, 2000* (5th ed.). Washington, DC.

[USDHHS] U.S. Department of Health and Human Services. 1996. *Physical Activity and Health: A Report of the Surgeon General.* Atlanta, GA: U.S. Department of Health and

Human Services, Centers for Disease Control and Prevention, National Center for Chronic Disease Prevention and Health Promotion.

[USDHHS] U.S. Department of Health and Human Services. 2000. *Healthy People 2010* (017-001-00547-9). Washington, DC.

Williams, C.L., L.L. Hayman, S.R. Daniels, T.N. Robinson, J. Steinberger, S. Paridon, and T. Bazzarre. 2002. Cardiovascular Health in Childhood: A Statement for Health Professionals from the Committee on Atherosclerosis, Hypertension, and Obesity in the Young (AHOY) of the Council on Cardiovascular Disease in the Young, American Heart Association. *Circulation* 106:143–60.

PART VI

Type 2 Diabetes in Childhood and Adolescence

CHAPTER 15

The Epidemiology and Management of Type 2 Diabetes in Children and Adolescents

Eva Tsalikian and Michael Tansey

The epidemic of childhood obesity in the United States and the rest of the world over the last two or three decades is well documented (World Health Organization 1994). In recent years, there has also been a dramatic increase in the prevalence of type 2 diabetes in children and adolescents (Fagot-Campagna et al., 2000). Traditionally, diabetes in children and adolescents was considered to be of autoimmune origin known as type 1 diabetes. Diabetes of non-autoimmune origin, type 2 diabetes, has historically been thought to be present almost exclusively in overweight adults, frequently occurring later in life and associated with sedentary lifestyle and a family history of type 2 diabetes. Type 2 diabetes is most commonly found in children and adolescents from minority groups, although the incidence of diabetes is increasing in obese children of all ethnic backgrounds (Sayeed et al., 1997; Kitagawa et al., 1998).

Type 2 diabetes in adults is responsible for severe long-term complications of micro- and macroangiopathy. Cardiovascular and renal disease as well as neuropathy and retinopathy are common in adults with type 2 diabetes. Their prevalence is the result of many etiologic factors including diabetes control, genetic factors, and duration of disease. Obese children with type 2 diabetes manifest many of the metabolic changes commonly seen in adults with type 2 diabetes, such as hypertension and hyperlipidemia. The long-term implications of developing this disease at a very young age are not yet known. However, the public health implications of the increased incidence of diabetes in children and adolescents are enormous and suggest the need for much greater pressure to eliminate childhood obesity and its deleterious consequences.

DEFINITION OF DIABETES

A diagnosis of diabetes either type 1 or 2 is made if symptoms of diabetes such as polyuria, polydipsia, and fatigue are present and random plasma glucose is over 200 mg/dL. A fasting plasma glucose over 126 mg/dL is also diagnostic of diabetes, as is an oral glucose tolerance test plasma glucose over 200 mg/dL at 2 hours after glucose load. Since the most common type of diabetes in children and adolescents is of autoimmune origin (type 1), markers of this type of diabetes such as islet cell antibodies, insulin autoantibodies, and glutamic acid decarboxylase (GAD) antibodies are usually present in these children at diagnosis. In children with type 2 diabetes, however, these antibodies are not usually present. Furthermore, in type 2 diabetes, fasting and stimulated or postprandial insulin and c-peptide levels are normal or elevated, in contrast to the low levels detected in children with type 1 diabetes. Although rare in adults with type 2 diabetes, initial presentation with ketonuria or in diabetic ketoacidosis has been observed in children with type 2 diabetes.

METABOLIC SYNDROME

A common pre-type 2 diabetes syndrome that has been well-characterized in adults has now been detected in obese children and adolescents. These patients exhibit central obesity, mild dyslipidemia, hypertension, and insulin resistance with impaired glucose metabolism that has not yet resulted in hyperglycemia. This syndrome of insulin resistance has been also called *syndrome X*, or *metabolic syndrome*, and has been shown to predispose patients to the development of type 2 diabetes (Fig. 15.1). The syndrome was first described in adults with hyperinsulinemia and insulin resistance (Reaven, 1988) and this hyperinsulinemia was considered to be the etiology for the development of the other characteristics of the syndrome such as the lipid impairment and cardiovascular involvement, as in hypertension.

Although the exact mechanism for this aggregate of metabolic characteristics and their interrelationships has not yet been elucidated, recent estimates of the prevalence of this syndrome in the adult population are very high—up to 24% in the U.S. In the adolescent population examined in the National Health and Nutrition Examination Survey III (NHANES III), 30% of the overweight and 4% of all adolescents met criteria for the metabolic syndrome (Cook et al., 2003). The specific criteria for the diagnosis of the metabolic syndrome in children and adolescents have not been defined. For the purposes of the NHANES III study, the adult criteria for metabolic syndrome were modified. Even for adults

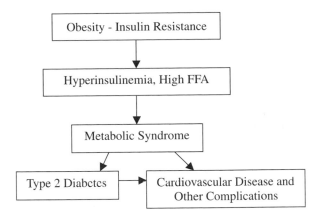

FIGURE 15.1
The sequence of events in obesity. Insulin resistance and hyperinsulinemia as well as hyperlipidemia, particularly high free fatty acids (FFA), lead to the metabolic syndrome and type 2 diabetes, and then to cardiovascular disease and other complications.

there are two sets of criteria for the metabolic syndrome those developed by the World Health Organization (WHO) and the National Cholesterol Education Program (NCEP).

The etiology of the syndrome is not known but most probably includes genetic, metabolic, and environmental factors. In children, our understanding of the metabolic syndrome is still evolving. In a multiethnic cohort of 167 obese children and adolescents given an oral glucose tolerance test, only four adolescents, all of minority descent, were diagnosed with diabetes, whereas 25% of the children (ages 4 to 10) and 21% of the adolescents (ages 11 to 18) were observed to have insulin resistance without hyperglycemia, therefore the diagnostic criteria for diabetes were not met (Sinha et al., 2002). These young individuals with impaired glucose tolerance are considered to be at high risk for the development of type 2 diabetes.

Intensive efforts are now being made in adults to secure early identification of individuals with impaired glucose tolerance and to intervene with lifestyle changes and pharmacologic agents to avoid the development of type 2 diabetes (Tuomilehto et al., 2001; Diabetes Prevention Program Research Group, 2002). It is not known whether similar intensive efforts to secure lifestyle changes would prevent the development of diabetes in obese children identified as having insulin resistance. Nevertheless, it is important that such an intervention is recommended and a diet and exercise program is in place, and only if such a program does not appear to be successful in improving metabolic parameters or if worsening is evident should a pharmacologic approach be considered. A recent study of obese adolescents with impaired glucose tolerance and family history of type 2 diabetes demonstrated improvement of fasting plasma glucose and insulin levels following treatment with metformin (Freemark and Bursey, 2001). Metformin treatment is very well tolerated by adolescents but the very long–term effects of the use of this pharmacologic agent in these young individuals is not known, particularly since we do not know at this time if the treatment will need to continue indefinitely. In addition, treatment of children for the other components of the metabolic syndrome such as dyslipidemia and hypertension that are now considered the precursors of cardiovascular disease in adults (Freedman et al., 1999) has not been adequately addressed. Lifestyle intervention is considered an appropriate approach for the management of these components of the metabolic syndrome. Therefore this should be the cornerstone of management of children with obesity, impaired glucose tolerance, and cardiovascular risk factors that constitute the entity of the metabolic syndrome.

■ EPIDEMIOLOGY OF TYPE 2 DIABETES IN CHILDREN AND ADOLESCENTS

The prevalence of type 2 diabetes in children and adolescents is on the rise (Table 15.1) in the United States (Pinhas-Hamiel et al., 1996; American Diabetes Association, 2000; Fagot-Campagna et al., 2000). Reports from Canada, Japan, Australia, New Zealand, Libya, and Bangladesh have also reported an increase in the prevalence of type 2 diabetes in children and adolescents (Owada et al., 1990; Braun et al., 1996; Harris et al., 1996; Kadiki et al., 1996; Sayeed et al., 1997; McGrath et al., 1999). In Japan, for instance, the incidence of type 2 diabetes in children increased from 7.3 to 13.9 per 100,000/year between the periods of 1976 to 1980 and 1991 to 1995 (Kitagawa et al., 1998). In the United States the prevalence of type 1 and type 2 diabetes is reported to be 4.1 per 1000 (13 diabetes cases out of 2867 12- to 19-year-olds), based on NHANES III data. The earlier NHANES II data reported 2.0 per 1000 in the same age group. In recent years, the prevalence in 15- to 19-year-old Pima Indians in Arizona was estimated to be 50.9 per 1000 (Knowler et al., 1990). This represents a dramatic increase during the last 20 years. Only six cases of type 2 diabetes were reported among Pima Indian adolescents between 1965 and 1979, however, by 1986, 120 cases had been documented, and by 1997, 201 cases had been documented (Indian Health Service, 1998).

A study examining type 2 diabetes in 10 to 19 year olds in Cincinnati, Ohio, reported that the incidence increased from 0.7 per 100,000/year in 1982 to 7.3 per 100,000/year in 1994 (Pinhas-Hamiel et al., 1996). Many other studies focusing on Caucasian (Rosenbloom et al., 1999), African-American (Willi et al., 1998), Hispanic (Haffner et al., 1990), American Indian (Knowler et al., 1993), and First Nation People groups throughout the United States and Canada (Dean, 1998) have demonstrated the increasing prevalence of type 2 diabetes in children and adolescents. Even with the documented increases, these estimates of

TABLE 15.1

Epidemiology of obesity and type 2 diabetes in children and adolescents

Study Group or Finding	Reference
Worldwide prevalence of obesity	World Health Organization, 1998; Strauss, 2002
In the United States, 22% of preschool children were overweight and 10% were obese in 2000.	Scott et al., 1997; Rocchini, 2002
The prevalence of type 2 diabetes in children and adolescents is on the rise in the United States.	Pinhas-Hamiel et al., 1996; American Diabetes Association, 2000; Fagot-Campagna et al., 2000
In the United States, the prevalence of type 1 and type 2 diabetes is reported to be 4.1 in 1000.	National Health and Nutrition Examination Survey III
The incidence of type 2 diabetes in 10- to 19-year-olds in Cincinnati, Ohio, went from 0.7 per 100,000 per year in 1982 to 7.3 per 100,000 per year in 1994	Pinhas-Hamiel et al., 1996
Prevalence in Caucasian children	Rosenbloom et al., 1999
Prevalence in African-American children	Willi et al., 1998
Prevalence in Hispanic children	Haffner et al., 1990
Prevalence in Pima Indians of Arizona	Knowler et al., 1990; Indian Health Service, 1998
Prevalence in American Indians	Knowler et al., 1993
Prevalence in First Nation People groups throughout the United States and Canada	Dean, 1998
Prevalence in countries other than the United States	Owada et al., 1990; Braun et al., 1996; Harris et al., 1996; Kadiki et al., 1996; Sayeed et al., 1997; McGrath et al., 1999; Kitagawa et al., 1998

the incidence and prevalence of type 2 diabetes in children and adolescents are likely to be underestimates because of the nonsymptomatic onset of disease and the lack of direct sequelae early in the disease process.

This dramatic increase in type 2 diabetes among children and adolescents has paralleled the dramatic increase in the prevalence of obesity in children (Scott et al., 1997). Multiple studies have shown that there is an epidemic of childhood obesity in many parts of the world (World Health Organization, 1998). This worldwide epidemic seems to be due to the higher caloric intake and the decreased activity levels of children, which in turn seem to be characteristics of many modern societies (Strauss, 2002). In children, adolescents and adults, obesity increases insulin resistance and disturbs lipid metabolism. This metabolic syndrome is a precursor of glucose intolerance and type 2 diabetes.

■ RISK FACTORS

Many studies confirm that obesity is commonly observed in children and adolescents with type 2 diabetes. For example, 96% of children and adolescents diagnosed with type 2 diabetes in a pediatric tertiary care center in Arkansas between 1988 and 1995 had a body mass index (BMI) at diagnosis that was higher than the 85th percentile for age and sex (Scott et al., 1997). As age at diagnosis increased in that cohort, the BMI percentile also increased. Obesity is also well documented as a risk factor associated with increased insulin resistance in both adults and children. Obesity, specifically visceral fat, in children and adolescents is associated with higher circulating insulin levels and decreased insulin sensitivity (Steinberger et al., 1995; Arslanian and Suprasongsin, 1996a; Caprio et al., 1996). This association has been shown in both Caucasian and African-American children and adolescents. Increased physical activity has been shown to increase insulin sensitivity. Independent of obesity, decreased physical activity in individuals of similar weight has been shown to be associated with increased insulin resistance (Folsom et al., 1996). Both obesity and decreased physical activity, therefore, create the conditions of insulin resistance that promote the development of type 2 diabetes.

The exact role of genetic factors in type 2 diabetes is not yet clear, although intensive research efforts to define precisely the role of genetics in this disease are presently under way. It is clear that family history is strongly associated with type 2 diabetes in children and adolescents. Studies have demonstrated that as many as 74% to 100% of children and adolescents with type 2 diabetes have a first- or second-degree relative with type 2 diabetes (Fagot-Campagna et al., 2000). Among Pima Indian youth the disease occurs almost exclusively in those individuals who have at least one parent with diabetes (Knowler et al., 1990). A family history of one first- or second-degree relative with the disease was present in 87% of Mexican-American children and adolescents with type 2 diabetes (Glaser, 1997). In several studies of African-American youth diagnosed with type 2 diabetes, over 95% had at least one relative with type 2 diabetes and often several generations were affected (Pinhas-Hamiel et al., 1996; Scott et al., 1997; Willi et al., 1998).

Puberty is also a risk factor for type 2 diabetes in children and adolescents. Puberty and the hormones associated with it have been shown to increase insulin resistance (Amiel et al., 1986; Cook et al., 1993; Moran et al., 1999). Most of the cases of type 2 diabetes in children are diagnosed during puberty between the ages of 12 and 14 years. Along with the sex hormones, growth hormone has been postulated to be a major factor in the insulin resistance associated with puberty. Growth hormone peaks have higher frequency and amplitude during adolescence (Hindmarsh et al., 1988).

Sex may also be a risk factor, since the prevalence of type 2 diabetes is slightly higher in adult women, and studies of adolescents also show a higher prevalence in females. Overweight adolescent females may have polycystic ovary syndrome, which is associated with an increased risk for developing type 2 diabetes because of severe hyperinsulinemia and impairment of glucose disposal in muscle and other tissues (Ehrmann et al., 1995; Legro et al., 1999). Hyperandrogenism and polycystic ovary syndrome in adolescent females may be a risk factor that accounts in part for the higher prevalence of type 2 diabetes in females than in males.

Race appears to be a risk factor for type 2 diabetes. The increased prevalence of this disease among African-Americans seems to be related to the fact that insulin sensitivity is lower in African-American children, adolescents and adults, than in Caucasian individuals of the same weight (Arslanian and Suprasongsin, 1996b; Danadian et al., 1998, 1999). Similarly, the increased incidence of type 2 diabetes in Pima Indians and Mexican-Americans seems to be related to decreased insulin sensitivity in the members of these groups. In the United States, ethnic predisposition is an important risk factor for the development of type 2 diabetes in young and older individuals alike. Nevertheless, the increased prevalence of type 2 diabetes in countries such as Japan, Libya, and Bangladesh, with racial or ethnic groups different from the groups having a predisposition to type 2 diabetes in the United States, calls into question the extent to which race or ethnicity is itself a true or significant risk factor.

■ DIAGNOSIS

The American Diabetes Association has adopted formal guidelines for identifying those individuals who should be screened for type 2 diabetes (American Diabetes Association, 2000). Individuals who are obese (BMI >85th percentile for age and sex, weight for height >85th percentile, or weight >120% of ideal body weight) and those individuals who have any other risk factor should be screened. The other risk factors include having a family history of type 2 diabetes in a first- or second-degree relative, membership in a high risk ethnic group (American Indian, African-American, Hispanic-American, Asian/South Pacific Islander), signs of insulin resistance, such as acanthosis nigricans (hyperpigmentation and thickening of skin folds around the neck and axilla), hypertension, dyslipidemia, or polycystic ovary syndrome. Children who are 10 years of age and older or pubertal should also be screened if they are obese and have at least one risk factor. These high-risk individuals continue to be at risk even if the first test is normal, and they should be screened again at 2-year intervals.

▓ TESTING FOR TYPE 2 DIABETES IN CHILDREN

A fasting plasma glucose and/or a 2-hour postprandial glucose may be used to screen for type 2 diabetes. Fasting is defined as no food or drink for at least 8 hours prior to the test. The diagnosis of diabetes in children or adolescents can be made when there are symptoms of diabetes, such as polyuria, polydipsia, weight loss and a casual or a 2-hour postprandial plasma glucose >200 mg/dL, or a fasting plasma glucose >126 mg/dL. There are only limited circumstances in which an oral glucose tolerance test is necessary for the diagnosis. If an oral glucose tolerance test is performed, the appropriate glucose load recommended for children, is 1.75 g/kg and no more than 75 g.

▓ TREATMENT OF TYPE 2 DIABETES IN CHILDREN AND ADOLESCENTS

Goals of treatment of type 2 diabetes in children and adolescents are weight control, normoglycemia, and normal HbA1c level (a measure of blood glucose control over the preceding 6- to 8-week period). The comorbidities of hypertension and hyperlipidemia should also be treated along with diabetes in children and adolescents. In adults a more aggressive approach to management of hypertension and hyperlipidemia is recommended for individuals with type 2 diabetes than that for nondiabetic individuals. It is likely that this approach would also be beneficial for adolescents with type 2 diabetes. The long-term goal of treatment is to prevent or decrease the frequency of micro and macrovascular complications of diabetes. These complications are responsible for the high diabetes morbidity and mortality observed after only a few years duration of the disease. All studies on the long-term complications of diabetes have been conducted in adults. The UK Prospective Diabetes Study (UKPDS) presented strong evidence that good control of blood sugar is associated with lower rates of microvascular complications (UKPDS Group, 1998) and a substudy of this group also showed a decrease in the cardiovascular complications in individuals with type 2 diabetes that were well controlled. The early age of onset of diabetes in children and adolescents poses a particularly difficult problem, since long-term complications are known to be directly related to duration of the disease and to hyperglycemia.

At diagnosis, type 2 diabetes in children and adolescents may present with a wide spectrum of symptoms or disease severity, from asymptomatic presentation to diabetic ketoacidosis or nonketotic coma. The latter two conditions are associated with high morbidity and mortality and should be immediately managed by medical professionals experienced with their treatment. In patients who are not ill at presentation nonpharmacologic treatment should be considered as the first and preferred treatment. Appropriate dietary intake and increased physical activity are the initial recommendations. All children and adolescents diagnosed with type 2 diabetes should receive comprehensive self-management education. Self-monitoring of blood glucose is an important part of this education. Blood glucose self-monitoring should include both fasting and postprandial blood glucose measurements with a frequency that will be determined by the health care team and will be based on the severity of disease and method of treatment. Dietary education should be done by a dietetic professional familiar and experienced with the dietary needs of children with diabetes. Dietary recommendations should be culturally appropriate, sensitive to the family resources, and provided to all caregivers. Dietary restrictions have to be very carefully implemented in a growing child. Young children need to be monitored for appropriate growth during periods of dietary restrictions. Specific recommendations for a healthy dietary intake and increased physical activity by a child or adolescent must be implemented by the family as a whole. Studies have shown that the extent of family participation in the treatment of children and adolescents with type 2 diabetes tends to accurately predict the success or failure of such treatment (Birch and Fisher, 1998).

Success in the treatment of type 2 diabetes is defined as cessation of weight gain with normal linear growth, near-normal fasting blood glucose (upper range of normal 125 mg/dL) and near-normal HbA1c (upper range of normal 6%). Some patients with type 2 diabetes may need to lose weight to achieve an appropriate BMI. If nonpharmacologic treatment is not successful, monotherapy with one of the oral hypoglycemic agents may be warranted. There are five types of pharmacologic agents that are usually prescribed for adults with type 2 diabetes. Sulfonylureas (insulin secretagogues) have been available for several decades. They have not been used in children and are not the appropriate agent because they do not address the main problem encountered in adolescent type 2 diabetes, that of insulin resistance. Glucosidase inhibitors, which usually work by slowing down absorption of carbohydrates, are usually not well tolerated by children and adolescents because of the gastrointestinal symptoms common with use of these agents.

The more recently developed insulin sensitizers come under three different categories: biguanides, meglitinide, and thiazolidinediones. Among these insulin-sensitizing agents, only metformin, one of the biguanides, is approved for adolescents over 12 years of age. Metformin is the agent most frequently prescribed for type 2 diabetes in children and adolescents and is usually well tolerated at a dose of 500 to 1500 mg daily. The action of the biguanides is manifested by decreasing hepatic glucose production and output and enhancing primarily hepatic and also muscle insulin sensitivity without direct effect on β-cell function. The American Diabetes Association recommends metformin for treatment of type 2 diabetes in children and adolescents, although rather limited evidence exists for its effectiveness and safety in young patients.

The newest insulin sensitizers available, the thiazolidinediones (TZDs), improve peripheral insulin sensitivity. One of these agents (troglitazone) has been associated with fatal hepatic failure and is not currently available. None of the rest of the TZDs has been proven safe and effective in young patients, however, studies are presently under way. If monotherapy fails to achieve the goals of normoglycemia and/or improved HbA1c, combination therapy with one of the insulin sensitizers and one of the secretagogues (promote insulin secretion, i.e., sulfonylureas) may need to follow monotherapy. However, the effectiveness and safety of these combinations of oral hypoglycemic agents in children and adolescents have not yet been investigated. Pharmacologic treatment of type 2 diabetes in children and adolescents should only be initiated in consultation with a pediatric specialist.

If during the course of treatment the patient's hyperglycemia becomes severe or the patient is symptomatic or ketotic or indicates evidence of type 1 diabetes by the presence of autoimmune markers, insulin treatment should be started. Insulin can be given in any of the therapeutic schemes that may be used for the treatment of type 1 diabetes. In addition to insulin, oral pharmacologic agents such as insulin sensitizers can be helpful.

In children and adolescents with type 2 diabetes, it is very important to treat comorbidities of hypertension and hyperlipidemia. In patients with diabetes and microalbuminuria, angiotensin-converting enzyme (ACE) inhibitors are the agents of choice for the treatment of hypertension, as they are shown to have beneficial effects in preventing diabetic nephropathy. Other agents for control of hypertension such as α blockers, calcium antagonists, and low-dose diuretics may also be used (see Chapter 10).

In children who have hyperlipidemia, weight loss, increased activity and improvement of blood glucose control often results in improvement in lipid profiles. If the above measures and added dietary modifications do not succeed in normalizing lipid profiles, bile acid–sequestering agents or HMG-CoA reductase inhibitors (statins) may be prescribed (see Chapter 7). However, statins are contraindicated during pregnancy, so adolescent females of childbearing age should be accordingly counseled.

Finally, prevention of type 2 diabetes in children and adolescents may be the best way to avoid the consequences of this disease. Guidelines for the prevention of diabetes in children should not be different from those for adults. Prevention of obesity through lifestyle changes is probably the first step in the prevention of diabetes. Lifestyle changes focusing on weight management and increasing physical activity should be promoted in all children at high risk for the development of type 2 diabetes. These changes will be most successful if the child's family incorporates them into their routine and, ideally, if the community the child lives in, including school or neighborhood, embraces them.

■ SUMMARY

- The increased prevalence of type 2 diabetes in children and adolescents may be the most serious consequence of the obesity epidemic.

• Type 2 diabetes in older adults is associated with life-limiting macro- and microvascular as well as cardiovascular and neuropathic complications.
• Most of the complications clearly depend on the duration of diabetes and glycemic control, although many other factors (e.g., genetic) appear to be involved.
• As a result, the onset of type 2 diabetes in children and adolescents creates a major public health problem for a cohort of individuals who are likely to suffer serious life-limiting complications during their mid-adulthood years.

■ REFERENCES

American Diabetes Association. 2000. Type 2 Diabetes in Children and Adolescents. *Diabetes Care* 23:381–9.

Amiel, S.A., R.S. Sherwin, D.C. Simeson, A.A. Lauritano, and W.V. Tamborlane. 1986. Impaired Insulin Action in Puberty. *N Engl J Med* 315:215–9.

Arslanian, S., and A. Suprasongsin. 1996a. Insulin Sensitivity, Lipids and Body Composition in Children: Is "Syndrome X" Present? *J Clin Endocrinol Metab* 81:1058–62.

Arslanian, S., and C. Suprasongsin. 1996b. Differences in the in vivo Insulin Secretion and Sensitivity in Healthy Black versus White Adolescents. *J Pediatr* 129:440–4.

Birch, L.L., and J.O. Fisher. 1998. Development of Eating Behaviors among Children and Adolescents. *Pediatrics* 101:539–49.

Braun, B., M.B. Zimmerman, N. Kretchmer, R.M. Spargo, R.M. Smith, and M. Gracey. 1996. Risk Factors for Diabetes and Cardiovascular Disease in Young Australian Aborigines. *Diabetes Care* 19:472–9.

Caprio, S., M. Bronson, R.S. Sherwin, F. Rife, and W.V. Tamborlane. 1996. Co-existence of Severe Insulin Resistance and Hyperinsulinemia in Preadolescent Obese Children. *Diabetologia* 39:1489–97.

Cook, J.S., R.P. Hoffman, M.A. Steine, and J.R. Hansen. 1993. Effects of Maturational Stage on Insulin Sensitivity during Puberty. *J Clin Endocrinol Metab* 77:725–30.

Cook, S., M. Weitzman, P. Auinger, M. Nguyen, and W.H. Dietz. 2003. Prevalence of a Metabolic Syndrome Phenotype in Adolescents. *Arch Pediatr Adolesc Med* 157:821–7.

Danadian, K., G. Balasekaran, V. Lewry, M. Meza, R. Robertson, and S.A. Arslanian. 1999. Insulin Sensitivity in African-American Children with and without Family History of Type 2 Diabetes. *Diabetes Care* 22:1325–9.

Danadian, K., V. Lewy, C. Suprasongsin, M. Meza, and S. Arslanian. 1998. Central Adiposity and Insulin Sensitivity in Healthy African-American Children. *Pediatr Res* 43:73A.

Dean, H. 1998 . NIDDM-Y in First Nation Children in Canada. *Clin Pediatr* 39:89–96.

Diabetes Prevention Program Research Group. 2002. Reduction in the Incidence of Type 2 Diabetes with Lifestyle Intervention or Metformin. *N Engl J Med* 346:393–403.

Ehrmann, D.A., J. Sturis, M.M. Byrne, T. Karrison, R.L. Rosenfield, and K.S. Polonsky. 1995. Insulin Secretory Defects in Polycystic Ovary Syndrome. Relationship to Insulin Sensitivity and Family History of Non-Insulin-Dependent Diabetes Mellitus. *J Clin Invest* 96:520–7.

Fagot Campagna, A., D.J. Pettitt, M.M. Engelgau, N.R. Burrows, L.S. Geiss, R. Valdez, G.L.A. Beckles, J. Saaddine, E.W. Gregg, D.F. Williamson, and K.M.V. Narayan. 2000. Type 2 Diabetes among North American Children and Adolescents: An Epidemiologic Review and a Public Health Perspective. *J Pediatr* 136:664–72.

Folsom, A.R., D.R. Jacobs, Jr., L.E. Wagenknecht, S.P. Winkhart, C. Yunis, J.E. Hilner, P.J. Savage, D.E. Smith, and J.M. Flack. 1996. Increase in Fasting Insulin and Glucose over Seven Years with Increasing Weight and Inactivity of Young Adults. The CARDIA Study. Coronary Artery Risk Development in Young Adults. *Am J Epidemiol* 144:235–46.

Freedman, D.S., W.H. Dietz, S.R. Srinivasan, and G.S. Berenson. 1999. The Relation of Overweight to Cardiovascular Risk Factors among Children and Adolescents: The Bogalusa Heart Study. *Pediatrics* 103:1175–82.

Freemark, M., and D. Bursey. 2001. The Effects of Metformin on Body Mass Index and Glucose Tolerance in Obese Adolescents with Fasting Hyperinsulinemia and a Family History of Type 2 Diabetes. *Pediatrics* 107:E55.

Glaser, N.S. 1997. Non-Insulin-Dependent Diabetes Mellitus in Childhood and Adolescence. *Pediatr Clin North Am* 44:307–37.

Haffner, S.M., M.P. Stern, B.D. Mitchell, H.P. Hazuda, and J.K. Patterson. 1990. Incidence of Type II Diabetes in Mexican Americans Predicted by Fasting Insulin and Glucose Levels, Obesity and Body Fat Distribution. *Diabetes* 39:283–8.

Harris, S.B., B.A. Perkins, and E. Whalen-Brough. 1996. Non-Insulin-Dependent Diabetes Mellitus among First Nations Children. *Can Fam Phys* 42:869–76.

Hindmarsh, P., L. Di Silvio, P.J. Pringle, A.B. Kurtz, and C.G.D. Brook. 1988. Changes in Serum Insulin Concentration during Puberty and Their Relationship to Growth Hormone. *Clin Endocrinol* 28:381–8.

Indian Health Service. 1998. Trends in Indian Health. Rockville, MD: U.S. Department of Health and Human Services, Indian Health Service, Office of Planning, Evaluation, and Legislation, Division of Program Statistics.

Kadiki, O.A., M.R.S. Reddy, and A.A. Marzouk. 1996. Incidence of Insulin-Dependent Diabetes (IDDM) and Non-Insulin Dependent Diabetes (NIDDM) (0–34 Years at Onset) in Benghazi, Libya. *Diabetes Res Clin Pract* 32:165–73.

Kitagawa, T., M. Owada, T. Urakami, and K. Yamauchi. 1998. Increased Incidence of Non-Insulin-Dependent Diabetes Mellitus among Japanese Schoolchildren Correlates with an Increased Intake of Animal Protein and Fat. *Clin Pediatr* 37:111–5.

Knowler, W.C., D.J. Pettitt, M.F. Saad, and P.H. Bennett. 1990. Diabetes Mellitus in the Pima Indians: Incidence, Risk Factors and Pathogenesis. *Diabetes Metab Rev* 6:1–27.

Knowler, W.C., M.F. Saad, D.J. Pettitt, R.G. Nelson, and P.H. Bennett. 1993. Determinants of Diabetes Mellitus in the Pima Indians. *Diabetes Care* 16:216–27.

Legro, R.S., A.R. Kunselman, W.C. Dodson, and A. Dundaif. 1999. Prevalence and Predictors of Risk for Type 2 Diabetes Mellitus and Impaired Glucose Tolerance in Polycystic Ovary Syndrome: A Prospective, Controlled Study in 254 Affected Women. *J Clin Endocrinol Metab* 84:165–9.

McGrath, N.M., G.N. Parker, and P. Dawson. 1999. Early Presentation of Type 2 Diabetes Mellitus in Young New Zealand Maori. *Diabetes Res Clin Pract* 43:205–9.

Moran, A., D.R. Jacobs, Jr., J. Steinberger, C-P. Hong, R. Prineas, R. Luepker, and A.R. Sinaiko. 1999. Insulin Resistance during Puberty. *Diabetes* 48:2039–44.

Owada, M., Y. Hanaoka, Y. Tanimoto, and T. Kitagawa. 1990. Descriptive Epidemiology of Non-Insulin-Dependent Diabetes Mellitus Detected by Urine Glucose Screening in School Children in Japan. *Acta Paediatr Jpn* 32:716–24.

Pinhas-Hamiel, O., L.M. Dolan, S.R. Daniels, D. Standiford, P.R. Khoury, and P. Zeitler. 1996. Increased Incidence of Non-Insulin-Dependent Diabetes Mellitus among Adolescents. *J Pediatr* 128:608–15.

Reaven, G.M. 1988. Banting Lecture 1988: Role of Insulin Resistance in Human Disease. *Diabetes* 37:1595–1607.

Rocchini, A.P. 2002. Childhood Obesity and a Diabetes Epidemic. *N Engl J Med* 346:854–5.

Rosenbloom, A.L., J.R. Joe, R.S. Young, and W.E. Winter. 1999. Emerging Epidemic of Type 2 Diabetes in Youth. *Diabetes Care* 22:345–54.

Sayeed, M.A., M.Z. Hussain, A. Banu, M.A.K. Rumi, and A.K.A. Khan. 1997. Prevalence of Diabetes in a Suburban Population of Bangladesh. *Diabetes Res Clin Pract* 34:149–55.

Scott, C.R., J.M. Smith, M.M. Cradock, and C. Pihoker. 1997. Characteristics of Youth-onset Non-Insulin-Dependent Diabetes Mellitus and Insulin-Dependent Diabetes Mellitus at Diagnosis. *Pediatrics* 100:84–91.

Sinha, R., G. Fisch, B. Teague, W.V. Tamborlane, B. Banyas, K. Allen, M. Savoye, V. Rieger, S. Taksali, G. Barbetta, R.S. Sherwin, and S. Caprio. 2002. Prevalence of Impaired Glucose Tolerance among Children and Adolescents with Marked Obesity. *N Engl J Med* 346:802–10.

Steinberger, J., C. Moorehead, V. Katch, and A.P. Rocchini. 1995. Relationship between Insulin Resistance and Abnormal Lipid Profile in Obese Adolescents. *J Pediatr* 126:690–5.

Strauss, R.S. 2002. Childhood Obesity. *Pediatr Clin North Am* 49:175–201.

Tuomilehto, J., J. Lindstrom, J.G. Eriksson, T.T. Valle, H. Hamalainen, P. Ilanne-Parikka, S. Keinanen-Kiukaanniemi, M. Laakso, A. Louheranta, M. Rastas, V. Salminen, and M. Uusitupa. 2001. Prevention of Type 2 Diabetes Mellitus by Changes in Lifestyle among Subjects with Impaired Glucose Tolerance. *N Engl J Med* 344:1343–50.

UKPDS Group. 1998. Intensive Blood Glucose Control with Sulphonylureas or Insulin Compared with Conventional Treatment and Risk of Complications in Patients with Type 2 Diabetes (UKPDS 33). *Lancet* 352:837–53.

Willi, S.M., A. Kennedy, B. Wojciechowski, and T. Garvey. 1998. Insulin Resistance and Defective Glucose Insulin Coupling in Ketosis-Prone Type 2 Diabetes in African-Americans. *Diabetes* 47:A306.

World Health Organization. 1994. *Prevention of Diabetes Mellitus*. Geneva: World Health Organization.

World Health Organization. 1998. *Obesity: Preventing and Managing the Global Epidemic*. Geneva: World Health Organization.

PART VII

Smoking Prevention and Cessation among Youth

CHAPTER 16

Prevalence of and Risk Factors for Cigarette Smoking among Youth

Cynthia M. Goody, John B. Lowe, Mary Lober Aquilino, and Esther M. Baker

Every day, more than 2000 young people under the age of 18 become regular smokers (Substance Abuse and Mental Health Services Administration [SAMHSA], 2003). In fact, over 80% of adult smokers begin using cigarettes during their teen years (Centers for Disease Control and Prevention [CDC], 2004a). Smoking is associated with significant health consequences in the adolescent and young adult years including respiratory problems, cardiovascular disease, substance abuse, and mental disorders (U.S. Department of Health and Human Services [USDHHS], 1994). Adolescent smokers report increased coughing, wheezing, shortness of breath, and sputum production. They experience more respiratory infections that last longer and are more severe than youth who do not smoke. Lung function is diminished and atherosclerotic lesions have been noted in deceased smokers as young as 15 years of age (USDHHS, 1994; also see Chapter 1). Serum lipid profiles indicate increased low-density lipoprotein cholesterol and decreased high-density lipoprotein cholesterol levels in youth who smoke (USDHHS, 1994). Adolescent smokers are also more likely to use other drugs than nonsmokers (Myers, 1999; Jacobsen et al., 2001). They are three times more likely than nonsmokers to use alcohol, eight times more likely to use marijuana, and 22 times more likely to use cocaine. Smoking is also associated with poor general health and may be a marker for underlying mental health problems such as depression (USDHHS, 1994). Additional health problems, including chronic obstructive pulmonary disease, heart disease, stroke, and lung cancer, tend to be manifested in future decades (Breslau and Peterson, 1996; Chassin et al., 1996; Chen and Millar, 1998;

Skurnik and Shoenfeld, 1998). Coronary heart disease and stroke are the first and third leading causes of death in the United States, and are the primary types of cardiovascular disease caused by smoking (USDHHS, 2004). Over one-third of the more than 440,000 smoking-related deaths that occur in the United States each year involve cardiovascular disease (CDC, 2002). Chronic obstructive pulmonary disease is the fourth leading cause of death in the United States, resulting in more than 118,000 deaths per year. Smoking is the cause of approximately 90% of all deaths due to chronic obstructive pulmonary disease (USDHHS, 2004).

Regular cigarette smoking inflicts significant health burdens on individuals and society. Given current smoking trends among youth, about 5 million of today's teens, or one-third of children who become regular smokers, will die prematurely from a disease attributed to smoking (CDC, 1996). In fact, smoking kills more people annually than AIDS, alcohol, drug abuse, auto accidents, murders, suicides, and fires combined (CDC, 2004b). These figures become even more disturbing when one takes into account that smoking-related disease and death are preventable.

Current cigarette smoking trends among youth will affect the future health of individuals and communities. This chapter discusses two sets of factors influencing the prevalence of cigarette smoking and the trends related to the initiation of youth cigarette smoking. First, demographic (nonmodifiable) factors that influence the prevalence of youth smoking will be briefly outlined. Second, modifiable risk factors (social and environmental) or concomitant behaviors that also contribute to youth smoking prevalence will be discussed. An understanding of these risk factors will aid health professionals in developing prevention and treatment programs to assist youth who use cigarettes and may desire to quit smoking.

▪ PREVALENCE OF SMOKING BY HIGH SCHOOL STUDENTS

Overall, about one in five students in high school are current smokers, defined as a student who has had a cigarette in the past 30 days. While 6 in 10 students have experimented with tobacco on an occasional basis, less than half are never smokers (Table 16.1). Many of these students experimenting with tobacco believe they can control the use and the addiction until a time after high school. Unfortunately, this does not seem to be the case for many as they go on to become daily smokers—that is, smoking at least one cigarette every day in the past 30 days.

▪ NONMODIFIABLE RISK FACTORS

Use of cigarettes during the high school years varies considerably by age and grade level, sex, and race/ethnicity (Tables 16.2 and 16.3). Socioeconomic status is also associated with youth smoking.

TABLE 16.1
Prevalence of youth cigarette smoking, grades
9–12 in the United States, Youth Risk Behavior
Surveillance System, 2003

Category	%
Never smoker	41.6
Ever smoker[*]	58.4
Current smoker[†]	21.9
Current frequent smoker[‡]	9.7
Daily smoker[**]	15.8

[*]Ever tried cigarette smoking, even one or two puffs.
[†]Smoked cigarettes on at least 1 of the 30 days preceding the survey.
[‡]Smoked cigarettes on at least 20 of the 30 days preceding the survey.
[**]Smoked one or more cigarettes every day for 30 days.
Source: CDC (2004c).

Age and Grade Level

Age or grade level is a key variable influencing the initiation of cigarette smoking (Table 16.2). During the period from 1991 to 2003, overall smoking prevalence among high school students declined from 27.5% to 21.9%. The onset of smoking increases with grade level to 12th grade (CDC, 2004c).

Sex

Data from the Youth Risk Behavior Surveillance System (YRBSS) (CDC, 2003) suggest that while there was once a sex differential in smoking rates for males and females during middle school, rates are now similar at both the middle school and high school levels. However, young females and males tend to differ in their reasons for smoking cigarettes. One study indicates that both young males and females view the act of smoking cigarettes positively (Lewis et al., 2001) while other studies suggest that a positive image is more predictable among boys than girls (Dinh et al., 1995; Skara et al., 2001; Soldz and Cui, 2001). Pierce et al. (1993) concluded that boys expected more benefits from smoking than did girls, and that the relationship between the expected number of benefits and susceptibility to smoking was stronger among boys than among girls.

TABLE 16.2

Percentage of high school students who ever used cigarettes, currently smoked, or were daily smokers, by grade and sex, Youth Risk Behavior Surveillance System, 2003

	9th Grade			10th Grade			11th Grade			12th Grade		
Category	M	F	T	M	F	T	M	F	T	M	F	T
Ever smoker*	53.0	50.9	50.2	59.0	57.7	58.3	60.1	59.8	60.0	64.7	65.9	65.4
Current smoker[†]	16.0	18.9	17.4	21.7	21.9	21.8	23.2	24.0	23.6	29.0	23.3	26.2
Daily smoker[‡]	11.4	11.6	11.5	14.3	15.8	15.0	17.8	18.4	18.1	21.0	18.3	19.8

F, females; M, males; T, total.

*Ever tried cigarette smoking, even one or two puffs.

[†]Smoked cigarettes on at least 1 of the 30 days preceding the survey.

[‡]Ever smoked one or more cigarettes every day for 30 days.

Source: CDC (2004).

TABLE 16.3

Trends in percentage of high school students who reported current smoking* by sex and race/ethnicity, Youth Risk Behavior Surveillance System, United States, 1991–2003

Category	1991	1993	1995	1997	1999	2001	2003
Current	27.5	30.5	34.8	36.4	34.8	28.5	21.9
Sex							
Females	27.3	31.2	34.3	34.7	34.9	27.7	21.9
Males	27.6	29.8	35.4	37.7	34.7	29.2	21.8
Race/Ethnicity							
White, non-Hispanic	30.9	33.7	38.3	39.7	38.6	31.9	24.9
Females	31.7	35.3	39.8	39.9	39.1	31.2	26.6
Males	30.2	32.2	37.0	39.6	38.2	32.7	23.3
Black, non-Hispanic	12.6	15.4	19.2	22.7	19.7	14.7	15.1
Females	11.3	14.4	12.2	17.4	17.7	13.3	10.8
Males	14.1	16.3	27.8	28.2	21.8	16.3	19.3
Hispanic	25.3	28.7	34.0	34.0	32.7	26.6	18.4
Females	22.9	27.3	32.9	32.3	31.5	26.0	17.7
Males	27.9	30.2	34.9	35.5	34.0	27.2	19.1

*Smoked cigarettes on at least 1 of the 30 days preceding the survey.
Source: CDC (2004d).

Race/Ethnicity

Well-documented differences exist in the cigarette smoking practices of youth from varying racial and ethnic backgrounds. From 1991 to 2003, white, non-Hispanic (white), high school males reported the highest current cigarette use and black, non-Hispanic (black) high school females reported the lowest rate (CDC, 2004d) (Table 16.3). While the prevalence of cigarette smoking among black and white adolescents has increased, the rate has remained consistently lower among black adolescents than their white or Hispanic counterparts (Faulkner and Merritt, 1998; CDC, 2003, 2004c). The National Survey Results on Drug Abuse suggests that white youth have the highest rate of cigarette smoking (39.7%), followed by Hispanics (34%) and blacks (22.7%) (Johnston et al., 1999). Further, the National Youth Tobacco Survey (NYTS) and YRBSS data indicate that black, Hispanic, and white middle school students smoke less than their high school counterparts (CDC, 2003, 2004c; American Legacy Foundation, 2004).

By stages of cigarette use for 12th grade students, Flay et al. (1998) found that black 12th grade students were more likely to remain never-users (59.6%); white 12th grade students were more likely to be regular smokers (18.4%); and white and Hispanic 12th grade students were more likely to be experimenters (34.6% and 36.1%, respectively). No significant differences existed among these three race/ethnicity groups in terms of the percentage of students in the 12th grade who had ever used cigarettes.

When examining cigarette use by race and sex, the YRBSS data (CDC, 2004c) indicate that at the high school level, Hispanic males had the highest use in the categories of lifetime cigarette use and current cigarette use, white males had the highest use among current users, and black females had the lowest use across all categories of cigarette use. For all race and sex groups, the highest percentage of cigarette use occurred in the ever-used-cigarettes category. Beyond this for all race and sex groups, a lower percentage of cigarette use occurred in the currently smoked-cigarettes and daily-cigarette-use categories (Table 16.3).

■ Socioeconomic Status

Evidence suggests that low socioeconomic status increases youth risk for smoking. Conrad et al. (1992) noted from 11 studies that smoking initiation was substantially more likely among youth from a low socioeconomic background than among youth with middle to high socioeconomic background. Other studies have suggested that low socioeconomic status places girls at a higher risk than boys for smoking cigarettes (Chassin et al., 1992). Harrell et al. (1998) followed youth from the third and fourth grades through the eighth and ninth grades and found that adolescents from low socioeconomic backgrounds were more likely to experiment with cigarette smoking and to smoke cigarettes. They also noted that white youth as well as youth from low socioeconomic backgrounds were more likely to experiment with cigarettes.

■ MODIFIABLE RISK FACTORS

Researchers attribute smoking initiation and continuation of smoking by youth to a multitude of interconnected behavioral, social and environmental factors. These include poor scholastic achievement, peers, parental modeling and expectations, depression and low self-esteem, substance abuse, and physical inactivity.

■ Scholastic Achievement

Students with below-average performances in school, regardless of gender, are more likely than the better than average students to be current or former cigarette users (Hu et al., 1998). Predictors of cigarette smoking for girls include performance on reading tests and for boys, grade point average (Brunswick and Messeri, 1984).

Using the longitudinal data from the Teenage Attitudes and Practices Survey (TAPS, 1989–1993), Distefan et al. (1998) found that youth with average or below-average school performance at baseline were 1.34 (95% CI 1.11–1.63) times more likely to have ever tried cigarettes at follow-up as those with above-average scholastic performance. Youth with below-average school performance were 1.68 (95% CI 1.14–2.48) times more likely to transition from experimentation to established smoking compared to their counterparts with above-average academic performance. Some studies indicate that girls' commitment to school is higher than that of boys and that lack of commitment increases the incidence of cigarette smoking (Chassin et al., 1984; Waldron et al., 1991).

Adolescents' lack of commitment to scholastic obligations corresponds to youths' onset and progression of cigarette smoking (Conrad et al., 1992). In one longitudinal study, investigators found no gender-specific differences in the effect while other studies suggested that commitment to school affects girls more strongly than it affects boys (Hibbett and Fogelman, 1990; Waldron et al., 1991; Skinner and Krohn, 1992). Because of conflicting findings, no conclusion can be drawn about the gender-specific differences related to commitment to scholastic achievement and youth cigarette smoking.

Peers

Adolescents who smoke influence their peers to use cigarettes (Meijer et al., 1996; Gritz et al., 1998). Peer smoking was predictive of some phase of smoking in all but 1 (Newcomb et al., 1989) of 16 longitudinal studies reviewed by Conrad et al. (1992). Adolescents who had close friendships with others who smoked or had involvement with peers who smoked were more likely to experiment with or use cigarettes regularly (Pierce et al., 1993). Girls may be more influenced by peer smoking than boys (Pirie et al., 1991; Waldron et al., 1991). Further, results from Flay et al. (1998) suggest that friends' smoking significantly predicts experimental and regular cigarette use for both males and females. Friends' smoking also predicted youths' experimentation with cigarettes, but only among females.

Parental Modeling and Expectations

Youth are about two times more likely to smoke if one or both parents engage in cigarette smoking (Green et al., 1991; Conrad et al., 1992; Jackson and Henriksen, 1997). However, Distefan et al. (1998) found that smoking status of parents did not influence teens' experimentation with or regular use of cigarettes. This finding might reflect differing parental attitudes and behavior toward their child smoking. When adolescents perceived parental attitudes toward smoking as positive, teen cigarette smoking increased (Wang et al.,

1996; Jackson and Henriksen, 1997). Parental approval of adolescent cigarette smoking contributed to increased experimentation with and regular use of cigarettes among youth (Palmer, 1970; Hunter et al., 1982). Several studies determined that parental demands prompted adolescents not to smoke (Kandel and Wu, 1995; Chassin et al., 1998). Specific practices such as parent—child discussion of smoking, punishment for using cigarettes, and rules against adolescent smoking influence youth to smoke less (Kandel and Wu, 1995; Noland et al., 1996; Jackson and Henriksen, 1997; Chassin et al., 1998). Importantly, adolescents are about one-third less likely to use cigarettes when their parents stopped smoking (Farkas et al., 1999).

Depression and Low Self-Esteem

Adolescents with low self-esteem may be more likely to begin smoking cigarettes, especially if they believe such an action will enhance their image. In some longitudinal studies, adolescents with low self-esteem were more likely than those with high self-esteem to initiate cigarette smoking in the next year (Ahlgren et al., 1982; Simon et al., 1995). Other longitudinal studies observed no relationship between low-self esteem and the initiation of cigarette smoking (Brunswick and Messeri, 1983–1984; Winefield et al., 1992).

Best et al. (1995) noted that girls who scored high on personal dissatisfaction were more likely to smoke than girls who appeared to be more satisfied. This relationship between personal dissatisfaction and cigarette smoking was not observed in boys. Similar findings from another study suggested that self-esteem might be a factor in smoking behavior among middle school girls, but not among boys in any grade (Abernathy et al., 1995). Feelings of sadness, euphoria or depression among adolescents may be a consequence of smoking. In one study, girls were no more likely than boys to smoke for relief from problems and to control negative feelings (Novacek et al., 1991). Further supporting this are findings from a study suggesting that teenage girls of all ages and younger teenage boys who smoke do so to cope with anxiety and depression (Patton et al., 1996).

Substance Abuse

The 2002 National Household Survey on Drug Abuse, conducted among adolescents age 12 through 17 years, indicates that youth who use drugs, including alcohol, are much more likely to smoke cigarettes (SAMHSA, 2003). Whether tobacco or other drugs provide the gateway to expanded substance abuse has not been determined. Data from the National Health Interview Survey indicate that smoking aggregates with binge drinking and marijuana use among black, Hispanic, and white males and females (Escobedo et al., 1997).

Physical Activity

Involvement in physical activities may divert adolescents' attention away from cigarette smoking. Researchers have consistently reported that adolescents who are less active are more likely to be smokers than those who are more active (Escobedo et al., 1993; Winnail et al., 1995; Davis et al., 1997). The number of sports a student plays is inversely related to the chances of being a smoker (Escobedo et al., 1993; Davis et al., 1997). Winnail et al. (1995) support World Health Organization findings suggesting that a high level of physical activity may protect against cigarette use.

SUMMARY

- Over one-half of high school students have ever tried cigarettes.
- Cigarette use during adolescence varies with age, sex, and race/ethnicity. During the teen years, the prevalence of smoking increases with age for both females and males.
- Hispanic and white students at the high school level have a higher prevalence of cigarette smoking than black students at the same level.
- Many interconnected factors, behaviors, and predictors contribute to smoking initiation and continuation during adolescence. The concomitant behaviors and predictors attributed to youth cigarette smoking include poor scholastic achievement, peers, parental modeling and expectations, depression and low self-esteem, substance abuse, and physical activity.
- The evidence-based research about the patterns and determinants of cigarette smoking among youth may assist health professionals in developing prevention and treatment programs for youth who smoke cigarettes. Continued efforts of examining cigarette smoking among youth will promote further understanding of numerous ever-changing factors, suggest issues for future research, and guide decision makers in the policy arena as they attempt to reduce the burden of tobacco use.

REFERENCES

Abernathy, T., L. Massad, and L. Romano-Dwyer. 1995. The Relationship between Smoking and Self-Esteem. *Adolescence* 30:899–907.

Ahlgren, A., A.A. Norem, M. Hochhauser, and J. Garvin. 1982. Antecedents of Smoking among Pre-Adolescents. *J Drug Educ* 12:325–40.

American Legacy Foundation. 2004. *Cigarette Smoking Among Youth: Results from the 2002 National Youth Tobacco Survey.* Retrieved January 2006, from http://www.americanlegacy .org/americanlegacy/skins/alf/home.aspx.

Best, J.A., K.S. Brown, R. Cameron, S.M. Manske, and S. Santi. 1995. Gender and Predisposing Attributes as Predictors of Smoking Onset: Implications for Theory and Practice. *J Health Educ* 26(Suppl 2):S52–S60.

Breslau, N., and E.L. Peterson. 1996. Smoking Cessation in Young Adults: Age of Initiation of Cigarette Smoking and Other Suspected Influences. *Am J Public Health* 86:214–20.

Brunswick, A.F., and P.A. Messeri. 1983—1984. Causal Factors in Onset of Adolescents' Cigarette Smoking: A Prospective Study of Urban Black Youth. *Adv Alcohol Subst Abuse* 3:35–52.

Brunswick, A.F., and P.A. Messeri. 1984. Origins of Cigarette Smoking in Academic Achievement, Stress, and Social Expectations: Does Gender Make a Difference? *J Early Adolesc* 4:353–70.

[CDC] Centers for Disease Control and Prevention. 1996. Projected Smoking-Related Deaths among Youth—United States. *Morb Mortal Wkly Rep* 45:1971–4.

[CDC] Centers for Disease Control and Prevention. 2002. Annual Smoking-Attributable Mortality, Years of Potential Life Lost, and Economic Costs-United States, 1995–1999. *Morb Mortal Wkly Rep* 51:300–3.

[CDC] Centers for Disease Control and Prevention. 2003. Tobacco Use among Middle School and High School Students—United States, 2002. *Morb Mortal Wkly Rep* 52: 1096–8.

[CDC] Centers for Disease Control and Prevention. 2004a. Tobacco Information and Prevention Source. Retrieved January 2006, from http://www.cdc.gov/tobacco/issue.htm

[CDC] Centers for Disease Control and Prevention. 2004b. Tobacco-Related Mortality. Retrieved January 2006, from http://www.cdc.gov/tobacco/factsheets/Tobacco_Related_Mortality_factsheet.htm

[CDC] Centers for Disease Control and Prevention. 2004c. Youth Risk Behavior Surveillance—United States, 2003. *Morb Mortal Wkly Rep* 53(No.SS-2):1–100.

[CDC] Centers for Disease Control and Prevention. 2004d. Cigarette Use among High School Students—United States, 1991–2003. *Morb Mortal Wkly Rep* 53:499–502.

Chassin, L., C. Clark, S.J. Presson, E. Corty, and R.W. Olshavsky. 1984. Predicting the Onset of Cigarette Smoking in Adolescents: A Longitudinal Study. *J Appl Soc Psychol* 14:224–43.

Chassin, L., C.C. Presson, J.S. Rose, and S.J. Sherman. 1996. The Natural History of Cigarette Smoking from Adolescence to Adulthood: Demographic Predictors of Continuity and Change. *Health Psychol* 15: 478–84.

Chassin, L., C.C. Presson, S.J. Sherman, and D.A. Edwards. 1992. Parent Education Attainment and Adolescent Cigarette Smoking. *J Subst Abuse* 4:219–34.

Chassin, L., C.C. Presson, M. Todd, J.S. Rose, and S.J. Sherman. 1998. Maternal Socialization of Adolescent Smoking: The Intergenerational Transmission of Parenting and Smoking. *Dev Psychol* 34:1189–201.

Chen, J. and W.J. Millar. 1998. Age of Smoking Initiation: Implications for Quitting. *Health Rep* 9:39–46.

Conrad, K.M., B.R. Flay, and D. Hill. 1992. Why Children Start Smoking Cigarettes: Predictors of Onset. *Br J Addict* 87:1711–24.

Davis, T.C., C. Arnold, I. Nandy, J.A. Bocchini, A. Gottlieb, R.B. George, and H. Berkel. 1997. Tobacco Use among Male High School Athletes. *J Adolesc Health* 21:97–101.

Dinh, K.T., I.G. Sarason, A.V. Peterson, and L.E. Onstad. 1995. Children's Perceptions of Smokers and Nonsmokers: A Longitudinal Study. *Health Psychol* 14:32–40.

Distefan, J.M.. E.A. Gilpin. W.S. Choi, and J.P. Pierce. 1998. Parental Influences Predict Adolescent Smoking in the United States, 1989–1993. *J Adolesc Health* 22:466–74.

Escobedo, L.G., S.E. Marcus, D. Holtzman, and G.A. Giovino. 1993. Sports Participation, Age at Smoking Initiation, and the Risk of Smoking among US High School Students. *JAMA* 269:1391–5.

Escobedo, L.G., M. Reddy, and R.H. DuRant. 1997. Relationship between Cigarette Smoking and Health Risk and Problem Behaviors among US Adolescents. *Arch Pediatr Adolesc Med* 151:66–71.

Farkas, A.J., J.M. Distefan, W.S. Choi, E.A. Gilpin, and J.P. Pierce. 1999. Does Parental Smoking Cessation Discourage Adolescent Smoking? *Prev Med* 28:213–8.

Faulkner, D.L., and R.K. Merritt. 1998. Race and Cigarette Smoking among United States Adolescents: The Role of Lifestyle Behaviors and Demographic Factors. *Pediatrics* 101:E4.

Flay, B.R., F.B. Hu, and J. Richardson. 1998. Psychosocial Predictors of Different Stages of Cigarette Smoking among High School Students. *Prev Med* 27:A9–A18.

Green, G., S. Macintyre, P. West, and R. Ecob. 1991. Like Parent Like Child? Associations between Drinking and Smoking Behavior of Parents and Their Children. *Br J Addict* 86:745–58.

Gritz, E.R., A.V. Prokhorov, K.S. Hudmon, R.M. Chamberlain, W.C. Taylor, C.C. DiClemente, D.A. Johnston, S. Hu, L.A. Jones, M.M. Jones, C.K. Rosenblum, C.L. Ayars, and C.I. Amos. 1998. Cigarette Smoking in a Multiethnic Population of Youth: Methods and Baseline Findings. *Prev Med* 27:365–84.

Harrell, J.S., S.I. Bangdiwalam, S. Deng, J. Webb, and C. Bradley. 1998. Smoking Initiation in Youth. *J Adolesc Health* 23:271–9.

Hibbett, A., and K. Fogelman. 1990. Future Lives of Truants: Family Formation and Health-Related Behaviour. *Br J Educ Psychol* 60:171–9.

Hu, T., Z. Lin, and T.E. Keeler. 1998. Teenage Smoking, Attempts to Quit, and School Performance. *Am J Public Health* 88:940–3.

Hunter, S.M., J.G. Baugh, L.S. Webber, M.C. Sklov, and G.S. Berenson. 1982. Social Learning Effects on Trial and Adoption of Cigarette Smoking in Children: The Bogalusa Heart Study. *Prev Med* 11:29–42.

Jackson, C. and L. Henriksen. 1997. Do as I Say: Parent Smoking, Antismoking Socialization, and Smoking Onset in Children. *Addict Behav* 22:107–14.

Jacobson, P.D., P.M. Lantz, K.E. Warner, J. Wasserman, H.A. Pollack, and A.K. Ahlstrom. 2001. *Combating Teen Smoking: Research and Policy Strategies.* Ann Arbor: University of Michigan Press.

Johnston, L.D., P.M. O'Malley, and J.G. Bachman. 1999. National Survey Results on Drug Abuse: The Monitoring the Future Study, 1975–1998. Rockville, MD: National Institute on Drug Abuse, NIH Publication 98–4346.

Kandel, D.B., and P. Wu. 1995. The Contribution of Mothers and Fathers to the Intergenerational Transmission of Cigarette Smoking in Adolescence. *J Res Adolesc* 5:225–52.

Lewis, P.C., J.S. Harrell, C. Bradley, and S. Deng. 2001. Cigarette Use in Adolescents: The Cardiovascular Health in Children and Youth Study. *Res Nurs Health* 24:27–37.

Meijer, B., D. Branski, K. Knol, and E. Kerem. 1996. Cigarette Smoking Habits among Schoolchildren. *Chest* 110:921–6.

Myers, M.G. 1999. Smoking Intervention with Adolescent Substance Abusers: Initial Recommendations. *J Subst Abuse Treat* 16:289–98.

Newcomb, M.D., W.J. McCarthy, and P.M. Bentler. 1989. Cigarette Smoking, Academic Lifestyle, and Social Impact Efficacy: An Eight-Year Study from Early Adolescence to Young Adulthood. *J Appl Soc Psychol* 19:251–81.

Noland, M.P., R.J. Kryscio, J. Hinkle, R.S. Riggs, L.H. Linville, V.Y. Ford, and T.C. Tucker. 1996. Relationship of Personal Tobacco-Raising, Parental Smoking and Other Factors to Tobacco Use among Adolescents Living in a Tobacco-Producing Region. *Addict Behav* 21:349–61.

Novacek, J., R. Raskin, and R. Hogan. 1991. Why Do Adolescents Use Drugs? Age, Sex, and User Differences. *J Youth Adolesc* 20:475–92.

Palmer, A.B. 1970. Some Variables Contributing to the Onset of Cigarette Smoking among Junior High School Students. *Soc Sci Med* 4:359–66.

Patton, G.C., M. Hibbert, M.J. Rosier, J.B. Carlin, J. Caust, and G. Bowes. 1996. Is Smoking Associated with Depression and Anxiety in Teenagers? *Am J Public Health* 86:225–30.

Pierce, J., A. Farkas, N. Evans, C. Barry, W. Choi, B. Rosbrook, M. Johnson, and D.G. Bal. 1993. Tobacco Use in California 1992: A Focus on Preventing Uptake in Adolescents. Sacramento, CA: California Department of Health Services.

Pirie, P.L., D.M. Murray, and R.V. Luepker. 1991. Gender Differences in Cigarette Smoking and Quitting in a Cohort of Young Adults. *Am J Public Health* 81:324–7.

Simon, T.R., S. Sussman, C.W. Dent, D. Burton, and B.R. Flay. 1995. Prospective Correlates of Exclusive or Combined Adolescent Use of Cigarettes and Smokeless Tobacco: A Replication-Extension. *Addict Behav* 20:517–24.

Skara, S., S. Sussman, and C.W. Dent. 2001. Predicting Regular Cigarette Use among Continuation High School Students. *Am J Health Behav* 25:147–56.

Skinner, W.F., and M.D. Krohn. 1992. Age and Gender Differences in a Social Process Model of Adolescent Cigarette Use. *Sociol Inq* 62:56–82.

Skurnik, Y., and Y. Schoenfeld. 1998. Health Effects of Cigarette Smoking. *Clin Dermatol* 16:545–56.

Soldz, S., and X. Cui. 2001. A Risk Factor Index Predicting Adolescent Cigarette Smoking: A 7-Year Longitudinal Study. *Psychol Addict Behav* 15: 33–41.

[SAMHSA] Substance Abuse and Mental Health Services Administration. 2003. Results from the 2002 National Survey on Drug Use and Health: National Findings. Rockville, MD: Office of Applied Studies. NHSDA Series H-22, DHHS Publication No. SMA 03–3836.

[USDHHS] U.S. Department of Health and Human Services. 1994. *Preventing Tobacco Use Among Young People: A Report of the Surgeon General.* Atlanta, GA: U.S. Department of Health and Human Services, Public Health Service, Centers for Disease Control and Prevention, National Center for Chronic Disease Prevention and Health Promotion, Office on Smoking and Health.

[USDHHS] U.S. Department of Health and Human Services. 2004. *The Health Consequences of Smoking: A Report of the Surgeon General.* Atlanta, GA: U.S. Department of Health and Human Services, Public Health Service, Centers for Disease Control and Prevention, National Center for Chronic Disease Prevention and Health Promotion, Office on Smoking and Health.

Waldron, I., D. Lye, and A. Brandon. 1991. Gender Differences in Teenage Smoking. *Women Health* 17:65–90.

Wang, Q., E. Fitzhugh, J. Eddy, and R.C. Westerfield. 1996. Attitudes and Beliefs of Adolescent Experimental Smokers: A Smoking Prevention Perspective. *J Alcohol Drug Educ* 41:1–12.

Winefield, H.R., A.H. Winefield, and M. Tiggemann. 1992. Psychological Attributes of Young Adult Smokers. *Psychol Rep* 70:675–81.

Winnail, S., R. Valois, R. McKeown, R. Saunders, and R. Pate. 1995. Relationship between Physical Activity Level and Cigarette, Smokeless Tobacco, and Marijuana Use among Public High School Adolescents. *J School Health* 65:438–42.

CHAPTER 17

Prevention and Management
of Youth Cigarette Smoking

Mary Lober Aquilino and John B. Lowe

Cigarette smoking behavior during the teen and early adult years has been char-acterized as a sequence of developmental stages (Hirschman et al., 1984; Mayhew et al., 2000). Initiation or uptake of smoking and progression from one stage to another is influenced by economic, physiological, psychologic, environmental, and social factors. An understanding of the stages of acquisition of smoking behavior, the phenomenon of nicotine addiction and withdrawal, and the fac-tors that influence these variables is critical to designing and delivering tobacco dependence interventions.

■ STAGES OF YOUTH SMOKING

Mayhew et al. (2000) suggest six stages of adolescent smoking development includ-ing precontemplation, contemplation or preparatory, initiation, experimentation, regular smoking, and established or daily smoking (Table 17.1). Adolescents can maintain the experimentation stage for months, only smoking in specific social or environmental situations. A person's self-image as a smoker develops during this stage, which immediately precedes regular smoking. *Regular smoking* is defined as smoking on a consistent, yet still infrequent basis. Once a person progresses to the sixth stage of established or daily smoking, quitting becomes more difficult. For smoking behavior to be viewed on a continuum, two additional stages, cessation and relapse, are necessary. In fact, many smokers who attempt to quit move back and forth on the continuum several times before permanent cessation is achieved.

TABLE 17.1
Six stages of adolescent smoking progression

Stage	Characterization
Precontemplation	Never smoked
	Never considered smoking
	No desire to start smoking in the near future
	Unaware of positive reasons to start smoking
	Ignore or resist pressures to smoke
Contemplation (preparatory, pre-experimentation)	Begin to think about smoking
	Notice smoking more in society
	Attend to cigarette advertising
Initiation	Onset of tobacco use
	First few cigarettes tried
Experimentation	Sporadic tobacco use
	Gradual increase in smoking
	Increase in the variety of situations in which cigarettes are used
Regular smoking	Smoking on a consistent, yet infrequent basis
Established smoking (habituation, dependence, addiction)	Daily smoking

Source: Mayhew et al. (2000).

▪ NICOTINE DEPENDENCE AND WITHDRAWAL

Many teens are addicted to tobacco and most teens who smoke want to quit (Rojas et al., 1998; Colby et al., 2000). Of adolescents who have smoked at least 100 cigarettes in their lifetime, most of them report that they would like to quit but are not able to do so (CDC, 2001). Adolescents experience varying rates of tobacco dependence and withdrawal, with 20% to 68% of adolescents classified as dependent, and at least 60% reporting some form of withdrawal upon cutting back or quitting smoking. Daily smokers appear to have higher dependence and withdrawal prevalence than nondaily smokers, and daily smokers, who smoke more cigarettes per day, are more dependent than lighter smokers (Colby et al., 2000). People who begin smoking between the ages of 14 and 16 years are more likely to become nicotine dependent than are those who start smoking at a later age (Breslau et al., 1993).

Cigarette smoking is the most prevalent form of nicotine addiction in the United States. Most cigarettes in the United States market contain 10 mg or more of nicotine. Through inhaling smoke, the average smoker takes in 1 to 2 mg of nicotine per cigarette. Nicotine is absorbed through the skin and mucosal lining of the mouth and nose or by inhalation in the lungs. Nicotine can reach peak blood levels within 10 seconds of inhalation. Compulsive drug seeking and use, even in the face of negative health consequences, characterize addiction. Most smokers identify tobacco use as harmful and express a desire to reduce or stop using it (Benowitz, 1998).

Nicotine is a naturally occurring substance and is 1 of over 4000 chemicals found in tobacco smoke. Identified in the early nineteenth century, nicotine has been shown to be one of the most addictive drugs and to produce a number of complex and often unpredictable effects on humans. Nicotine acts as both a stimulant and a sedative and affects most organ systems of the body. Through the action of nicotine, the adrenal glands discharge epinephrine resulting in a sudden release of glucose and an increase in blood pressure, respiration, and heart rate. At the same time, nicotine suppresses pancreatic secretion of insulin, leaving smokers in a constant hyperglycemic state (National Institute of Drug Abuse [NIDA], 2001). Of primary importance to its addictive nature are findings that nicotine activates the brain pathways that regulate feelings of pleasure by increasing the level of dopamine. The acute effects of nicotine dissipate in several minutes, causing smokers to continue dosing frequently to maintain the drug's pleasurable effects and prevent symptoms of withdrawal (Benowitz, 1998; NIDA, 2001). In fact, smokers in the beginning stages of nicotine addiction smoke to gain pleasure, while those who are addicted refrain from quitting smoking to avoid the negative consequences of withdrawal. Chronic exposure to nicotine results in addiction, and repeated exposure to nicotine results in the development of tolerance (Benowitz, 1998).

Cessation of nicotine use is followed by withdrawal symptoms that can last up to a month. These symptoms include irritability, craving, cognitive and attentional deficits, sleep disturbances, and increased appetite. The dramatic changes in the brain's pleasure pathways that occur during withdrawal from chronic nicotine use are comparable in magnitude and duration to similar changes observed during the withdrawal of other abused drugs such as cocaine, opiates, amphetamines, and alcohol (NIDA, 2001).

For most individuals who smoke, tobacco dependence is more than nicotine addiction. The social and psychological aspects of dependence are less universal and more difficult to measure than the biological aspects. Therefore, current measures for diagnosing tobacco dependence focus on nicotine addiction. Table 17.2 presents two well-known clinical measures for diagnosing addiction: the *Diagnostic and Statistical Manual of Mental Disorders, Fourth Edition* (DSM-IV; American Psychiatric Association [APA], 1994) and the *International Classification of Diseases and Related Health Problems, Tenth Revision* (ICD-10; World Health Organization [WHO], 1992). The most widely used brief self-report measure of nicotine dependence is the Fagerstrom Tolerance Questionnaire (FTQ) (Fagerstrom, 1978) or the revised version, the Fagerstrom Test for Nicotine Dependence (FTND) presented in Table 17.3 (Heatherton et al., 1991). While used routinely in research, these measures may also be used in clinical practice.

TABLE 17.2
DSM-IV and ICD-10 descriptions of nicotine abuse and
tobacco dependence

Label	DSM-IV Nicotine abuse	ICD-10 Tobacco dependence
Definition	A destructive pattern of nicotine use, leading to significant social, occupational, or medical impairment	A mental and behavioral disorder attributable to the use of psychoactive substances
Diagnostic criteria	Nicotine tolerance Nicotine withdrawal symptoms Greater use of nicotine than intended Unsuccessful efforts to decrease or control nicotine use Great deal of time spent using nicotine Nicotine-caused reduction in social, occupational, or recreational activities Continued use of nicotine, despite knowing harmful effects Presence of three or more of these conditions signifies dependence	Increased tolerance Physical withdrawal state Strong desire to take drug Difficulty controlling use Higher priority given to drug than to other activities and obligations Using drug despite harmful consequences

Source: DSM-IV descriptions from American Psychiatric Association (1994), and ICD-10 descriptions from World Health Organization (1992).

Behavioral factors can also affect the severity of withdrawal symptoms. The feel, smell, and sight of a cigarette and the ritual of obtaining, handling, lighting, and smoking the cigarette are all associated with the pleasurable effects of smoking and can impede cessation efforts (NIDA, 2001). Smoking is a learned response to a number of thoughts and feelings. A smoker learns that the drug nicotine and the act of smoking can continue to provide relief from life stressors. The longer a person uses tobacco, the stronger the links to nicotine and the more difficult it is to quit. Similarly, the longer a person smokes, the more habitual the act of smoking becomes and the harder it is to break the habit (NIDA, 2001).

PREVENTION AND TREATMENT
OF YOUTH SMOKING

There are four points of potential impact for managing youth smoking behavior: (1) preventing smoking initiation, (2) minimizing cigarette use, (3) provid-

TABLE 17.3
Fagerstrom Test for Nicotine Dependence

Questions	Responses	Points
1. How soon after you wake do you smoke your first cigarette?	Within 5 minutes	3
	6 to 30 minutes	2
	31 to 60 minutes	1
	After 60 minutes	0
2. Do you find it difficult to refrain from smoking in places where it is forbidden?	Yes	1
	No	0
3. Which cigarette would you most hate to give up?	The first one in the morning	1
	All others	0
4. How many cigarettes per day do you smoke?	10 or less	0
	11 to 20	1
	21 to 30	2
	31 or more	3
5. Do you smoke more frequently during the first hours after waking than during the rest of the day?	Yes	1
	No	0
6. Do you smoke if you are so ill that you are in bed most of the day?	Yes	1
	No	0

*Scoring: 0 to 2, very low dependence; 3 to 4, low dependence; 5, medium dependence; 6 to 7, high dependence; 8 to 10, very high dependence.
Source: Heatherton et al. (1991).

ing smoking cessation treatment, and (4) providing follow-up to prevent relapse (Table 17.4). Discussion of related strategies for each intervention point follows.

■ Preventing Initiation of Smoking

Intervention should focus on preventing or delaying the initial smoking experience for youth who have never used tobacco (nonusers, pre-experimenters). Approaches to prevention should be targeted at the various factors that influence initiation of tobacco use and continuation of tobacco addiction (Lynch and Bonnie, 1994; Jacobson et al., 2001). Effective strategies keep youth from assuming that tobacco use is the peer group or community norm. These strategies include helping parents and other household members quit; advocating for smoke-free schools, workplaces, sports venues, restaurants, and other public facilities; providing counter—tobacco media messages; and increasing the price of tobacco through excise taxes (Farkas et al., 2000; Patel and Greydanus; 2000; Jacobson et al., 2001). Such measures can also lead to decreased availability of and access to tobacco products, particularly when individuals close to youth do not smoke.

TABLE 17.4
Managing youth smoking behavior: intervention points

Intervention Points	Strategies
Deterring or delaying initiation of cigarette use during the teen and early adult years	Helping parents to quit Advocating for smoke-free public facilities Providing and supporting counter-tobacco media messages Advocating for product regulation and access restriction Supporting tobacco excise taxes
Minimizing cigarette use to prevent progression to regular smoking behavior and subsequent tobacco dependence	Ask about tobacco use at every encounter Strongly advise children or youth to quit Provide information on the health risks of smoking and nicotine addiction
Smoking cessation intervention	Follow the National Cancer Institute* and Agency for Healthcare Research and Quality† clinical practice guidelines for smoking intervention with behavioral and pharmacologic approaches
Relapse prevention	Follow up by phone or office visit within weeks of the quit date Continue monitoring progress on a regular basis up to 1 year after quitting

*National Cancer Institute (http://www.cancer.gov/cancertopics/tobacco/quitting-and-prevention).
†Agency for Healthcare Research and Quality (http://www.ahrq.gov/path/tobacco.htm).

Minimizing Cigarette Use

Limiting Product Availability and Creating Positive Social Norms

Tobacco control policies alter the legal, social, economic, and physical environments that support smoking behavior. They are designed to limit youth exposure to tobacco promotion, decrease access to tobacco products, and alter the social norm of tobacco use. Approaches to prevention of youth smoking include social marketing campaigns, tax increases, and restrictions on where smokers can smoke.

Policies related to restricted advertising, sale and use of tobacco have been shown to have a significant impact on cigarette smoking. The tobacco industry continues marketing to children in youth-oriented magazines, in stores, and through sporting event sponsorships (King and Siegel, 2001). Increased susceptibility to smoking and the onset of smoking experimentation have been found to be associated with receptivity to tobacco advertising and the use of promotional items (Perez-Stable and Fuentes-Afflick, 1998). In fact, children buy the most heavily advertised cigarette brands and are three times more sensitive to advertising than adults (CDC, 2001). Policies restricting such tobacco industry influence in both schools and the general community decrease youth exposure to tobacco advertising (Perez-Stable and Fuentes-Afflick, 1998). Countermarketing messages substantially influence public support for tobacco control intervention and build a supportive climate for school and community efforts (CDC, 2001).

Increasing the Price of Tobacco

Access can also be restricted by taxation of tobacco products. Tobacco consumption is inversely related to price. Increasing the cost of cigarettes by taxation not only helps finance tobacco education but also decreases access to tobacco by youth. Those youth who actually purchase cigarettes are more sensitive to price increases than adults (Lynch and Bonnie, 1994).

Establishing Smoke-Free Venues

Restriction of places where smoking is allowed is becoming much more pervasive in the United States. Currently, most government buildings, schools and health care facilities have banned indoor smoking and, to varying degrees, smoking within a designated distance of buildings. The current focus of smoking bans is in the workplace, in an effort to protect employees such as those working in bars, restaurants, and casinos and on airplanes. It is anticipated that such bans will not only protect the health of workers, but may also have a secondary effect on smoking rates.

Occasional Smoking

A critical time in the development of smoking behavior is the experimental or occasional user stage. This is typical of the youth who smokes only on weekends or in conjunction with certain events. Occasional users are not generally chemically addicted to tobacco but are beginning to form the social associations that often make smoking cessation more difficult. These youth approach smoking as a "bridge" behavior to get them through the adolescent years, and they report planning to quit after high school or college or, if female, when pregnancy occurs. The focus of intervention during the experimentation stage is to prevent progression to regular use and subsequent habituation and addiction. One approach to minimizing tobacco use is to frame smoking in the context of all health behaviors, both positive and negative. Thus, programs may need to shift the approach to tobacco use away from coping with life events and toward dealing with drug use. It could be speculated that this will need to occur not only in the school environment but through the establishment of 100% smoke free venues frequented by youth.

▪ Providing Smoking Cessation Treatment

Once a person has progressed to regular tobacco use (current user, dependent, addicted), most individuals exhibit some level of physical and psychological dependence. Initial symptoms of nicotine dependence can occur for some adolescents within 4 weeks of initiating monthly smoking (DiFranza et al., 2000). Two-thirds of teenagers who smoke have attempted to quit. To quit, the individual must make a conscious choice to refrain from tobacco use. While it is possible for some people to quit smoking without external support, many smokers require both physical and psychological support. Social pressures, emotional dependence, and physiologic addiction are barriers to quitting, while health-oriented values are highly associated with quit attempts (Pletcher and Schwartz, 2000).

For most individuals, smoking cessation should be a gradual process because withdrawal symptoms are less severe in those who quit gradually than in those who quit all at once. Rates of relapse are highest in the first few weeks and months and diminish considerably after 3 months. In fact, 90% of people who try to quit smoking cigarettes relapse or return to smoking within 1 year, with the majority relapsing within a week. Pharmacologic treatments can double the odds of success. A combination of behavioral and pharmacologic treatments further improves the chances of smokers being successful in quitting (NIDA, 2001).

Behavioral Cessation Interventions

Behavior interventions, used alone or in conjunction with pharmacologic interventions, include group sessions, social support networks, or individual counseling, and can be school, community, or clinic based. Formats range from informal contacts with peer or professional counselors to regularly scheduled intensive cessation programs. Newer initiatives include the use of telephone counseling and Web-based interactions. While telephone counseling has been shown to be an effective strategy for adult smoking cessation, there are no reported evaluations of Web-based interventions (Stead et al., 2003).

Pharmacologic Cessation Interventions

Although there are several types of pharmacologic cessation aids, their use with adolescents has not been well investigated. The clinical practice guidelines (Fiore et al., 2000) recommend that "since there is no evidence that buproprion HCL (Zyban) or nicotine replacement is harmful for adolescents, clinicians should consider their use when tobacco dependence is obvious. However, because of the behavioral aspects of smoking in adolescents, clinicians should be confident of the patient's tobacco dependence and intention to quit before instituting pharmacotherapy. Factors such as degree of dependence, number of cigarettes per day and body weight should be considered" (Fiore et al., 2000, p. 102).

Nicotine replacement therapy (NRT) is commonly used to relieve nicotine withdrawal symptoms in adults. NRT is believed to produce less severe physiologic alterations than tobacco delivery systems and provide users with lower overall nicotine levels than what they receive while smoking. An added benefit is that these pharmacologic forms of nicotine have little abuse potential because they do not produce the pleasurable effects of tobacco products, nor do they contain the carcinogens and gases associated with tobacco smoke. NRT is available in four, equally effective forms: chewing gum, transdermal patch, nasal spray, and inhaler (NIDA, 2001). Adverse side effects noted from users of NRT include headaches, dizziness, nausea, weakness, blurred vision, vivid dreams, and diarrhea. Patch users also report mild itching and irritation of the skin under the patch site (Patel and Greydanus, 2000). Evidence of NRT abuse is essentially nonexistent (Benowitz, 1998).

Only two nonrandomized, clinical trials have examined the effectiveness of NRT with teen smokers. In the first, a sample of 22 subjects with a mean smoking rate of 23.3 cigarettes per day and 2.6 mean years of smoking achieved a quit rate of 4.5% at 6 months using NRT (Smith et al., 1996). In a larger study of 101 adolescents who smoked an average of 20 cigarettes per day, brief counseling in combination with NRT resulted in a quit rate of 10.9% at 6 weeks and 5% at 6 months (Hurt et al., 2000). According to Patten (2000), ethical considerations and issues of acceptability, convenience, compliance, social approval, cost, and availability also need to be studied. In addition, nicotine replacement products are not available to persons under 18 years of age without a prescription. NRT use in adolescents needs further study (Patten, 2000).

Zyban (bupropion HCL) is used in the adult population to aid smoking cessation. Zyban, an antidepressant, is a relatively weak inhibitor of the neuronal uptake of norepinephrine, serotonin, and dopamine, and does not inhibit monoamine oxidase. While the mechanism by which it enhances an individual's ability to abstain from smoking is unknown, it is thought to control nicotine craving or thoughts about cigarette use. Zyban requires a prescription and the recommended adult dosage is 150 mg twice a day. The safety and efficacy of the drug has not been established for individuals less than 18 years of age. The most commonly reported side effects are dry mouth and insomnia. Other adverse effects include headache, decreased appetite, dizziness, sweating, nausea, increased pulse, irregular pulse, agitation, and anxiety (Patel and Greydanus, 2000; NIDA, 2001; GlaxoSmithKlein, 2002).

Cost is a potential deterrent to the use of nicotine replacement products and other smoking cessation aids and should be a consideration in recommending such products. While third-party payers will usually cover the cost of nicotine inhalers, nasal sprays, and Zyban, nicotine gum and patches are not generally reimbursed. Currently, nicotine gum and nicotine patches cost between $30 and $50 per week. Until the cost of NRT equals the immediate price of smoking cigarettes, the cost will be a substantial deterrent.

■ Providing Follow-up to Prevent Relapse

Typically, a person desiring to quit smoking will make several attempts before being successful. Once successful, the chances of a lapse or relapse back to smoking are high. A *lapse* is defined as a slip when the smoker may have a puff once a day but not for more than 6 days, and a *relapse* is when this smoking behavior continues to increase or lasts more than a week (Ossip-Klein et al., 1986). Relapse appears to lead back into regular smoking unless an effort is put forward to alter the smoking behavior (Lowe et al., 1997). During the initial weeks of abstinence and up to a year after quitting, the ex-smoker is at risk of having a cigarette. Therefore, maintaining involvement with individuals who have recently quit smoking for at least a full year following a quit attempt is essential, since relapse is most likely to occur during this time period.

■ HEALTH CARE PROVIDERS' ROLE
IN CLINIC-BASED INTERVENTIONS

Health care providers should send a strong message to youth who do not smoke and to their parents regarding the importance of abstaining from tobacco use. Where there is evidence of nicotine addiction and a desire to quit smoking, counseling and behavioral and pharmacologic interventions, shown to be effective with adults, should be considered and modified as necessary for use with youth. There are no specific guidelines for their use with youth in the initiation or experimentation stage of tobacco use.

Physician- or nurse-mediated interventions to promote smoking cessation among adults have been developed, implemented, and tested in randomized control designs. Moderate effects on biochemically proven smoking cessation have been achieved in diverse clinical settings, ranging from 5% to 15% abstinence at 1 year. The Tobacco Use and Dependence Guideline Panel (Fiore et al., 2000) has developed guidelines for treating adults, and similar recommendations have been developed by the National Cancer Institute (NCI) that are targeted to clinicians caring for children (Table 17.5). Providers should monitor risk for smoking in the preteen and teenage years and ask youth about their smoking behavior as early as 8 years of age. Anticipatory guidance should also be offered to parents and other caretakers regarding risk factors, including the effect of their own smoking on the child's likelihood to try cigarettes. Both adults and youth should be advised to quit. Depending on readiness, they should be provided motivational information and assisted in making a quit attempt. Systematic follow-up to this intervention is crucial to quitting and prevention of relapse.

In addition to providing individual treatment, clinicians should support and participate in school and community efforts to decrease youth initiation of smoking and offer youth-specific cessation programs. This participation includes overt

TABLE 17.5

Tobacco intervention guidelines for children and youth*

- *Anticipate* the child's or youth's risk for smoking, and provide preventive guidance to caretakers and child.
- *Ask* about the child's or youth's experimentation regularly from 8 years of age on, about household member smoking, and about other sources of environmental tobacco smoke exposure.
- *Advise* the child or youth and caretakers who smoke to quit using clear, personal, and relevant messages.
- *Assess* the child's or youth's and caretakers' readiness to commit to cessation activities.
- *Assist* those indicating readiness to develop a quit plan and provide self-help literature, specific techniques, nicotine replacement therapy, and/or referral to community programs. Provide those who are not ready with motivational information.
- *Arrange* for follow-up appointments or phone calls to reinforce quitting or address relapse.

*Based on Agency for Healthcare Research and Quality clinical practice guidelines for adults (http:/ /www.ahrq.gov/path/tobacco.htm), and the National Cancer Institute guidelines for children (http://www.cancer.gov/cancertopics/tobacco/quitting-and-prevention).

support of local policies restricting smoking in public places and distribution of tobacco products to minors and promotion of taxation of tobacco products.

■ IMPORTANCE OF PROVIDER TRAINING

Most health care providers have the opportunity to offer tobacco use education and counseling, yet few receive specific training in this area (Schubiner et al., 1998; Stein et al., 2000). In a stratified random survey of family physicians and pediatricians, more than 40% indicated that they do not have the skills required to counsel children and adolescents, with a significantly higher proportion of pediatricians (54.8%) than family physicians (24.9%) citing this as a barrier to counseling (Kaplan et al., 2004). A feasibility study showed that pediatric residents trained to use the NCI program raised tobacco issues more often, counseled adolescents about smoking cessation more frequently, and reported the use of more effective techniques than a nonrandomized comparison group who failed to attend teaching seminars (Klein et al., 1995). Klein et al. (2001) concluded that physicians familiar with smoking cessation guidelines were more likely to provide tobacco cessation counseling to adolescents. There are numerous venues for a practicing health care provider to update their knowledge and skill in providing tobacco use counseling. Continuing education programs are offered through professional organizations and government sponsors such as the American Lung Association (http://www.lungusa.org) and the American Heart Association (http://www.americanheart.org), in a variety of formats such as Web-based courses.

■ CLINICAL MANAGEMENT GUIDELINES
FOR YOUTH SMOKING

Table 17.6 provides a brief overview of clinical management for youth smoking, including significant findings on patient history and examination, anticipatory guidance considerations, and intervention for parents or youth who smoke. Smoking should be treated as a vital sign that is monitored at each patient encounter. Children as young as 8 years of age should be assessed for knowledge about and risk for tobacco use and current behavior as indicated by history or examination. Parental and other household member smoking should also be assessed and appropriate counseling offered. If adult household members who smoke are present at the visit, they should be informed about risks of smoking for them and other household members and be advised to quit.

■ FUTURE CONSIDERATIONS IN TREATING
YOUTH WHO SMOKE

Research in two areas holds promise for prevention and treatment of youth smoking. A nicotine vaccine is being developed to prevent youth in the early stages of smoking from progressing to regular smoking, and genetic researchers are attempting to identify genetic susceptibility to nicotine addiction.

■ Nicotine Vaccine

A nicotine vaccine is being developed to reduce the amount of nicotine that reaches the brain so as to reduce its effects and help keep people from becoming addicted (Patel and Greydanus, 2000). Human testing, funded by the National Institute of Drug Abuse, is currently under way at the University of Nebraska Medical Center (UNMC, 2004).

■ Genetic Susceptibility

There is increasing evidence that smoking initiation, dependence, and subsequent difficulty in quitting may be due in part to an inherited vulnerability (genetic susceptibility) to nicotine addiction (Moolchan et al., 2000; Zickler, 2000). Recent research offers evidence of a genetic explanation for as much as half of the propensity to become a smoker and half of the apparent inability of some smokers to quit (Pomerleau, 1995; Jacobson et al., 2001). Greater insight into gene—behavior interaction effects will provide the opportunity to develop individual-specific interventions for those at greater risk for developing tobacco dependence. Of importance in dealing with this potential ability to identify susceptible popu-

TABLE 17.6
Clinical management guidelines for youth smoking

History and Examination

- Family members who smoke or have smoked
- Family history of CVD, COPD, lung cancer
- Current smokers in household (second-hand exposure; cigarette availability)
- Number of friends who smoke
- Previous or current cigarette use
- Previous quit attempts
- Associated health problems (e.g., frequent respiratory infections, bronchitis, persistent cough, shortness of breath, asthma, low LDL cholesterol)
- Tobacco odor on clothing
- Tobacco odor on breath
- Brownish staining on tongue

Treatment

- Provide age-appropriate anticipatory guidance for parents, caregivers, and youth
- Counsel other family and household members who smoke on environmental exposure, cigarette access, and role modeling
- For youth who smoke, assess readiness to quit

  If they are not ready to consider smoking cessation

    Strongly advise youth to quit smoking
    Provide information on the effects of smoking and the benefits of smoking cessation

  If they are considering smoking cessation

    Strongly advise youth to quit smoking
    Discuss and reinforce reasons for desiring to quit
    Provide information on smoking cessation options, benefits of quitting, and potential barriers

  If they are ready to quit smoking

    Assist in setting a quit date
    Assist in developing a quit plan incorporating behavioral and pharmacologic aids as appropriate
    Contact the youth by phone within one week of quit date
    Arrange a follow-up appointment to discuss progress within one month of quit date, or sooner if therapy warrants

- For youth who have quit smoking within the last year

    Encourage continued abstinence
    Discuss relapse prevention
    Consider return visits or phone calls as necessary

CVD, cardiovascular disease; COPD, chronic obstructive pulmonary disease; LDL, low-density lipoprotein.

lations will be prevention of fatalistic attitudes on the part of those vulnerable individuals.

■ SUMMARY

- The majority of adults who smoke regularly began smoking during late childhood and adolescence.
- Despite considerable public emphasis on the health risks of smoking, youth continue to smoke at high rates. The etiology and significance of smoking initiation and continuance vary greatly in this age group.
- Smoking acquisition and cessation are generally unstable behaviors during the teen and young adult years, providing both opportunity and challenges for prevention and treatment. While there is evidence that multiple psychological, physical, environmental, and social factors influence the initiation of cigarette use, tobacco dependence in adolescence is not well explained. In addition, an extremely limited number of prevention and cessation interventions for this population have clearly demonstrated effectiveness.
- Sustained smoking prevention and cessation programming on multiple levels, taking into account the developmental status of the individual or target group, is the most promising strategy for decreasing cigarette addiction. A combination of behavioral and pharmacologic approaches appears to have the greatest potential for sustained cessation.
- Continued research with methodologic rigor is essential for determining the best practices for prevention and management of youth smoking. The magnitude of this public health problem warrants continued commitment to policy initiatives designed to reduce youth access to cigarettes and *their* desire to smoke.

■ REFERENCES

American Psychiatric Association. 1994. *Diagnostic and Statistical Manual of Mental Disorders, 4th ed.* Washington, DC: American Psychiatric Association.
Benowitz, N.L. (ed.). 1998. *Nicotine Safety and Toxicity.* New York: Oxford University Press.
Breslau, N., N. Fenn, and E.L. Peterson. 1993. Early Smoking Initiation and Nicotine Dependence in a Cohort of Young Adults. *Drug Alcohol Depend* 33:129–37.
[CDC] Centers for Disease Control and Prevention. 2001. *Youth Tobacco Surveillance— United States, 2000.* Retrieved January 2006, from http://www.cdc.gov/mmwr/preview/mmwrhtml/ss5004a1.htm.
Colby, S.M., S.T. Tiffany, S. Shiffman, and R.S. Niaura. 2000. Are Adolescent Smokers Dependent on Nicotine? A Review of the Evidence. *Drug Alcohol Depend* 59(Suppl 1):S83–S95.
DiFranza, J.R., N.A. Rigotti, A.D. McNeill, J.K. Ockene, J.A. Savageau, D. St Cyr, and M. Coleman. 2000. Initial Symptoms of Nicotine Dependence in Adolescents. *Tob Control* 9:313–9.

Fagerstrom, K.O. 1978. Measuring the Degree of Physical Dependence to Tobacco Smoking with Reference to Individualization of Treatment. *Addict Behav* 3:235–41.

Farkas, A.J., E.A. Gilpin, M.M. White, and J.P. Pierce. 2000. Association between Household and Workplace Smoking Restrictions and Adolescent Smoking. *JAMA* 284:717–22.

Fiore, M.C., W.C. Bailey, S.J. Cohen, S.F. Dorfman, M.G. Goldstein, E.R. Gritz, R.B. Heyman, C.R. Jaen, T.E. Kottke, H.A. Lando, R.E. Mecklenburg, P.D. Mullen, L.M. Nett, L. Robinson, M.L. Stitzer, A.C. Tommasello, L. Villejo, and M.E. Wewers. 2000. *Treating Tobacco Use and Dependence: A Clinical Practice Guideline.* Rockville, MD: Department of Health and Human Services, Public Health Service, Publication AHRQ 00–0032.

GlaxoSmithKlein. 2002. Prescribing Information. http://us.gsk.com/products/assets/us_zyban.pdf

Heatherton, T.F., L.T. Kozlowski, R.C. Frecker, and K.O. Fagerstrom. 1991. The Fagerstrom Test for Nicotine Dependence: A Revision of the Fagerstrom Tolerance Questionnaire. *Br J Addict* 86:1119–27.

Hirschman, R.S., H. Leventhal, and K. Glynn. 1984. The Development of Smoking Behavior: Conceptualization and Supportive Cross-Sectional Survey Data. *J Appl Soc Psychol* 14:184–206.

Hurt, R.D., G.A. Croghan, D. Beede, T.D. Wolter, I.T. Croghan, and C.A. Patten. 2000. Nicotine Patch Therapy in 101 Adolescent Smokers. *Arch Pediatr Adolesc Med* 154:31–7.

Jacobson, P.D., P.M. Lantz, K.E. Warner, J. Wasserman, H.A. Pollack, and A.K. Ahlstrom. 2001. *Combating Teen Smoking: Research and Policy Strategies.* Ann Arbor: University of Michigan Press.

Kaplan, C.P., Perez-Sable, E.J., Fuentes-Afflic, E., Gildengorin, V., Millstein, S., and Juarez-Reyes, M. 2004. Smoking Cessation Counseling with Young Patients: The Practice of Family Physicians and Pediatricians. *Arch Pediatr Adolesc Med* 158:83–90.

King, C, and M. Siegel. 2001. The Master Settlement Agreement with the Tobacco Industry and Cigarette Advertising in Magazines. *N Engl J Med* 345:504–11.

Klein, J.D., L.J. Levine, and M.J. Allan. 2001. Delivery of Smoking Prevention and Cessation Services to Adolescents. *Arch Pediatr Adolesc Med* 155:597–602.

Klein, J.D., M. Portilla, A. Goldstein, and L. Leininger. 1995. Training Pediatric Residents to Prevent Tobacco Use. *Pediatrics* 96:326–30.

Lowe, J.B., R. Windsor, K.P. Balanda, and L. Woodby. 1997. Smoking Relapse Prevention Method for Pregnant Women: A Formative Evaluation. *Am J Health Promot* 11:244–6.

Lynch, B.S., and R.J. Bonnie (eds.). 1994. *Growing up Tobacco Free: Preventing Nicotine Addiction in Children and Youths.* Institute of Medicine. Washington, DC: National Academy Press.

Mayhew, K.P., B.R. Flay, and J.A. Mott. 2000. Stages in the Development of Adolescent Smoking. *Drug Alcohol Depend* 59(Suppl):S62–S81.

Moolchan, E., M. Ernst, and J.E. Henningfield. 2000. A Review of Tobacco Smoking in Adolescents: Treatment Implications. *J Am Acad Child Adolesc Psychiatry* 39:682–93.

[NIDA] National Institute of Drug Abuse. 2001. *Research Report Series: Nicotine Addiction.* Rockville, MD: U.S. Department of Health and Human Services, National Institutes of Health, NIH Publication 01-4342.

Ossip-Klein, D.J., G. Bigelow, S.R. Parker, S. Curry, S. Hall, and S. Kirkland. 1986. Classification and Assessment of Smoking Behavior. *Health Psychol* 5(Suppl):3–11.

Patel, D.R., and D. Greydanus. 2000. Office Interventions for Adolescent Smokers. *Adolesc Med* 11:577–89.

Patten, C.A. 2000. A Critical Review of Nicotine Replacement Therapy for Teenage Smokers. *J Child Adolesc Subst Abuse* 9:51–75.

Perez-Stable, E.L., and E. Fuentes-Afflick. 1998. Role of Clinicians in Cigarette Smoking Prevention. *West J Med* 169:23–9.

Pletcher, J.R., and D.F. Schwartz. 2000. Current Concepts in Adolescent Smoking. *Curr Opin Pediatr* 12:444–9.

Pomerleau, O.F. 1995. Individual Differences in Sensitivity to Nicotine: Implications for Genetic Research on Nicotine Dependence. *Behav Genet* 25:161–77.

Rojas, N.L., J.D. Killen, K.F. Haydel, and T.N. Robinson. 1998. Nicotine Dependence among Adolescent Smokers. *Arch Pediatr Adolesc Med* 152:151–6.

Schubiner H.A., A. Herrold, and R. Hurt. 1998. Tobacco Cessation and Youth: The Feasibility of Brief Office Interventions for Adolescents. *Prev Med* 27:A47–A54.

Smith, T.A., R.F. House, I.T. Croghan, T.R. Gauvin, R.C. Colligan, K.P. Offord, L.C. Gomez-Dahl, and R.D. Hurt. 1996. Nicotine Patch Therapy in Adolescent Smokers. *Pediatrics* 98:659–67.

Stead, L.F., T. Lancaster, and R. Perera. 2003. Telephone Counseling for Smoking Cessation. *Cochrane Database of Syst Rev* 1.

Stein, R.J., C.K. Haddock, K.K. O'Byren, N. Hymowitz, and J. Schwab. 2000. The Pediatrician's Role in Reducing Tobacco Exposure in Children. *Pediatrics* 106:1–17.

University of Nebraska Medical Center. Press release, March 22, 2004. Retrieved January 2006, from http://app1.unmc.edu/PublicAffairs/newsarchive/view_art.cfm?article_id=866&sstring=smoking.

World Health Organization (WHO). 1992. *International Classification of Diseases and Related Health Problems (ICD-10), 10th Revision*. Geneva: World Health Organization.

Zickler, P. 2000. *Evidence Builds that Genes Influence Cigarette Smoking*. Rockville, MD: National Institute of Drug Abuse, U.S. Department of Health and Human Services, National Institutes of Health, 15:1.

PART VIII

Promoting Health
in the School Setting

CHAPTER 18

Policy and Practice: Changing the Home, School, and Community Environment to Promote Health

Russell V. Luepker and Leslie A. Lytle

The aim of health promotion is to reduce or prevent health-impairing behaviors. While individual choice and familial and genetic factors play important roles in these behaviors, the physical and social environment is highly influential, as it determines what is available and acceptable. This is most apparent in three of the major health-impairing behaviors: eating patterns, physical activity, and tobacco use. Although each of these factors has important elements of individual choice, these choices are heavily influenced by the surrounding environment of the media, community, family, and peers. The role of the environment is particularly apparent among youth, as lifetime habits are formed and reinforced at this age.

In this chapter we will discuss the home or family environment, which sets and constrains many health behaviors by parental example, parental choices, and physical surroundings. Also addressed is the school environment, which comprises a substantial portion of the day for school-age children and is where learning and socialization with peers take place. The policies, practices, and examples set by schools and teachers play an important role in their students' developing health habits. Finally, we will discuss the community environment, which controls policy and regulations as well as availability of healthy products, and sets an example through its leaders.

In each of these areas there is a commitment to promoting healthier lifestyles and preventing disease. However, there are also strong commercial interests that seek to limit restrictive policies and to promote their products. These conflicts are increasingly recognized as cigarette advertising targets youth, fast-food vendors serve school cafeterias, and restructuring of schools leads to reduced time for physical activity.

This chapter describes some of these issues and the scientific work that underlies environmental policy recommendations. Methods of creating a healthier environment for youth are also suggested.

■ NUTRITION: HOW DOES THE SCHOOL FOOD ENVIRONMENT AFFECT STUDENTS' NUTRITIONAL HEALTH?

Besides families, the physical and social environment of schools may play the most significant role in the eating habits and dietary intake of school-age youth. In the United States, more than 95% of 5- to 17-year-olds are enrolled in school, spending more than 6 hours daily for at least 9 months of the year and consuming at least one meal each day within the school or with peers from school. Ten percent of youth in the United States get two meals daily from their schools (Dwyer, 1995). The influence of the school environment is widespread and occurs through the types of foods and beverages available in the school cafeteria, in school stores, in vending machines, at school events, and even in classrooms. In addition to food being available in the physical environment, the school is a dominant scene for youth to learn and practice the social side of eating. The role modeling of peers and adults in the school and the use of food as incentive and reinforcement provide important learning opportunities about food choices.

There is some regulation of the schools' physical environment through U.S. food policy. The policy side of the school food environment starts with the meal programs regulated by the U.S. Department of Agriculture (USDA). In 1946, Congress passed the National School Lunch Act, and in 1966 Congress passed the School Breakfast Program, with the goal of providing healthy meals to youth in schools through a federally subsidized meal program. In 1995, the School Meals Initiative for Healthy Children (USDA, 1994) was passed by Congress with the goal of improving the nutritional content of meals served as part of the National School Lunch Program (NSLP) and the School Breakfast Program (SBP) and to ensure that meals served were consistent with the Dietary Guidelines for Americans, the national nutritional guidance document produced by the USDA, and the U.S. Department of Health and Human Services (USDHHS).

To be eligible for federal money to subsidize the cost of offering free and reduced meals to students, school districts must document that the meals they serve meet federal requirements. The content of meals served as part of the NSLP and the SBP must limit the proportion of energy from fat and saturated fat to no more than 30% and less than 10%, respectively, and must meet the Recommended Dietary Allowances for calories, protein, calcium, iron, vitamin A, and vitamin C. School food service departments documenting that they provide meals with these nutritional levels get cash reimbursements for every child receiving a meal (Eisinger, 1998). In fiscal year 2003, nearly 29 million children were participating daily in the NSLP and nearly 9 million were participating in the SBP for a combined annual cost of approximately 9 billion dollars (USDA, 2005). Data from the USDA suggest that youth who participate in the NSLP and SBP eat healthier diets than those of youth who do not participate in these programs at school. Children in these programs consume less sugar, more milk and vegetables, less soda and sweetened fruit drinks, and higher intakes of key vitamins (USDA, 2001a).

While the NSLP and SBP, as federal food policy, contribute to the nutritional health of American youth, they have a limited range. The nutritional standards that apply to the NSLP and the SBP do not apply to foods offered in the school outside of those programs. The only federal regulation of foods and beverages sold outside of the NSLP and SBP is that the sale of "foods of minimal nutritional value" (which include carbonated soft drinks, chewing gum, water ices, and candies made primarily from sweeteners) is prohibited during school meal periods (Wechsler et al., 2001). That exception allows school administrators and the food service a great deal of discretion in offering other foods in the cafeteria during mealtime. In addition, there is no restriction of any foods or beverages sold outside of the cafeteria at any time of the school day and no federal policy that addresses other food-related issues in schools, such as foods used as fund-raisers, foods used as incentives or rewards, the withholding of access to food as punishment, or school staff eating practices and rules during class time.

The effect of food and beverage options in schools that are beyond the purview of the policy instituted by the USDA and USDHHS's Healthy School Meal Initiative is of great concern. The practice of offering a wide variety and always-available source of food in schools is ubiquitous across the United States. Findings from the School Nutrition Dietary Assessment Study (USDA, 2001b) show that more than 90% of schools offered an à la carte line at lunchtime; 76% of high schools, 55% of middle schools, and 15% of elementary schools had vending machines available for student use. In addition, 41% of high schools, 35% of middle schools, and 9% of elementary schools had school stores, snack bars, or canteens that sold food or drinks. The School Health Policies and Programs Study (SHPPS) of 2000, conducted by the Centers for Disease Control and Prevention (CDC) and including data from all 50 states and the District of Columbia, confirmed these findings. The SHPPS data indicate that 43% of elementary schools, 74% of middle and junior high schools, and 98% of high schools have vending machines, school stores, canteens, or snack bars (Wechsler et al., 2001).

Compounding the concern about the easy access students have to foods in the school environment is the poor nutritional content of the foods available in these alternative or competitive venues. The SHPPS study showed that of the middle and junior high schools that had vending machines, school stores, canteens, or snack bars, 84% offered soft drinks, sport drinks, or fruit drinks, compared to 20% offering low-fat or skim milk; and 61% offered cookies, crackers, cakes, and pastries, whereas only 38% offered lower-fat versions of cookies, crackers, cakes, and pastries (Wechsler et al., 2001). Other research has produced similar findings (Story et al., 1996; Harnack et al., 2000; USDHHS, 2000; French et al., 2003; U.S. General Accounting Office, 2003).

Easy access to foods and beverages during the school day impacts the nutritional intake of adolescents across the entire day. Kubik et al. (2003) considered the effect of the presence of an à la carte line and of snack and beverage vending machines in middle schools on students' daily intake of fruits, vegetables, and energy from total fat and saturated fat. Youth who attended schools that did not have an à la carte line consumed significantly more servings of fruits and vegetables and significantly less energy from total fat and saturated fat compared to students attending schools with à la carte lines. In addition, fewer snack vending machines in the school was significantly related to a higher intake of fruits (Kubik et al., 2003). These results show the power of the physical environment and suggest that students do not compensate for foods consumed during the school day by changing what they eat outside of school.

There are also other school food policy issues that affect the social environment related to eating and have an impact on students' dietary intakes. Policies and practices that influence what students hear, see, and experience as normative behaviors around food choices may be powerful for impressionable youth. The SHHPS study showed that nearly one-quarter of schools allowed candy, foods from fast-food restaurants, and soft drinks to be promoted on the school campus, and only 25% of schools surveyed in the study had a school policy discouraging or preventing faculty and school staff from using junk food as a reward for good behavior or academic performance. In addition, in 82% of the schools, school clubs or organizations sold food at school or in the community to raise money. Most commonly, the foods sold were chocolate candy, cookies, pastries, and baked goods. Only 28% of the schools sold fruits and vegetables as fund-raisers (Wechsler et al., 2001).

Social norms around eating may also be modeled and reinforced through school staff practices. As part of the Teens Eating for Energy and Nutrition in School (TEENS) study (Lytle and Perry, 2001; Lytle et al., 2004), middle school teachers were surveyed in 16 schools in the Midwest. They were asked to give their opinions about the school food environment, their classroom rules for eating, and their own eating patterns at school (Kubik et al., 2002). Seventy percent of the teachers asked to participate in the one-time survey completed the survey ($n = 476$). Overall, they supported a healthier food environment in the school. Nearly 70% of respondents agreed that vending machines at school should offer only healthy food and beverage items and only 13% agreed with the statement that students should be able to buy soft drinks and candy at school. At the same time, more than one-half of the sample (53%) allowed students to eat in the classroom and one-fourth permitted consumption of soft drinks in class. Most teachers (73%) used candy as an incentive or reward for students and 62%

of teachers reported using beverage vending for their own use, purchasing primarily sweetened soft drinks or fruit drinks.

A number of national documents with recommendations for improving the health of the school environment have been released. These include the CDC's *Guidelines for School Health Programs to Promote Lifelong Healthy Living* (1996), the *Surgeon General's Call to Action to Prevent and Decrease Overweight and Obesity* (USDHHS, 2001) and *Fit, Healthy and Ready to Learn* (Bogden, 2000). These documents have spurred a great deal of interest in food-related policy and practice for schools. We are just beginning to see movement toward more school food policy at the local and state levels. Some states, including West Virginia, California, and New York, are leading the charge in attempting to pass state policy that restricts the availability of competitive foods, or foods that compete with other foods offered as part of the reimbursable meal plan. West Virginia has regulated the sale of all foods during the instructional day, established nutritional guidelines for sugar, and required that foods sold as à la carte sales must include only those that could be sold as part of the NSLP or the SBP. In other states such as California and New York, where legislation is pending to limit or eliminate the availability of competitive foods in schools, time will tell if the strength and reach of what finally is passed are adequate, and whether states have the ability to regulate and monitor the policies and laws.

■ PHYSICAL ACTIVITY: HOW DOES THE SCHOOL ENVIRONMENT AFFECT STUDENTS' PHYSICAL ACTIVITY LEVELS?

Fueled by the epidemic of obesity and the unprecedented increase in type 2 diabetes among youth, there is increasing national concern about youth levels of physical activity. Current recommendations suggest that preadolescent children should have at least 60 minutes of physical activity a day (Corbin and Pangrazi, 1998; Biddle et al., 1998); however, research suggests that most children do not reach these levels (USDHHS, 2000). In addition, an age-related decline of 26% to 37% in total physical activity occurs during adolescence (Aaron et al., 2002). This age-related decline is more evident in girls than in boys (Kimm et al., 2000), and socioeconomic differences are seen for levels of structured and unstructured leisure-time physical activity. The Youth Media Campaign Longitudinal Survey, conducted in a nationally representative sample of 9- to 13-year-olds, found that non-Caucasian youth and youth whose parents had lower education and income levels were significantly less likely to participate in organized or free-time physical activity outside of the school day than were their peers (CDC, 2003).

Schools have the opportunity to reduce these gaps and to increase students' levels of physical activity by instituting school policy and practices that provide time for being active during the school day, ensuring quality experiences that promote moderate to vigorous physical activity, and promoting a lifestyle that embraces being active. Most schools have failed to take advantage of this opportunity. Daily enrollment in physical education (PE) classes dropped from 42% to 25% among high school students between 1991 and 1995. Both the quantity and the quality of school PE have slipped over the last decade (USDHHS, 2000). Often PE is not required in high school and enrollment in PE classes decreases alarmingly from 9th to 12th grade among girls (81% to 39%) and boys (81% to 45%). Approximately 89% of secondary schools allow students to be exempt or excused from PE classes (USDHHS, 2000).

Unlike the nutrition programs in schools where some federal policy is in place for regulating the healthfulness of at least an element of the school food environment, there are no enforced federal policies or regulations on the school environment for physical activity. There are a number of recommendations related to students' opportunities to be active that have been endorsed and promoted by the federal government. *Healthy People 2010* (USDHHS, 2000) includes four objectives for improving the nation's health that directly address youths' opportunities for physical activity: (1) increase the proportion of the nation's public and private schools that require daily PE for all students; (2) increase the proportion of adolescents who participate in daily school PE; (3) increase the proportion of adolescents who spend at least 50% of school PE class time being physically active; and (4) increase the proportion of the nation's public and private schools that provide access to their physical activity spaces and facilities for all persons outside of normal school hours (i.e., before and after the school day, on weekends, and during summer and other vacations). In addition, the CDC's (1997) research-based Guidelines for School and Community Programs to Promote Lifelong Physical Activity Among Young People recommend the following: (1) quality, daily PE; (2) classroom health education that complements PE through knowledge and self-management skills to maintain a healthy lifestyle; (3) daily recess periods for elementary school students; and (4) extracurricular physical-activity programs including sports, extramurals, and activity clubs (CDC, 1997; Burgeson et al., 2001). Other sources including the 1996 *Surgeon General's Report on Physical Activity and Health* (USDHHS, 1996) and recommendations from the National Association for Sport and Physical Education (NASPE 1995, 1998, 2001, 2002) and the National Association of State Boards of Education (NASBE) (Bogden, 2000) herald the need to increase and improve opportunities for students to be physically active in school and in after-school activities.

While no federal regulations for physical activity exist, states, school districts, and individual schools are monitored to examine their policies and practices relating to physical activity. In 2000, the CDC conducted its second School Health Policies and Programs Study (SHPPS) to document physical activity— related policies and practices in schools (kindergarten through grade 12) at the state, district, school, and classroom levels. The authors found that most states require elementary schools (78.4% of states), middle and junior high schools (85.7% of states), and senior high schools (82.4% of states) to teach PE, and likewise, most school districts require that schools teach PE. However, schools have discretion on the amount of PE offered to students. The SHHPS study showed that approximately one-half of the nation's schools required some PE for students in grades 1 to 5. However, only 32.2% of schools required 6th graders to take PE, and by the time students reached 9th and 12th grade, the proportion of schools requiring PE decreased to 13.3% and 5.4%, respectively (Burgeson et al., 2001). *Healthy People 2010* (USDHHS, 2000), the CDC (1997), the NASPE (1995), and Bogden (2000) recommend daily PE for students, defined as at least 150 minutes per week for elementary school students and at least 225 minutes per week for middle or junior and senior high students, yet the SHPPS study (Burgeson et al., 2001) found few schools, nationwide, meeting these requirements. Among schools that required PE, only 8.0% of elementary schools, 6.4% of middle and junior high schools, and 5.8% of senior high schools provided daily PE for all students for the entire school year, meeting the minimal time requirements (Burgeson et al., 2001).

Healthy People 2010 goals also speak to the quality of PE classes and include recommendations for PE classes to provide at least 50% of moderate to vigorous physical activity. While the SHPPS study did not allow for examination of activity time in PE classes state-, district-, or school-wide, other data suggest that PE classes are not meeting recommendations to achieve active time. In the National Institute of Child Health and Human Development (NICHD) Study (NICHD, 2003), representing 814 youth in the third grade from 10 locations around the country, youth were observed in their PE class, and the System for Observing Fitness Instruction Time (SOFIT) methodology was used to obtain objective, observed activity levels and lesson content at the class level (McKenzie at al., 1991). Overall, PE classes lasted about 32.5 minutes and included about 5 minutes of very active time and 12 minutes of moderate to vigorous physical activity (or 15% and 37% of total class time, respectively). In addition, boys were engaged in moderate to vigorous physical activity for about 38% of lesson time whereas girls were engaged in moderate to vigorous physical activity only 36% of lesson time. Nearly one-third of PE classes were spent in management and knowledge activities that were largely sedentary activities for the students. The study also noted wide variation among schools, indicating that state-, district-, and school-level policies and practices are highly variable (NICHD, 2003).

Although a plethora of guidelines and recommendations exist to support increased amounts of quality physical activity for students during the school day, without strong federal or state policies that support, mandate, and regulate implementation of these guidelines, they are not likely to be widely institutionalized in our nation's schools. Unless guidelines and recommendations become enforced and supported policies, it is likely that PE classes and other opportunities for students to be active will be "on-the-fence" issues. If budgets are flush and school-level academic goals are being reached, PE and physical activity for students are likely to be supported. But in times of financial uncertainty and increased accountability for academic achievement goals, opportunities for PE and

physical activity are likely to suffer. Given what we know about the relation between activity and learning (Pellegrini et al., 1995; Pellegrini and Bjorklund, 1998)
and activity and student health (CDC, 1997; Biddle et al., 1998;) these are likely
to be poor trade-offs.

▉ TOBACCO USE

Cigarette smoking is one of the most widely practiced health-damaging behaviors. Commonly beginning as experimentation among youth ages 12 to 14, the
addicting effects of nicotine result in lifelong dependency. In addition, youth
are exposed to environmental tobacco smoke beginning in utero and subsequently by smoking peers and adults, including their parents. For several decades,
schools have been a predominant focus of anti-smoking education. In addition,
the education system recognizes the role of the social and physical environment
in the initiation and maintenance of cigarette smoking behavior. Policies on
nonsmoking in schools have developed worldwide. Finally, the prohibition of
tobacco sales to youth, often by weakly enforced laws, have provided another
method of discouraging cigarette smoking among the young.

▉ Origins of Youth Smoking

In 1994, the Surgeon General's report described the natural history of smoking
initiation and addiction among youth (USDHHS, 1994). Although it varies by
country and setting, most cigarette smoking begins in the early teenage years (12
to 14 years old). It is a product of multiple forces, but particularly those related
to the environment. Peer pressure is a leading source of initiation. Friends who
have begun smoking encourage others to share the habit. It often occurs in the
setting of adult and parental smoking, including that of teachers in their schools.
The mass media provide a backdrop for smoking with ads that encourage youth
to smoke by portraying smoking as glamorous, exciting, and adult (DiFranza
et al., 1991; Warner et al., 1992).

   These events occur at a unique developmental stage in the life of young people.
The teen years are a time of assertion of independence and rebelliousness. Acting
in opposition to the wishes of adults is prominent. In a society where most adults
do not smoke and discourage youth from smoking, cigarette use is one sign of this
rebelliousness. Children seeking to be perceived as adults are reinforced in this
perception by the environment created by cigarette advertising.

   While the past two decades have seen ebbs and flows in cigarette smoking
among youth, it continues to be common and is the major source of new smokers. A Legacy Foundation—CDC survey in 1999 found that 12.8% of middle
school students and 34.8% of high school students had smoked one or more
cigarettes during the previous 30 days (CDC, 2000). Although the tobacco in-

dustry has increasingly targeted young adults (ages 18 and above) to smoke, most smokers indicate that their initial experiences and subsequent addiction began in their school years.

Role of the Education System

The influential role of peers, the educational role of the school system, and the fact that youth spend a substantial portion of their days in school led naturally to schools focusing on discouraging cigarette smoking. Antismoking programs became an integral part of health education in most school districts decades ago. Early programs focused on harm done by cigarettes (Thompson, 1978). Health professionals, frequently parent or hospital volunteers, would lecture students on the health effects of smoking, including emphysema, lung cancer, and heart disease. This would be reinforced by pictures of actual specimens of lungs damaged by cigarette smoke. Children naturally recoiled from this gross demonstration of harm. Unfortunately, subsequent study demonstrated that this strategy had no effect on youth. To them, these were diseases of aging and had no relevance to their lives. Most believed that they could quit smoking upon reaching adulthood and could thus avoid any harmful effects (USDHHS, 1994). Subsequent work recognized the important role of social influences such as peers, parents, teachers, and the mass media (Botvin and Wills, 1985). These programs emphasized the short-term consequences of cigarette smoking, such as cough, shortness of breath, and reduced athletic performance. Such programs met with considerable early success and regular cigarette smoking dropped in many school districts.

However, the crucial role of other aspects of the environment was neglected. Teacher-led smoking prevention and cessation programs were followed by breaks in the teacher's lounge, which was clouded by tobacco smoke. The tobacco industry recognized the threat to their market and developed sophisticated advertising strategies to encourage cigarette smoking among youth. The ready availability of cigarettes for youth through vending machines and compliant sellers allowed wide access to children despite laws to the contrary. It became increasingly apparent that classroom educational programs alone were not adequate to reduce the smoking burden among youth.

Social and Physical Environment

The social and physical environment plays a crucial role in youths' access to cigarettes and their opportunity to smoke. A number of strategies to control youth smoking have been pursued along with broader community policies to control public tobacco use. The schools are a favored site for programs to limit smoking because youth spend a considerable portion of each day there and school behaviors are heavily influenced by peers. In addition, because cigarette sales to youth are illegal, efforts have focused on restricting access.

The first environmental approaches to school smoking were the development of tobacco bans, or smoke-free schools (Heckert and Matthews, 2000). Initially these were aimed at students and eliminated smoking areas, both within the school and on school grounds. As these policies developed, the contradiction of allowing teachers to smoke while forbidding addicted teenagers to smoke resulted in a total ban on cigarette smoking for both students and faculty in many places. The development of these bans led to the need for clearly articulated and written policies with associated disciplinary action. It was in this area of enforcement that ambiguous policies and vague practices were most problematic (Bowen et al., 1995; O'Hara Tompkins et al., 1999). These policies nonetheless became widespread and more formalized. The Synar amendment, part of a U.S. national drug policy, states zero tolerance for tobacco in schools (Pentz et al., 1997). The CDC developed a set of recommendations to be applied at both the school and community levels, including development of local policies and enforcement of smoke-free schools. The CDC also endorsed restrictions on local advertising of cigarettes and made recommendations for prevention and cessation programs (O'Hara Tompkins et al., 1999).

At the same time, communities and schools advocated stricter control of access to cigarettes (Rigotti et al., 1997; Forster et al., 1998). Such programs reflected prior regulations passed into law that prohibited cigarette purchase by individuals under 18 years of age. However, these were rarely enforced because cigarette sales constituted an important source of profits for many small businesses. Nonetheless, increasingly, more rigorous enforcement with substantial penalties to shop owners and clerks became more common. In addition, out of concern that cigarette machines made tobacco readily available at any age, some communities banned these machines while others placed them under closer surveillance. Limiting access to cigarettes has become part of a comprehensive smoking prevention program for youth.

Increasing the price of cigarettes through increased taxes is widely believed to be most effective among youth. Given their limited income, youth are more price-sensitive than other groups. The raising of cigarette taxes is associated with reduced youth smoking in the context of a broader community program (Sly et al., 2001).

Most experts agree that effective programs to prevent and limit cigarette smoking among youth must contain many elements. In the community context, limiting of smoking areas in public buildings and workspaces helps set the environment, while youth access to cigarettes is a complimentary strategy. Finally, clearly articulated school policies for smoke-free schools, coupled with education and cessation programs, are now widely recommended.

In summary, significant progress has been made in social, environmental, and policy programs to limit youth access to tobacco and initiation of a tobacco habit. Nonetheless, successes are not universal and the tobacco industry continues to look for new ways to engage young smokers.

■ IMPLEMENTING POLICY AND ENVIRONMENTAL CHANGE: EXAMPLES FROM RESEARCH

■ Environmental and Policy Interventions to Improve Dietary Behaviors in Youth: The TEENS Study

The Teens Eating for Energy and Nutrition at School (TEENS) study evaluated the effectiveness of a school-based intervention to increase middle school students' consumption of fruits, vegetables, and lower-fat foods in order to decrease their future risk for cancer (Lytle et al., 2004). The TEENS study was conducted in 16 middle or junior high schools in the Midwest and included a 2-year intervention with a cohort of students as they moved from seventh to eighth grade. The TEENS intervention included a classroom curriculum in both seventh and eighth grade with an emphasis on experiential learning with a behavioral focus, a family component that was delivered as part of the classroom curriculum, and an environment change component that focused on positively influencing the availability and promotion of fruits, vegetables, and lower-fat snack options in the school cafeteria and throughout the school building (Lytle and Perry, 2001). In addition, the environment change component included the initiation of School Nutrition Advisory Councils (SNACs) to consider school-wide food policy (Kubik et al., 2001). The primary outcome for TEENS was student-level consumption of fruits and vegetables and proportion of energy intake coming from total fat (Lytle et al., 2004); secondary outcomes evaluating the success of the environmental changes were also examined.

One of the primary TEENS strategies for changing the food environment included working with the school food service to improve the healthfulness of foods and beverages offered on the à la carte line. Thirteen of the 16 TEENS schools had à la carte lines. Eliminating this source of competitive foods in the schools was not an option; the school food service depended on the extra income that these lines provided to subsidize the cost of providing the lunches available from the federal NSLP and believed that students expected to have other lunch options besides the regular school lunch. The intervention began by assessing all the foods and beverages available to students on à la carte lines and classifying them as foods to promote and foods to limit. The first category consisted of fruits and vegetables; pretzels, bagels, and other low-fat grain items; low-fat milk; water; and any snack product that had fewer than 5 g of fat per serving (Table 18.1). Foods to limit included sweetened fruit drinks, candy bars, chips, cookies, and other snack items that had ≥5 g of fat per serving (Table 18.1). At baseline, between 17 and 233 (mean number per school = 75) items were offered on the 13 à la carte lines and 79% and 95% fell into the foods-to-limit category for intervention and control schools, respectively. Not surprisingly, student purchases of à la carte items (range of 276 to 6505 items; mean per school = 1306 items) also greatly favored foods in the foods-to-limit category (90% and 96% of sales from foods to limit in intervention and control schools, respectively) (Kubik et al., 2003).

TABLE 18.1
Sample of foods to promote and foods to limit on school snack lines

Foods to Promote	Foods to Limit
100% fruit juice	Soft drinks
Bottled water	Fruit drinks and sport drinks
Skim milk	Milk shakes
Low-fat* yogurt	French fries
Fresh fruits and vegetables	Nachos and cheese
Bagels	Pizza
Baked pretzels with low-fat* cheese	Candy bars
Low-fat* chips and salty snacks	Chips and salty snacks
Low-fat* packaged cookies and desserts	Packaged cookies and desserts
Low-fat* ice cream, frozen yogurt or frozen fruit bars	School-prepared higher fat desserts

*Fewer than 5 g of fat per serving.

The environmental intervention strategy involved working with the school food service to change the offerings, promote the healthier items, and consider new pricing strategies to encourage students to choose the healthier items. Training sessions were conducted with school food service staff from the eight intervention schools to provide the rationale for increasing healthier options on the à la carte line and, more importantly, to provide skills and resources to help them identify, purchase, and promote the healthier items in their schools. Many school food service staff had the perception that lower-fat foods (e.g., baked chips, lower fat cookies) did not taste good, would not be liked by students, and would not be purchased, resulting in lost revenue. As part of the training, taste testing was conducted with school food service, providing them with an opportunity to taste lower-fat snack products and with lists of products that met the fat criteria and distributors of the healthier products. In addition, the first case of the lower-fat product was purchased for the school so that any loss of revenue from an à la carte item that did not move on the line was absorbed by the research study. Training and guidance about product placement and presentation were provided, and the way that pricing affects sales was demonstrated.

At the end of the 2-year intervention period, the proportion of foods to promote, compared to that of foods to limit, offered to students changed in a favorable direction. Between baseline and follow-up, the proportion of items offered on the à la carte lines in intervention schools from the "foods-to-promote" category increased from 12% to 42% of all items, resulting in a statistically significant difference ($p = 0.04$) between treatment conditions. In addition, student purchases of items from the foods to promote increased from 10% at baseline to 36% at follow-up, approaching a statistically significant difference between conditions ($p = 0.07$). For both measures, secular trends and/or study contamination may have mitigated the opportunity to realize greater differences between treatment conditions. Since schools were randomized, not school districts, there is a good chance that information and suggestions given to school food service directors and staff in intervention schools were shared with school food service staff from control schools. Future evaluations of these types of environmental changes should consider randomizing by school district, rather than by school, to reduce the potential for study contamination.

▪ Environmental and Policy Interventions to Increase Physical Activity in Youth: The CATCH Study

The Child and Adolescent Trial for Cardiovascular Health (CATCH) was a multicenter, multicomponent, school-based intervention trial designed to evaluate the effectiveness of individual, family, and school—environmental intervention strategies to reduce youth risk for cardiovascular disease. The CATCH intervention trial occurred in 96 schools in four field centers from 1991 to 1994 and exposed a cohort of youth from the time they were in the third grade through the fifth grade to a variety of intervention strategies that promoted increased physical activity, consumption of diets that were low in total fat, saturated fat, and sodium, and abstinence from tobacco use (Perry et al., 1997).

While the primary outcome of CATCH was student serum cholesterol levels (Luepker et al., 1996), a variety of environmental outcomes were also assessed, including the dietary fat, saturated fat, and sodium content of meals offered to students (Osganian et al., 1996), school-level policies to make schools tobacco-free (Elder et al., 1996), and the content and structure of school PE (McKenzie et al., 1996). The discussion here will focus on the environmental strategies to positively affect levels of physical activity by changing policy and practice related to school PE.

The goals of the CATCH PE intervention component were to have schools provide at least 90 minutes of PE time each week for students and to increase the time spent in moderate to vigorous physical activity during PE to at least 40%. The minimal requirement for PE time was met as part of the school recruitment procedures. Schools agreeing to participate in the CATCH research study needed to agree to provide at least 90 minutes of PE to students if their school was randomized into the intervention condition.

In addition to schools' guarantee of 90 minutes of PE weekly, school staff involved in teaching CATCH PE participated in formal and informal training sessions. The formal CATCH PE training sessions were conducted by CATCH intervention staff and focused on positively affecting the structure and content of PE class to minimize sedentary management time; reduce time spent in giving instructions and disciplining students; maximize the number of students who are active during the class; and increase the amount of active time during class by providing more choices and fewer elimination games and finding ways to have students practice game and sports skills in a more active manner. In addition to more formal training sessions in which these ideas and CATCH PE materials were presented, role modeled, and practiced in group settings, CATCH PE interventionists also conducted on-site training sessions to help with school-specific problem solving and to offer continued support for delivering CATCH PE strategies.

The effectiveness of this practice-focused intervention strategy was evaluated through the SOFIT (System for Observing Fitness Instruction Time) method (McKenzie et al., 1991). This method is used to unobtrusively assess, at a class level, the type and intensity of students' activities and the behaviors of PE specialists or teachers in PE classes. At baseline, in intervention and control schools, 37% and 34% of PE class time, respectively, was spent in moderate to vigorous physical activity (on average about 10 minutes of a 30-minute class). After the 3-year CATCH intervention period, PE classes delivered in intervention schools were significantly more active than PE classes in the control schools (52% moderate to vigorous physical activity in intervention schools and 42% in control schools; $p = 0.002$) and surpassed the *Healthy People 2000* goals of more than 50% of class time spent in moderate to vigorous physical activity (Luepker et al., 1996; McKenzie et al., 1996). These changes translated into students in intervention schools having a higher estimated energy expenditure and higher energy expenditure rate per PE lesson compared to students in control schools. The CATCH study provided evidence that environmental change is possible through training and support of school staff who deliver PE to students and is effective in increasing student activity levels during the school day.

■ Environmental and Policy Interventions to Reduce Smoking Behaviors in Youth: Outcomes of Smoking Policies

Considerable research has been conducted on the effect of implementation of school-based smoking policies. Some authors believe that there is little evidence that tobacco control in the schools, such as bans and enforcements, work (Maes and Lievens, 2003; Aveyard et al., 2004a). Surveys of students have found that bans controlling smoking had an impact only on school grounds (Unger et al., 1999). The students believed that this had little effect on overall rates. In California, teenage smokers were aware of the policies and opposed them (Unger et al., 1999). They thought that students would find ways around the policy.

However, studies of other schools and districts demonstrate considerable success. Complete bans involving both students and teachers were best in reducing smoking rates among students (Heckert and Matthews, 2000; Maes and Lievens, 2003). In a large study, a clear and enforced written policy was most effective, resulting in a 9.5% student smoking rate compared to 30.1% in schools with no policy (Moore et al., 2001). Adjustment for student characteristics reduced but did not eliminate the differences. In another study of 166 secondary schools in the United Kingdom, a smoking policy with rigorous and authoritative implementation resulted in a relative risk of student smoking of 0.80 compared to 1.16 in the schools with no such policy (Aveyard et al., 2004b). Many authorities believe that a combination of clear and well-enforced policies along with educational programs for prevention and cessation are the most effective combination (Hamilton et al., 2003).

The effectiveness of broader community programs is less well studied. Perry and colleagues found substantial student smoking decreases in schools in a town undergoing a community-wide heart disease prevention program, compared to control communities (Perry et al., 1989). Similar findings were observed in Florida, where a media and access enforcement campaign showed apparent success (Sly et al., 2001). Positive results have also been observed in California, where an increased tobacco tax was coupled with a major media campaign.

■ CHALLENGES TO CHANGE IN ENVIRONMENTAL POLICY AND PRACTICE

The attempt to positively influence the school environment by changing policy or school-level practice is a new endeavor for health promotion work. In addition to the difficulties inherent to a new innovation, there are other unique elements of environmental change that pose significant challenges.

The largest challenge to changing the school environment might be the current societal environment in which our schools exist. Current emphasis on academic achievement standards is causing schools to reduce the amount of time students spend in "extras" such as PE, health education, and nutrition education. Federal and state governments and school districts are increasingly setting standards for school-level student academic achievement and pass rates. Consequences of poor performance by students may include school closings or budget restrictions. Many schools are responding to this threat by increasing the time that students spend studying academic subjects and frequently by reducing or eliminating all together PE and recess time. Beyond the school day, tight budgets mean increased student athletic fees for students who want to play on sports teams and a decrease in extracurricular and intramural programs.

Tight budgets also mean that many schools need to bring in extra money to support programming. Nationwide, schools receive approximately 750 million dollars per year from companies that sell snacks or processed foods in schools (Nestle, 2002). More than one-third of elementary schools, one-half of middle schools, and nearly three-quarters of high schools have a contract that gives a company rights to sell soft drinks at the school (Wechsler et al., 2001). As an example of how lucrative these contracts can be for schools, a major survey of vending contracts in the state of Texas, conducted by the Texas Department of Agriculture (2003), estimated that the total annual revenue from those contracts was approximately 54 million dollars. School-based health promotion efforts by public health professionals will continue to be stymied as long as schools face severe budget cuts and are presented with fiscal opportunities offered by the food industry. The cost of health promotion policies and practice will just be too dear.

At the practical level, getting organizations or agencies to institute environmental change is more complex than attempting change at the individual level, the previous focus of health promotion work. Behaviorial change strategies for individuals usually require motivation, instruction, development of skills and social supports, and practice and reinforcement of the new behavior. Policy or environmental change requires motivation and commitment of one or more policy makers and then adoption, implementation, and maintenance of the innovation by all other stakeholders. As an example, increasing the activity level of one individual is possible if sufficient motivation, incentives, and reinforcements for change are provided to the individual. Getting a school to adopt daily PE for all students all year, however, requires at least the following steps: (1) obtaining policy and practice support from the highest administrative level necessary; (2) working through all institutional barriers and procedures to approve the policy or practice; (3) articulating the policy, conditions, requirements, and ways that the policy will be monitored to other stakeholders; (4) training or assisting staff to implement the new policy (help find additional time in the school calendar, make necessary adjustments in staffing and scheduling, find additional resources for teachers or space) and; (5) implementing the new policy, monitoring it, retraining staff, and problem-solving barriers until the policy or practice is institutionalized.

Not only is the process of change more difficult but the time required to institute environmental or policy change is much longer and often indeterminable at the outset. Rarely can policy be put in place as part of a research study designed to evaluate effectiveness. As was the case in CATCH, a temporary change can be negotiated in school policy as an essential condition for participating in the research: schools must provide at least 90 minutes of PE time. However, for policy or practice to be sustained past a research period, the policy or practice must be rooted in the organization. That kind of committed change does not occur quickly. Research trials attempting environmental-level change must be prepared to build in additional time for intervention. The more stakeholders involved in the policy or practice change, the more time is needed for communication, organization, and integration of efforts.

Evaluation of the effectiveness of policy or environmental changes brings new study design and analysis challenges, and additional expense. In studies where the goal is environmental change, the unit of randomization and analysis becomes the institutions that are "receiving" the environmental change (not the individuals affected by the change). In school-based studies where interest is in examining the effectiveness of an environmental change, the school is the unit of randomization and analysis (Murray, 1998). This requirement means that more resources are required for both the intervention and evaluation costs. In addition, larger interventions for environmental change carry increased risks of study contamination. As evidenced in the example from TEENS, it is very difficult to control the naturally occurring spread of information and practice norms in the community.

Finally, measurement and assessment tools to evaluate change at the environmental level are just now being developed. In the past, measures of the environment were commonly considered process evaluation, often demanding less rigor as measurement tools than tools assessing outcome or impact evaluation (McGraw et al., 2000). But as environmental-level indicators move into the role of secondary outcomes, mediators of change or even primary outcomes in the importance of their validity and reliability will increase (Baranowski et al., 1997; Richter et al., 2000). If we truly consider the environment as an important factor in health and continue to develop and use theoretical models that include the environment as an important predictive and potentially mutable factor, then we must increase the quantity and quality of work done to develop valid and reliable methods and measures of environmental change (Lytle and Fulkerson, 2002).

■ SUMMARY

- School and community environment plays an important role in the health behaviors of youth. This is particularly true for those behaviors that increase the risk of cardiovascular disease: poor nutrition, physical inactivity, and cigarette smoking.
- Meals served at school are an important component of young people's diet. Federal policies and subsidies provide important recommendations for the food served in schools. However, empty-calorie snacks are still widely available through vending machines and alternative lunch lines. Promotion of unhealthy foods at schools is widespread.
- The epidemic of obesity and type 2 diabetes among youth is linked to physical inactivity. While there are national recommendations for physical activity in both quality and quantity, there are no national regulations. Most states require physical education classes but few say how many or how strenuous, leaving that to the district or individual school. Few schools follow the national recommendations for either intensity or duration of exercise. Competition for funds and time remains a crucial issue.
- The early teen years are when youth initiate cigarette smoking. Various aspects of their environment, including peer pressure, media, and schools, play important roles in their experimentation with cigarettes. In addition, access to cigarettes controls availability. Many schools are now smoke-free, banning both students and faculty from smoking on campus.
- Smoke-free schools are most effective in reducing youth smoking when the policies are clearly stated and consistently enforced.
- The recommendation that schools teach and practice health promotion is under considerable threat. The focus on academic achievement alone

endangers the offering of "extras" such as physical education and health education. Financial inducements by drink and snack providers provide an important supplemental income to schools facing budget reductions.

■ REFERENCES

Aaron, D.J., K.L. Storti, R.J. Robertson, A.M. Kriska, and R.E. LaPorte. 2002. Longitudinal Study of the Number and Choice of Leisure Time Physical Activity from Mid to Late Adolescence. *Arch Pediatr Adolesc Med* 156:1075–80.

Aveyard, P., W.A. Markham, and K.K. Cheng. 2004a. A Methodological and Substantive Review of the Evidence that Schools Cause Pupils to Smoke. *Soc Sci Med* 58:2253–65.

Aveyard, P., W.A. Markham, E. Lancashire, A. Bullock, C. Macarthur, K.K. Cheng, and H. Daniels. 2004b. The Influence of School Culture on Smoking among Pupils. *Soc Sci Med* 58:1767–80.

Baranowski, T., L.S. Lin, D.W. Wetter, K. Resnicow, and M. Davis Hearn. 1997. Theory as Mediating Variables: Why aren't Community Interventions Working as Desired? *Ann Epidemiol* S7:S89–S95.

Biddle, S., J. Sallis, and N. Cavell (eds). 1998. *Young and Active? Young People and Health-Enhancing Physical Activity: Evidence and Implications.* London: Health Education Authority.

Bogden, J.F. 2000. *Fit, Healthy and Ready to Learn, a School Health Policy Guide. Part I: Physical Activity, Healthy Eating, and Tobacco-Use Prevention.* Alexandria, VA: National Association of State Boards of Education.

Botvin, G.J., and T.A. Wills. 1985. Personal and Social Skills Training: Cognitive-Behavioral Approaches to Substance Abuse Prevention. In: *Prevention Research: Deterring Drug Abuse among Children and Adolescents.* Edited by C.S. Bell and R. Battjes. Bethesda, MD: U.S. Department of Health and Human Services, Public Health Service, Alcohol, Drug Abuse, and Mental Health Administration, National Institute on Drug Abuse. Monograph No. 63. DHHS Publication No. (ADM), 85–1334.

Bowen, D.J., S. Kinne, and M. Orlandi. 1995. School Policy in COMMIT: A Promising Strategy to Reduce Smoking by Youth. *J School Health* 65:140–4.

Burgeson, C.R., H. Wechsler, N.D. Brener, J.C. Young, and C.G. Spain. 2001. Physical Education and Activity: Results from the School Health Policies and Programs Study 2000. *J School Health* 71:279–93.

[CDC] Centers for Disease Control and Prevention. 1996. Guidelines for School Health Programs to Promote Lifelong Healthy Eating. *Morb Mortal Wkly Rep* 45(RR-9):1–41.

[CDC] Centers for Disease Control and Prevention. 1997. Guidelines for School and Community Programs to Promote Lifelong Physical Activity among Young People. *Morb Mortal Wkly Rep* 46(RR-6):1–36.

[CDC] Centers for Disease Control and Prevention. 2000. Tobacco Use among Middle and High School Students—United States, 1999. *Morb Mortal Wkly Rep* 49:49–53.

[CDC] Centers for Disease Control and Prevention. 2003. Physical Activity Levels among Children Ages 9–13 Years-United States, 2002. *Morb Mortal Wkly Rep* 52(33): 785–91.

Corbin, C.B., and R.P. Pangrazi. 1998. *Physical Activity for Children: A Statement of Guidelines.* Reston VA: National Association for Sport and Physical Education.

DiFranza, J.R., J.W. Richards, P.M. Paulman, N. Wolfe-Gillespie, C. Fletcher, R.D. Jaffe, and D. Murray. 1991. RJR Nabisco's Cartoon Camel Promotes Camel Cigarettes to Children. *JAMA* 266:3149–53.

Dwyer, J. 1995. The School Nutrition Dietary Assessment Study. *Am J Clin Nutr* 61(Suppl): 173S–7S.

Eisinger, P. 1998. *Toward an End to Hunger in America.* Washington, DC: Brookings Press.

Elder, J.P., C.L. Perry, E.J. Stone, C.C. Johnson, M. Yang, E.W. Edmundson, M.H. Smyth, T. Galati, H. Feldman, P. Cribb, and G.S. Parcel. 1996. Tobacco Use Measurement, Prediction, and Intervention in Elementary Schools in Four States: The CATCH Study. *Prev Med* 25:486–94.

Forster, J.L., D.M. Murray, M. Wolfson, T.M. Blaine, A.C. Wagenaar, and D.J. Hennrikus. 1998. The Effects of Community Policies to Reduce Youth Access to Tobacco. *Am J Public Health* 88:1193–8.

French, S., M. Story, J. Fulkerson, and A. Gerlach. 2003. Food Environment in Secondary Schools: A La Carte, Vending Machines, and Food Policies and Practices. *Am J Public Health* 93:1161–7.

Hamilton, G., D. Cross, T. Lower, K. Resnicow, and P. Williams. 2003. School Policy: What Helps to Reduce Teenage Smoking? *Nicotine Tob Res* 5:507–13.

Harnack, L., P. Snyder, M. Story, R. Holliday, L. Lytle, and D. Neumark-Sztainer. 2000. Availability of a la carte Food Items in Junior and Senior High Schools. *J Am Diet Assoc* 100:701–3.

Heckert, K.A., and K. Matthews. 2000. Toward Totally Smokefree Schools and Beyond: The Crown Public Health Smokefree Schools Grant Program. *Health Educ Behav* 27:328–38.

Kimm, S.Y.S., N.W. Glynn, A.M. Kriska, S.L. Fitzgerald, D.J. Aaron, S.L. Similo, R.P. McMahon, and B.A. Barton. 2000. Longitudinal Changes in Physical Activity in a Biracial Cohort during Adolescence. *Med Sci Sports Exer* 32:1445–54.

Kubik, M.Y., L.A. Lytle, P.J. Hannan, C.L. Perry, and M. Story. 2003. The Association of the School Food Environment with Dietary Behaviors of Young Adolescents. *Am J Public Health* 93:1168–73.

Kubik, M.Y., L.A. Lytle, P.J. Hannan, M. Story, and C.L. Perry. 2002. Food-Related Beliefs, Eating Behavior, and Classroom Food Practices of Middle School Teachers. *J School Health* 72:339–45.

Kubik, M.Y., L.A. Lytle, and M. Story. 2001. A Practical, Theory-Based Approach to Establishing School Nutrition Advisory Councils. *J Am Diet Assoc* 101:223–8.

Luepker, R.V., C.L. Perry, S.M. McKinlay, P.R. Nader, G.S. Parcel, E.J. Stone, L.S. Webber, J.P. Elder, H.A. Feldman, C.C. Johnson, S.H. Kelder, and M. Wu. 1996. Outcomes of a Field Trial to Improve Children's Dietary Patterns and Physical Activity. The Child and Adolescent Trial for Cardiovascular Health (CATCH). *JAMA* 275:768–76.

Lytle, L.A., and J.A. Fulkerson. 2002. Assessing the Dietary Environment: Examples from School-Based Nutrition Interventions. *Public Health Nutr* 5:893–9.

Lytle, L.A., D.M. Murray, C.L. Perry, M. Story, A.S. Birnbaum, M.Y. Kubik, and S. Varnell. 2004. School-Based Approaches to Affect Adolescents' Diets: Results from the TEENS Study. *Health Educ Behav* 31:270—87.

Lytle, L.A., and C.L. Perry. 2001. Applying Research and Theory in Program Planning: An Example from a Nutrition Education Intervention. *Health Promot Pract* 2:68–80.

Maes, L., and J. Lievens. 2003. Can the School Make a Difference? A Multilevel Analysis of Adolescent Risk and Health Behaviour. *Social Sci Med* 56:517–29.

McGraw, S.A., D. Sellers, E. Strong, K.A. Resnicow, S. Kuester, F. Fridinger, and H. Wechsler. 2000. Measuring Implementation of School Programs and Policies to Promote Healthy Eating and Physical Activity among Youth. *Prev Med* 31:S86–S97.

McKenzie, T.L., P.R. Nader, P.K. Strikmiller, M. Yang, E.J. Stone, C.L. Perry, W.C. Taylor, J.N. Epping, H.A. Feldman, R.V. Luepker, and S.H. Kelder. 1996. School Physical Education: Effect of the Child and Adolescent Trial for Cardiovascular Health. *Prev Med* 25:423–31.

McKenzie, T.L., J.F. Sallis, and P.R. Nader. 1991. SOFIT: System for Observing Fitness Instruction Time. *J Teach Phys Educ* 11:195–205.

Moore, L., C. Roberts, and C. Tudor-Smith. 2001. School Smoking Policies and Smoking Prevalence among Adolescents: Multilevel Analysis of Cross-Sectional Data from Wales. *Tob Control* 10:117–23.

Murray, D.M. 1998. *Design and Analysis of Group-Randomized Trials.* New York: Oxford University Press.

[NASPE] National Association for Sport and Physical Education. 1995. *Moving into the Future: National Standards for Physical Education.* Reston, VA.

[NASPE] National Association for Sport and Physical Education. 1998. *Physical Education Program Improvement and Self-Study Guide for High School.* Reston, VA.

[NASPE] National Association for Sport and Physical Education. 2001. *Opportunity to Learn Standards for Elementary Physical Education.* Reston, VA.

[NASPE] National Association for Sport and Physical Education. 2002. *2001 Shape of the Nation Report: Status of Physical Education in the United States.* Reston, VA: American Alliance for Health, Physical Education, Recreation and Dance.

[NICHD] National Institute of Child Health and Human Development Study of Early Child Care and Youth Development Network. 2003. Frequency and Intensity of Activity of Third Grade Children in Physical Education. *Arch Pediatr Adolesc Med* 157:185–190.

Nestle, M. 2002. *Food Politics.* Berkeley, CA: University of California Press.

O'Hara Tompkins, N., G.A. Dino, L.K. Zedosky, M. Harman, and G. Shaler. 1999. A Collaborative Partnership to Enhance School-Based Tobacco Control Policies in West Virginia. *Am J Prev Med* 16(3 Suppl):29–34.

Osganian, S.K., M.K. Ebzery, D.H. Montgomery, T.A. Nicklas, M.A. Evans, P.D. Mitchell, L.A. Lytle, M.P. Snyder, E.J. Stone, M.M. Zive, K.J. Bachman, R. Rice, and G.S. Parcel. 1996. Changes in the Nutrient Content of School Lunches: Results from the CATCH Eat Smart Food Service Intervention. *Prev Med* 25:400–12.

Pellegrini, A.D., and D.F. Bjorklund. 1998. The Role of Recess in Children's Cognitive Performance. *Educ Psychol* 32:35–40.

Pellegrini, A.D., P.D. Huberty, and I. Jones. 1995. The Effects of Recess Timing on Children's Classroom and Playground Behavior. *Am Educ Res J* 32:845–64.

Pentz, M.A., S. Sussman, and T. Newman. 1997. The Conflict between Least Harm and No-Use Tobacco Policy for Youth: Ethical and Policy Implications. *Addiction* 92:1165–73.

Perry, C.L., K.I. Klepp, and C. Sillers. 1989. Community-Wide Strategies for Cardiovascular Health: The Minnesota Heart Health Program Youth Program. *Health Educ Res* 4:87–101.

Perry, C.L., D. Sellers, C. Johnson, S. Pedersen, K. Bachman, G. Parcel, E. Stone, R.V. Luepker, M. Wu, P. Nader, and K.W. Cook. 1997. The Child and Adolescent Trial for Cardiovascular Health (CATCH): Intervention, Implementation, and Feasibility for Elementary Schools in the U.S. *Health Educ Behav* 24:716–35.

Richter, K.P., K.J. Harris, A. Paine-Andrews, S.B. Fawcett, T.L. Schmit, B.H. Lankenau, and J. Johnston. 2000. Measuring the Health Environment for Physical Activity and Nutrition among Youth: A Review of the Literature and Applications for Community Initiatives. *Prev Med* 31:S98–S111.

Rigotti, N.A., J.R. DiFranza, Y. Chang, T. Tisdale, B. Kemp, and D.E. Singer. 1997. The Effect of Enforcing Tobacco-Sales Laws on Adolescents' Access to Tobacco and Smoking Behavior. *N Engl J Med* 337:1044–51.

Sly, D.F., G.R. Heald, and S. Ray. 2001. The Florida "Truth" Anti-Tobacco Media Evaluation: Design, First Year Results, and Implications for Planning Future State Media Evaluations. *Tob Control* 10:9–15.

Story, M., J. Hayes, and B. Kalina. 1996. Availability of Foods in High Schools: Is There Cause for Concern? *J Am Diet Assoc* 96:123–6.

Texas Department of Agriculture. 2003. School District Vending Contract Survey. Retrieved January 2006, from http://www.squaremeals.org/fn/render/channel/items/0,1249,2348 _2515_0_0,00.h

Thompson, E.L. 1978. Smoking Education Programs 1960–1976. *Am J Public Health* 68:250–7.

Unger, J.B., L.A. Rohrbach, K.A. Howard, T.B. Cruz, C.A. Johnson, and X. Chen. 1999. Attitudes toward Anti-Tobacco Policy among California Youth: Associations with Smoking Status, Psychosocial Variables and Advocacy Actions. *Health Educ Res* 14:751–63.

[USDA] U.S. Department of Agriculture. June 10, 1994. *National School Lunch Program and School Breakfast Program Nutrition Objectives for School Meals* (7CFR 210.220). Federal Register 30218-051.

[USDA] U.S. Department of Agriculture, Food and Nutrition Service. 2001a. *Children's Diets in the Mid-1900s: Dietary Intake and its Relationship with School Meal Participation.* (CN-01-CDC), Alexandria, VA.

[USDA] U.S. Department of Agriculture. Food and Nutrition Service, Office of Analysis, Nutrition and Evaluation. 2001b. *School Nutrition Dietary Assessment Study-II: Summary of Findings.* Alexandria, VA: U.S. Department of Agriculture.

[USDA] U.S. Department of Agriculture. Retrieved January, 2006 National School Lunch Program Fact Sheet http://www.fns.usda.gov/cnd/lunch/AboutLunch/NSLPFactSheet .htm.

[USDHHS] U.S. Department of Health and Human Services. 1994. *Preventing Tobacco Use among Young People: A Report of the Surgeon General.* Atlanta, GA: U.S. Department of Health and Human Services, Public Health Service, Centers for Disease Control and Prevention, National Center for Chronic Disease Prevention and Health Promotion, Office on Smoking and Health.

[USDHHS] U.S. Department of Health and Human Services. 1996. *Physical Activity and Health: A Report of the Surgeon General.* Atlanta, GA: Centers for Disease Control and Prevention, U.S. Department of Health and Human Services.

[USDHHS] U.S. Department of Health and Human Services. 2000. *Healthy People 2010: Understanding and Improving Health,* 2nd ed. Washington, DC: U.S. Government Printing Office.

[USDHHS] U.S. Department of Health and Human Services. 2001. *The Surgeon General's Call to Action to Prevent and Decrease Overweight and Obesity.* Rockville, MD: Public Health Service, Office of the Surgeon General.

U.S. General Accounting Office. 2003. School *Lunch Program: Efforts Needed to Improve Nutrition and Encourage Healthy Eating.* Washington, DC: General Accounting Office. GAO Report Number 03-056.

Warner, K.E., L.M. Goldenhar, and C.G. McLaughlin. 1992. Cigarette Advertising and Magazine Coverage of the Hazards of Smoking. *N Engl J Med* 326:305–9.

Wechsler, H., N.D. Brener, S. Kuester, and C. Miller. 2001. Food Service and Foods and Beverages Available at School: Results from the School Health Policies and Programs Study 2000. *J School Health* 71:313–23.

EPILOGUE

C. Alex McMahan and Henry C. McGill, Jr.

A RISK SCORE FOR PRECLINICAL ATHEROSCLEROSIS IN YOUTH

The results presented in this book leave no doubt that atherosclerosis begins in childhood and that the risk factors for coronary heart disease derived from studies of adults not only are present in youth but also influence the progression of atherosclerosis. Controlled clinical trials, the gold standard of efficacy, have demonstrated that risk factor modification in adults reduces the probability of clinically manifest coronary heart disease and results in regression of advanced coronary artery atherosclerosis. However, no similar trial of risk factor reduction in youth has demonstrated that risk factor control in youth actually retards progression of atherosclerosis.

The Framingham Study developed a risk score that combined the effects of the various established risk factors to predict the probability of a clinically manifest coronary heart disease event within the following 10 years (Wilson et al., 1998). This risk score has proved useful in evaluating the risk status of adults for both physicians and their patients and in guiding their decisions regarding whether and how aggressively lifestyle modifications or drug treatment should be pursued to reduce that risk.

A physician will find it especially difficult to communicate the combined effects of the several risk factors to young patients because the end point is a lesion not apparent to the patient and the clinical manifestation is decades in the future. The physician may also have difficulty in deciding how aggressively to pursue lifestyle modification or possibly pharmacologic intervention. To aid in this decision, we have developed risk scores, based on the easily measured risk factors, that estimate the probability that a 15- to 34-year-old person has a significant atherosclerotic lesion in the coronary arteries or in the abdominal aorta (McMahan et al., 2005). Table E.1 shows the points given to each risk factor in the risk scores for the coronary arteries and for the abdominal aorta. Adding these

TABLE E.1
Risk scores for predicting target lesions in the coronary arteries
and the abdominal aorta

Risk Factor	Category		Points	
			Coronary Arteries	Abdominal Aorta
Age (years)	15–19*		0	0
	20–24		5	5
	25–29		10	10
	30–4		15	15
Sex	Men*		0	0
	Women		−1	1
Non-HDL cholesterol (mg/dL)	<130*		0	0
	130–159		2	1
	160–189		4	2
	190–219		6	3
	≥220		8	4
HDL cholesterol (mg/dL)	<40		1	0
	40–59*		0	0
	≥60		−1	0
Smoking	Nonsmoker*		0	0
	Smoker		1	4
Blood pressure	Normotensive*		0	0
	Hypertensive		4	3
Obesity (BMI, kg/m²)	Men	≤30*	0	0
		>30	6	0
	Women	≥30*	0	0
		>30	0	0
Hyperglycemia (glycohemoglobin, %)	< 8 *		0	0
	≥8		5	3

*Reference category.
Source: Reproduced from McMahan et al., *Archives of Internal Medicine*, 2005, volume 16s,
page 887. Copyright © 2005, American Medical Association. All rights reserved.

points for an individual's risk factor profile yields the risk score, and reference
to Figure E.1 gives the probability that the individual has an advanced atherosclerotic lesion (American Heart Association grade 4 or 5) in the left anterior
descending coronary artery, or more than 9% of the intimal surface of the right
coronary artery occupied by raised lesions, or more than 15% of the intimal
surface of the abdominal aorta occupied by raised lesions.

Coronary arteries

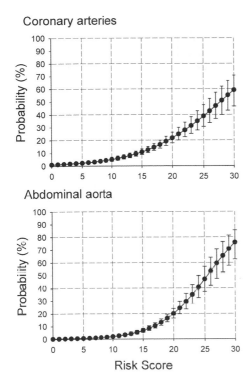

Abdominal aorta

Risk Score

FIGURE E.1

Estimated probability of target lesion in coronary arteries (upper panel) and the abdominal aorta (lower panel) by risk score. Error bars represent 95% confidence intervals. Modified from McMahan et al., *Archives of Internal Medicine*, 2005, volume 165, page 887. Copyright © 2005, American Medical Association. All rights reserved.

These risk scores have good discrimination, that is, the ability of a prediction model to separate subjects with target lesions from those without target lesions (*c*-indexes, 0.78 for the coronary arteries; 0.84 for the abdominal aorta). The *c*-index is the proportion of all pairs of subjects, one with and one without target lesions, in which the subject with the lesions has the higher predicted probability of lesions. A value of 0.50 for *c* indicates no discrimination (noninformative test) and a value of 1.0 indicates perfect discrimination. Coefficients for the risk factors are normalized so that each increase of 1 unit in the risk score is equivalent to the multiplicative change in the odds (additive change in the logarithm of the odds) due to a 1-year increase in age. Odds ratios for a 1-unit increase in the risk scores were 1.18 (95% confidence interval, 1.14–1.22) for the coronary arteries and 1.29 (95% confidence interval, 1.23–1.35) for the abdominal aorta.

Here is an example of how the risk score might be used. A male (0 points), age 17 (0 points), with non-HDL cholesterol 190–219 mg/dL (6 points), history of smoking (1 point), hypertension (4 points), and no other risk factors has a coronary artery risk score of 11, with all 11 of the points due to modifiable risk factors. Figure E.1 indicates that this individual has about a 6% probability of having a target coronary artery lesion. This low probability nevertheless indicates a young person at substantially increased risk relative to a person of similar age but without modifiable risk factors. However, if the same risk profile is maintained to age 30, the risk score becomes 26, and the probability of having a coronary artery target lesion is about 43%. Unlike risk scores for clinical events in adults, age makes a large contribution to the risk score in youth. Thus, it is important to establish and maintain control of the modifiable risk factors beginning in the teenage years.

Although these conclusions are based on observational data and we do not have proof of efficacy based on randomized controlled clinical trials, control of the cardiovascular risk factors has shown no adverse effects in either young persons or adults and is likely to have many beneficial effects other than retarding the progression of atherosclerosis—for example, reducing the risk of diabetes, hypertension, lung cancer, and chronic obstructive pulmonary disease, to name only a few of the more frequent consequences of obesity and tobacco use. It is time to start earlier to prevent adult coronary heart disease (McGill and McMahan 2003).

■ REFERENCES

McGill, H.C., Jr. and C.A. McMahan. 2003. Starting Earlier to Prevent Heart Disease. *JAMA* 290:2320–2.

McMahan, C.A., S.S. Gidding, Z.A. Fayad, A.W. Zieske, G.T. Malcom, R.E. Tracy, J.P. Strong, and H.C. McGill, Jr., for the Pathobiological Determinants of Atherosclerosis Research Group. 2005. Risk Scores Predict Atherosclerotic Lesions in Young People. *Arch Intern Med* 165:883–90.

Wilson, P.W.F., R.B. D'Agostino, D. Levy, A.M. Belanger, H. Silbershatz, and W.B. Kannel. 1998. Prediction of Coronary Heart Disease Using Risk Factor Categories. *Circulation* 97:1837–47.

INDEX

Acanthosis nigricans, 260, 301
Accelerometers, 278
ACE inhibitors, 201–204
Accidental death, youths/young adults
   atherosclerosis studies and, 8
Adiposity, 236–237, 255
Adiposity rebound, 240–241
Alcohol
   blood pressure and intake of, 199
   obese adolescent use of, 262
Alstrom syndrome, 243
Ambulatory blood pressure monitoring,
   187–188
American Academy of Pediatrics
   athletic participation with elevated
      blood pressure, 200
   recommendations for television
      watching, 201
American Diabetes Association
   metformin for treatment of type 2
      diabetes in children/
      adolescents, 303
   screening guidelines for type 2 diabetes,
      301
American Heart Association
   guidelines for cardiovascular risk
      reduction in children/
      adolescents, 135
   use of mercury manometers or aneroid
      devices, 185
Anorexia nervosa, 262
Anticholesterolemia drugs
   use in children/adolescents, 134–142
Antihypertensive drugs
   use in children/adolescents, 201–205
Antioxidants
   dietary intake and blood pressure, 33
Aorta. See Pathobiological Determinants of
   Atherosclerosis in Youth Study

Apolipoproteins
   biochemistry of, 109
   C-II
      familial hypertriglyceridemia, 127–
         128
   E
      levels in familial
         dysbetalipoproteinemia, 128
Atherogenic dyslipidemia, 128
Atherosclerosis. See also Cardiovascular
   disease
   animal models of, 28–29
   begins early in life, 3, 7, 21, 27, 64, 363
   cross-population studies of, 29–31
      American and Asian soldiers killed in
         battle, 30
      dietary lipid intake and, 30
      International Atherosclerosis
         Project, 30
      INTERSALT, 31, 33
      Kyushu-Minnesota autopsy study, 30
   fatty streaks vs. fibrous plaques, 3–4,
      125, 177
   composition of, 4
   geographic distribution, 29
   lesions
      progression/regression with use of
         cholesterol-lowering agents,
         130
   natural history of, 3–6, 27–28
      advanced lesion, 4–5
      fatty streak, 3–5
         in the aorta, 4
         in the coronary arteries, 4
      fibrous plaque, 4–5
      molecular biology of, 6
      raised fatty streak, 4
      rate of progression, 6
      vulnerable plaques, 5–6